Essential
Evidence-Based
Medicine

Dan Mayer

Albany Medical College

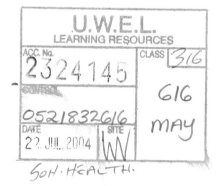
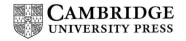

CAMBRIDGE
UNIVERSITY PRESS

PUBLISHED BY THE PRESS SYNDICATE OF THE UNIVERSITY OF CAMBRIDGE
The Pitt Building, Trumpington Street, Cambridge, United Kingdom

CAMBRIDGE UNIVERSITY PRESS
The Edinburgh Building, Cambridge CB2 2RU, UK
40 West 20th Street, New York, NY 10011–4211, USA
477 Williamstown Road, Port Melbourne, VIC 3207, Australia
Ruiz de Alarcón 13, 28014 Madrid, Spain
Dock House, The Waterfront, Cape Town 8001, South Africa

http://www.cambridge.org

First published 2004

Printed in the United Kingdom at the University Press, Cambridge

Typefaces Utopia 9/13 pt. and Dax   *System* LaTeX 2_ε [TB]

A catalog record for this book is available from the British Library

Library of Congress Cataloging in Publication data

Mayer, Dan.
  Essential evidence-based medicine/Dan Mayer.
    p.   cm.
  Includes bibliographical references and index.
  ISBN 0 521 83261 6 (hardback) – ISBN 0 521 54027 5 (paperback)
  1. Evidence-based medicine.   I. Title.
  [DNLM: 1. Evidence-Based Medicine. WB 102 M468e 2004]
R723.7.M396 2004
616–dc21   2003053202

ISBN 0 521 83261 6 hardback
ISBN 0 521 54027 5 paperback

Contents

In 1992 during a period of innovative restructuring of the medical school curriculum at Albany Medical College, Dr. Henry Pohl, then Associate Dean for Academic Affairs, asked me to develop a course to teach students how to become lifelong learners and how the health-care system works. This charge became the focus of a new longitudinal required four-year course initially called CCCS or Comprehensive Care Case Study. In 2000, the name was changed to Evidence Based Health Care (EBHC).

During the next ten years a formidable course was developed. It concentrates on teaching evidence-based medicine (EBM) and health-care systems operations to all medical students at Albany Medical College. The first syllabus was based on a course in critical appraisal of the medical literature intended for internal medicine residents at Michigan State University. This core has expanded by incorporating medical decision making and informatics. The basis for the organization of the book lies in the concept of the educational prescription proposed by Scott Richardson, M.D.

The goal of the text is to allow the reader, whether medical student, resident, allied health care provider, or practicing physician, to become a critical consumer of the medical literature. This textbook will teach you to read between the lines in a research study and apply that information to your patients.

For reasons I do not clearly understand many physicians are "allergic" to mathematics. It seems that even the simplest mathematical calculations drive them to distraction. Medicine is mathematics. Although the math content in this book is on a pretty basic level, most daily interaction with patients involves some understanding of mathematical processes. We may want to determine how much better the patient sitting in our office will do with a particular drug, or how to interpret a patient's concern about a new finding on their yearly physical. Far more commonly, we may need to interpret the information from the Internet that our patient brought in. Either way, we are dealing in probability. However, I have endeavored to keep the math as simple as possible.

This book does not require a working knowledge of statistical testing. The math is limited to simple arithmetic and a handheld calculator is the only computing instrument that is needed. Online calculators are available to do many of the calculations needed in the book and accompanying CD-ROM. They will be referenced and their operations explained.

The need for learning EBM is elucidated in the opening chapters of the book. The layout of the book is an attempt to follow the process outlined in the educational prescription. You will be able to practice your skills with the practice problems on the accompanying CD-ROM. The CD-ROM also contains materials for "journal clubs" (critical appraisal of specific articles from the literature) and PowerPoint slides.

A brief word about the CD-ROM

The attached CD-ROM is designed to help you consolidate your knowledge and apply the material in the book to everyday situations in EBM. There are four types of problems on the CD:

(1) **Multiple choice questions** are also called Self-assessment learning exercises. You will be given information about the answer after pressing "submit" if you get the question wrong. You can then go back and select the correct answer. If you are right, you can proceed to the next question. A record will be kept of your answers.

(2) **Short essay questions** are designed for one- to three-sentence answers. When you press "submit" you will be shown the correct or suggested answer for that question and can proceed to the next question. Your answer will be saved to a specified location in your computer.

(3) **Calculation and graphing questions** require you to perform calculations or draw a graph. These must be done off the program. You will be shown the correct answers after hitting the "submit" button. Your answer will not be saved.

(4) **Journal clubs** require you to analyze a real medical study. You will be asked to fill in a worksheet with your answers in short essay form. After finishing, a sample of correct and acceptable answers will be shown for you to compare with your answers.

Acknowledgements

There are many people who were directly or indirectly responsible for the publication of this book. Foremost, I want to thank my wife, Julia Eddy, without whose insight this book would never have been written. Her encouragement and suggestions at every stage during the development of the course, writing the syllabi, and finally putting them into book form, were the vital link in creating this work. At the University of Vermont she learned how statistics could be used to develop and evaluate research in psychology. She encouraged me to use the "scientific method approach" to teach medicine to my students, evaluating new research using applied statistics to improve the practice of medicine.

Next, I would like to acknowledge the help of all the students and faculty involved in the EBHC Theme Planning Group for the course since the start. This group of committed students and faculty has met monthly since 1993 to make constructive changes in the course. Their suggestions have been incorporated into the book and this invaluable input has helped me develop it from a rudimentary and disconnected series of lectures and workshops to what I hope is a fully integrated educational text.

I am indebted to the staff of the Office of Medical Education of the Department of Internal Medicine at the Michigan State University for the syllabus material that I purchased from them in 1993. This became the skeleton structure of the course on which this book is based. I think they had a great idea on how to introduce the uninitiated to critical appraisal. The structure of their original course can be seen in this work.

I would like to thank Sandi Pirozzo, M.D. and John Kaplan, Ph.D. for their chapters on searching and the ethical conduct of research respectively. I would especially like to thank the following faculty and students at Albany Medical College for their review of the manuscript: John Kaplan, Ph.D., Paul Sorum, M.D., Maude Dull, M.D. (AMC 2000), Kathleen Trapp, B.S., Peter Bernstein, B.S. (AMC 2002), Sue Lahey, M.L.S., Cindy Koman, M.L.S., and Anne Marie L'Hommedieu, M.L.S. Their editorial work over the past several years has helped me refine the ideas in this book. I would also like to thank Chase Echausier, Rachael Levet, and Brian Leneghan for their persistence in putting up with my foibles in the production of the manuscript, and my secretary, Line Callahan, for her Herculean effort in typing the manuscript. I also thank the creators of the CD-ROM, which was developed and executed by Tao Nyeu and my son, Noah Mayer. I owe a great debt to the staff at the Cambridge University Press for having the faith to publish this book. Specifically, I want to thank Senior Commissioning Editor for Medicine, Peter Silver, for starting the process. Of course, I am very thankful to my copy-editor, Hugh Brazier, whose expertise and talent made the process of editing the book actually pleasant.

Finally, this book is dedicated to my children, Memphis, Gilah, and Noah. Thanks for all of your patience.

A brief history of medicine and statistics

History is a pack of lies about events that never happened told by people who weren't there.
Those who cannot remember the past are condemned to repeat it.

George Santayana (1863–1952)

Learning objectives

In this chapter you will learn:
- a brief history of medicine and statistics
- the background to the development of modern evidence-based medicine
- how to put what we are doing into perspective

This is the beginning' of a process designed to make you a more effective reader of the medical research literature. This chapter will give you a historical perspective for learning how to use the best evidence in the practice of medicine.

Introduction

The American health-care system' is among the best in the world. Certainly we have the most technologically advanced system. We also spend the most money. Are we getting our money's worth? Are those of our citizens who have adequate access to health care getting the best possible care? What is the best possible health care and who defines it? These are some of the questions that we will be discussing in this book.

Evidence-based medicine is a new paradigm for the health-care system. It involves using the current evidence in the medical literature to provide the best possible care to patients. We search for the evidence needed to provide the best care for the patient. We measure the results by studying the health-care system and the specific outcomes of care given to patients. What follows is a brief history of medicine and statistics. This introduction will give you the historical basis and philosophical underpinnings of evidence-based medicine.

Table 1.1. The basis of healing systems in different civilizations

Civilization	Energy	Elements
Europe	Humors	Earth, air, choler (yellow bile), melancholia (black bile)
India	Chakras	Spirit, phlegm, bile
China	Qi	Earth, metal, fire, water, wood
Native America	Spirits	Earth, air, fire, water

Pre- and ancient history (dawn of civilization to about AD 1000)

Prehistoric man looked upon illness as a spiritual event. The ill person was seen as having a spiritual failing or being possessed by demons. Medicine practiced during this period and for centuries onward focused on removing these demons and cleansing the body (and/or spirit) of the ill person. Trephination (holes made in the skull to vent evil spirits or vapors) and religious rituals were the means to heal. With advances in civilization, healers focused on "treatments" that seemed to work. They used herbal (vegetable) medicines and became more skilled as surgeons.

About 4000 years ago, the Code of Hammurabi listed penalties for bad outcomes in surgery. The surgeon lost his hand if the patient died. The prevailing medical theories of this era and the next few millennia involved manipulation of various forms of energy passing through the body. Health required a balance of these energies. The energy had different names depending on where the theory was developed. It was *qi* in China, *chakras* in India, humors in Europe, and natural spirits among Native Americans. The forces achieving the balance of energy also had different names. Each civilization developed a healing method predicated on restoring the correct balance of these energies in the patient, as described in Table 1.1.

The ancient Chinese system of medicine was based upon the duality of the universe. Yin and yang represented the fundamental forces in a dualistic cosmic theory that bound the universe together. The *Nei Ching* (*Nei Jing*), one of the oldest medical textbooks, was written about the third century BC. Medical diagnosis was done by means of "pulse diagnosis" that measured the balance of *qi* in the body. This system included the 12 channels in which the *qi* flowed. Anatomic knowledge either corroborated the channels or was ignored. The first systematic study of human anatomy didn't occur until the mid eighteenth century. It consisted of the inspection of children who had died of plague and been torn apart by dogs. In addition to the five elements, there were also five planets, conditions of the weather, colors, and tones. Acupuncture as a healing art balanced yin and yang by insertion of needles into the energy channels at different points and manipulating the *qi*.

Medicine in ancient India was also very complex. Medical theory included seven substances: blood, flesh, fat, bone, marrow, chyle, and semen. From extant records, we know that surgical operations were performed in India as early as 800 BC, including kidney-stone removal and plastic surgery (replacement of amputated noses, the punishment for adultery). Diet and hygiene were crucial to curing in Indian medicine and clinical diagnosis was highly developed, depending as much on the nature of the life of the patient as on his symptoms. Other remedies included herbal medications, surgery, and the "five procedures": emetics, purgatives, water enemas, oil enemas, and sneezing powders. Inhalations, bleeding, cupping and leeches were also employed. Anatomy was learned from bodies that were soaked in the river for a week and then pulled apart. Indian physicians knew a lot about bones, muscles, ligaments, and joints, but not much about nerves, blood vessels, or internal organs.

The Greeks began to systematize medicine about the same time as the *Nei Ching* appeared in China. Although Hippocratic medical principles are considered archaic, his principles of the doctor–patient relationship are still followed today. In Rome, Galen created (incorrect) anatomical descriptions of the human body based primarily on the dissection of animals. The Middle (very dark) Ages saw the continued practice of Greek and Roman medicine. Most people turned to folk medicine that was usually performed by village elders (men or women) who healed using their experiences with local herbs. Arabic medicine introduced the use of chemical medications, the study of chemistry, and more extensive surgery.

Renaissance and industrial revolution

The first medical school was started in Salerno, Italy in the thirteenth century. The Renaissance led to revolutionary changes in the theory of medicine. In the fifteenth century, Vesalius repudiated Galen's incorrect anatomical theories and Paracelsus advocated the use of chemical instead of vegetable medicines. From the sixteenth-century development of the microscope (Janssen and Galileo get the credit although Leeuwenhoek and Hooke made it popular) to the seventeenth-century theory of the circulation of blood (Harvey), scientists learned about the actual functioning of the human body. The eighteenth century saw the development of modern medicines with the isolation of foxglove (digitalis) by Withering, the use of inoculation (against smallpox) by Jenner, and the postulation of the existence of vitamins (vitamin C, antiscorbutic factor) by Lind.

During the eighteenth century, medical theories were undergoing rapid and chaotic change. In Scotland, Brown theorized that health represented the conflict between strong and weak forces in the body. He treated imbalances with either opium or alcohol. Cullen preached a strict following of the medical orthodoxy of the time and recommended complex prescriptions to treat illness. Hahnemann was disturbed by the use of strong chemicals to cure, and developed the theory of homeopathy. Based upon the theory that like cures like, he prescribed medications in doses that were so minute that current atomic analysis cannot find even one molecule of the original substance in the solution. Benjamin Rush, the foremost physician of the century, was a strong proponent of bloodletting, a popular therapy of the time. He has the distinction of being the first physician in America who was involved in a malpractice suit (another story, and he won).

The birth of statistics

Prehistoric peoples had no concept of probability and the first mention is in the Talmud, written between AD 300 and 400. This alluded to the probability of two events being the product of the probability of each, but without explicitly using mathematical calculations. Among the ancients, the Greeks believed that the gods decided all life and therefore that probability did not enter into issues of daily life. The Greek creation myth involved a game of dice between Zeus, Poseidon, and Hades. The Greeks themselves turned to oracles and the stars instead.

The use of Roman numerals made any kind of complex calculation impossible. Numbers as we know them today, using the decimal system and the zero, probably originated around AD 500 in the Hindu culture of India. This was probably the biggest step towards being able to manipulate probabilities and determine statistics. The Arabic mathematician Khowarizmi defined rules for adding, subtracting, multiplying, and dividing in about AD 800. In 1202 the book of the abacus (*Liber abaci*) by Leonardo Pisano (known as Fibonacci) first introduced the numbers discovered by Arabic cultures to European civilization.

In 1494 Luca Paccioli defined basic principles of algebra and multiplication tables up to 60×60 in his book *Summa de arithmetica, geometria, proportioni e proportionalita*. He posed the first serious statistical problem of two men playing a game called balla, which is to end when one of them has won six rounds. However, when they stop playing A has only won five rounds and B three. How should they divide the wager? It would be another 200 years before this problem was solved.

In 1545 Girolamo Cardano wrote the books *Ars magna* (the great art) and *Liber de ludo aleae* (book on games of chance). This was the first attempt to use mathematics to describe statistics and probability, and accurately described the probabilities of throwing various numbers with dice. Galileo expanded on this by calculating probabilities using two dice. In 1619 a puritan minister, Thomas

Table 1.2. Probability of survival, 1660 and 1993

	Percentage survival to each age	
Age	1660	1993
0	100%	100%
26	25%	98%
46	10%	95%
76	1%	70%

Gataker, expounded on the meaning of probability by noting that it was natural laws and not divine providence that governed these outcomes.

Other famous scientists including Huygens (1657), Leibniz (1662), and Englishman John Graunt (1660) wrote further on norms of statistics, including the relation of personal choice and judgment to statistical probability. A group of Parisian monks at the Port Royal Monastery (1662) wrote an early text on statistics and were the first to use the word probability. Wondering why people were afraid of lightning even though the probability of being struck is very small, they stated that the "fear of harm ought to be proportional not merely to the gravity of the harm but also to the probability of the event."[1] This linked the severity, perception, and probability of the outcome of the risk for the person involved.

Blaise Pascal (1660) refined the theories of statistics and, with Pierre de Fermat, solved the balla problem of Paccioli. These all paved the way for modern statistics, which essentially began with the use of actuarial tables to determine insurance for merchant ships. This led to the foundation of Lloyds of London, which began its business of naval insurance in the 1770s. That was 100 years after Edward Lloyd opened his coffee shop in London at which merchant ship captains use to gather, trade their experiences, and announce the arrival of ships from various parts of the world.

John Graunt, a British merchant, categorized the cause of death of the London populace using statistical sampling, noting that "considering that it is esteemed an even lay, whether any man lived 10 years longer, I supposed it was the same, that one of any 10 might die within one year." He also noted the reason for doing this: to "set down how many died of each (notorious disease) . . . those persons may better understand the hazard they are in."[2] Graunt's statistics can be compared to recent data from the United States in 1993 in Table 1.2. As a result of this work, the government of the United Kingdom set up the first government-sponsored statistical sampling service.

[1] P. L. Bernstein. *Against the Gods: the Remarkable Story of Risk.* New York, NY: Wiley, 1998. p. 71.
[2] *Ibid.*, p. 82.

With the rise in statistical thinking, Jacob Bernoulli devised the law of large numbers, which stated that as the number of observations increased the actual frequency of an event would approach its theoretical probability. This is the basis of all modern statistical inference. In the 1730s, Daniel Bernoulli (Jacob's nephew) developed the idea of utility as the mathematical combination of the quantity and perception of risk.

Modern era (nineteenth century to today)

The nineteenth century saw the development of modern physiology (Bernard) anesthesia (Morton), antisepsis (Lister and Semmelweis), x-rays (Roentgen), the germ theory (Pasteur and Koch), and psychiatric theory (Freud). The growth of sanitary engineering and public health preceded this in the seventeenth and eighteenth centuries. This improvement had the greatest impact on human health through improved water supplies, waste removal, and living and working conditions. John Snow performed the first recorded modern epidemiological study in 1854 during a cholera epidemic in London. He found that a particular water pump (located on Broad Street) was the source of the epidemic and was being contaminated by sewage dumped into the River Thames. This type of data gathering in medicine was rare up to that time.

The twentieth century saw an explosion of medical technology. Specifics include the discovery of modern medicines (Erlich), antibiotics (sulfanilamide by Domagk and penicillin by Fleming), and modern chemotherapeutic agents to treat ancient scourges like diabetes (insulin by Banting, Best, and McLeod), cancer, and hypertension. The modern era of surgery has led to open-heart surgery, joint replacement, and organ transplantation. Advances in medicine continue at an ever-increasing rate.

Why weren't physicians using statistics in medicine? Before the middle of the twentieth century, advances in medicine and conclusions about human illness occurred mainly through the study of anatomy and physiology. The **case study** or **case series** was a common way to "prove" that a treatment was beneficial or that a certain etiology was the cause of an illness. The use of statistical sampling techniques took a while to develop. There were intense battles between those physicians who wanted to use statistical sampling and those who believed in the power of inductive reasoning from physiological experiments.

Pierre Simon Laplace (yes, the one of the famous law) put forward the idea (1814) that essentially all knowledge was uncertain and therefore probabilistic in nature. The work of Pierre Charles Alexandre Louis (1838) on typhoid and diphtheria showed that bleeding (the most important medical therapeutic tool of the time) was not beneficial in the treatment of these diseases. On the other side was Francois Double (1835) who felt that treatment of the individual was more important that knowing what happens to groups of patients. The art of medicine was defined as deductions from experience and induction from physiologic mechanisms. These were felt to be more important than the "calculus of probability." This debate continued for over 100 years in France, Germany, Britain, and the United States.

The rise of modern biomedical research

Most research done before the twentieth century was more anecdotal than systematic, consisting of descriptions of patients or pathological findings. James Lind, a Royal Navy surgeon, carried out the first recorded clinical trial in 1747. In looking for a cure for scurvy, he fed sailors afflicted with scurvy six different treatments and determined that a factor in limes and oranges (subsequently found to be vitamin C) cured the disease while other foods did not. His study was not blinded, but as a result (although not for 40 years) limes were stocked on all ships of the Royal Navy, and scurvy among sailors (limeys) became a problem of the past.

Research studies of physiology and other basic science research topics began to appear in large numbers in the nineteenth century. By the start of the twentieth century, medicine had moved from the empirical observation of cases to the scientific application of basic sciences to determine the best therapies and catalog diagnoses. Although there were some epidemiological studies that looked at populations, it was uncommon to have any kind of longitudinal study of large groups of patients. There was a 200-year gap from Lind's studies before the **controlled clinical trial** became the standard study for new medical innovations. It was only in the 1950s that the **randomized clinical trial** became the standard for excellent research.

There are three men (sorry, they were, and happened all to be British too) who made great contributions to the early development of the current movement in evidence-based medicine. Sir Ronald Fisher was the father of statistics. Beginning in the early 1900s, he developed the basis for most theories of modern statistical testing. Austin Bradford Hill was another statistician who in 1937 published a series of articles in the *Lancet* on the use of statistical methodology in medical research. In 1947 he published a simple commentary in the *British Medical Journal* calling for the introduction of statistics in the medical curriculum.[3] He called for physicians to be well versed in basic statistics and research study design in order to avoid the biases that were then so prevalent in what passed for medical research. Bradford Hill went on to direct the first true modern randomized clinical trial. He showed that streptomycin (antibiotic) therapy was superior to standard therapy for the treatment of pulmonary tuberculosis.

[3] A. Bradford Hill. Statistics in the medical curriculum? *Br. Med. J.* 1947; ii: 366.

Finally, Archie Cochrane was particularly important in the development of the current movement to perform systematic reviews of medical topics. He was a British general practitioner who did a lot of epidemiological work on respiratory diseases. In the late 1970s he published an epic work on the evidence for medical therapies in perinatal care. This was the first quality-rated systematic review of the literature on a particular topic in medicine. His book *Effectiveness and Efficiency* (1971) set out a rational argument for studying and applying EBM to the clinical situation.[4] Subsequently, groups working on systematic reviews spread through the United Kingdom and now they form a network in cyberspace throughout the world. In his honor they have been named the Cochrane Collaboration.

As Santayana said, it is important to learn from history so as not to repeat the mistakes that civilization has made in the past. The improper application of tainted evidence has resulted in poor medicine and increased cost without improving on human suffering. This book will give physicians the tools to evaluate the medical literature and pave the way for improved health for all. In the next chapter, we will begin where we left off in our history of medicine and statistics and enter the current era of evidence-based medicine.

---

[4] A. L. Cochrane. *Effectiveness & Efficiency: Random Reflections on Health Services.* London: Royal Society of Medicine, 1971.

2

What is evidence-based medicine?

The most savage controversies are those about matters as to which there is no good evidence either way.

Bertrand Russell (1872–1970)

Learning objectives

In this chapter you will learn:
- why you need to study evidence-based medicine
- the elements of evidence-based medicine
- how a good clinical question is constructed

What is so important about evidence

Evidence-based medicine (EBM) has been defined as "the conscientious, explicit, and judicious use of the best evidence in making decisions about the care of individual patients."[1]

In the 1980s there were several studies of the utilization of various operations by the health-care system in the northeastern USA. These showed that there were large variations in the amount of care delivered to similar populations. These studies found variations in rates of prostate surgery and hysterectomy of up to 300% between similar counties. The variation rate in the performance of cataract surgery was 2000%. The researchers concluded that physicians were using very different standards to decide which patients required surgery. Why were physicians using such different rules? Weren't they all reading the same textbooks and journal articles? In that case, shouldn't their practice be more uniform?

"Daily, clinicians confront questions about the interpretation of diagnostic tests, the harm associated with exposure to an agent, the prognosis of disease in a

---

[1] D. L. Sackett, W. M. Rosenberg, J. A. M. Gray, R. B. Haynes & W. S. Richardson. Evidence based medicine: what it is and what it isn't. *BMJ* 1996; 312: 71–72.

specific patient, the effectiveness of a preventive or therapeutic intervention, and the costs and clinical consequences of many other clinical decisions. Both clinicians and policy makers need to know whether the conclusions of a systematic review are valid, and whether recommendations in practice guidelines are sound."[2]

EBM stems from the physician's need to have *proven* therapies to offer patients. This is a paradigm shift that represents both a breakdown of the traditional hierarchical system of medical practice and the acceptance of the scientific method as the governing force in advancing the field of medicine. Simply stated, EBM is the application of the best evidence that can be found in the medical literature to the patient with a medical problem. It should result in the best possible care given to each patient. **Evidence-based clinical practice (EBCP)** is an approach to medical practice in which you (the clinician) are able to evaluate the strength of that evidence and use it in the best clinical practice for the patient sitting in your office.

Medical decision making: expert vs. evidence-based

the scientific basis of medical research, evidence-based medical practice been around for centuries. Its explicit application (as EBM) to problem ng in clinical medicine began simultaneously in the late 1980s at McMaster versity in Canada and at Oxford University in the United Kingdom. In response to high variability of practice, increasing costs, and complexity of medical care, systems were needed to define the best (and cheapest) treatments. Individuals trained in both clinical medicine and epidemiology collaborated to develop strategies to assist in the critical appraisal of clinical data from the biomedical journals.

In the past, a physician faced with a "clinical predicament" would turn to a senior physician (expert) for the definitive answer to this problem. This could take the form of an informal discussion on rounds with the senior attending (consultant) physician, or the referral of a patient to a specialist. The answer would come from the more experienced (and usually older) physician, and would be taken at face value by the younger (and more inexperienced) physician. It was usually based upon the many years of experience of the older physician, but was not necessarily ever tested empirically.

Steps in practicing evidence-based medicine

There are six steps in the process of EBM. These steps are also called the educational prescription[3], and they are as follows:

[2] McMaster University Department of Clinical Epidemiology and Biostatistics. Evidence-based clinical practice (EBCP) course, 1999.
[3] Based on: W. S. Richardson. *Educational prescription: the five elements.* University of Rochester.

(1) Craft a clinical question. This is the most important step since it sets the stage for a successful answer to the clinical predicament. It includes four parts:

The **patient** (population or clinical problem of interest)

The **intervention** (could be an exposure, test, or treatment)

The **comparison** (what you think the intervention is better or worse than)

The **outcome** of interest (ideally, the one of interest to the patient)

(2) Search the **medical literature** for those studies that are most likely to give the best evidence. This step requires good searching skills (**medical informatics**).

(3) Find the study that will best be able to answer this question, determine the magnitude (**effect size**) and precision of the final results.

(4) Perform a **critical appraisal** of the study to determine the **validity** of the results. Look for **sources of bias** that may represent a fatal flaw in the study.

(5) Determine how the results will help you in caring for your patient (**clinical application** or **external validity** of the study).

(6) Finally, you should **evaluate** the results in your patient or population.

With the rise of EBM, various groups have developed ways to package evidence to make it more useful to individual practitioners. These are the output of individual authors performing critical evaluation of clinically important questions. Various online databases around the world serve as repositories for these summaries of evidence. To date, most of the major centers for the dissemination of these have been in the United Kingdom.

The National Health Service sponsors the Centre for Evidence-Based Medicine based at Oxford University. This center is the home of various EBM resources. *Bandolier* is a summary of recent interesting evidence evaluated by the center and is published monthly. It is found at www.jr2.ox.ac.uk/bandolier, and is a wonderful blend of interesting medical information and uniquely British humor in an easy-to-read format. It is excellent for student use and free to browse. The center also has various other free and easily accessible features on its main site found at www.cebm.net. Other useful EBM websites are listed in the Bibliography.

Alphabet soup of critical appraisal of the medical literature

Several commonly used forms of critical appraisal are the Critically Appraised Topic (CAT), Disease Oriented Evidence (DOE), the Patient-Oriented Evidence that Matters (POEM), and the Journal Club Bank (JCB). The CAT format is developed by the Centre for Evidence-Based Medicine and many CATs are available online at the Center's website. CATs use the "User's guide to the medical literature" format (see Bibliography) to catalog reviews of clinical studies. DOEs and POEMs are a format developed for use by family physicians by the American Academy of Family Practice. The JCB is the format for the Evidence-Based Interest

Group of the American College of Physicians (ACP) and the Evidence Based Emergency Medicine group (www.ebem.org) working through the New York Academy of Medicine. Other organizations are beginning to use these formats to disseminate critical reviews on the web.

A DOE is a critical review of a study that shows that there is a change in the disease status when a particular intervention is applied. However, this disease-specific outcome may not make a difference to an individual patient. For example, it is clear that certain drugs (statins) lower cholesterol. However, it is not necessarily true that the same drugs reduce mortality from heart disease. Studies for some of these statin drugs have shown this correlation and therefore are POEMS. Another example is the PSA test for detecting prostate cancer. There is no question that the test can detect prostate cancer most of the time at a stage that is earlier than would be detected by a physician examination (positive DOE). However, it has yet to be shown that early detection using the PSA results in longer life span or an improved quality of life (not a positive POEM).

Other compiled sources of evidence are the American Society of Internal Medicine and American College of Physicians *ACP Journal Club*, published by the journal *Annals of Internal Medicine*, and the Cochrane Library, sponsored by the National Health Service in the United Kingdom. Both are available by subscription. The next step for the future use of EBM in this process is making the evidence easily available at the patient's bedside. This has been tried using an "evidence cart" containing a computer loaded with evidence-based resources during rounds.[4] Currently, PDAs and other handheld devices with large amounts of evidence downloaded onto them are being used at the bedside to fulfil this mission.

For many physicians, the most complex part of the process of EBM is the critical appraisal of the medical literature. Part of the perceived complexity with this process is a (natural) fear of statistics and consequent lack of understanding of statistical processes. The book will teach this in several steps. Each step will be reinforced on the CD-ROM with a series of practice problems and self-assessment learning exercises (SALEs) in which examples from the medical literature will be presented. This will also help you develop your skills of formulating clinical questions, and in time you will become a competent evaluator of the medical literature. This skill will serve you well for the rest of your career.

The clinical question: background vs. foreground

You can classify clinical questions into two basic types. **Background** questions are those which have been answered in the past and are now part of the "fiber

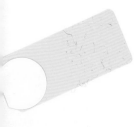

[4] D. L. Sackett & S. E. Straus. Finding and applying evidence during clinical rounds: the "evidence cart". *JAMA* 1998; 280: 1336–1338.

of medicine." Answers to these questions are usually found in medical textbook chapters. The learner must beware since the answers to these questions may be inaccurate or incorrect. They may not be based upon any credible evidence. Typical background questions relate to the nature of a disease or the usual cause, diagnosis, or treatment of common illnesses.

Foreground questions are those usually found at the cutting edge of medicine. They are questions about the most recent therapies, diagnostic tests, or current theories of illness causation. These are the questions that are the heart of the practice of EBM. The four-part clinical question is designed to provide for this information need.

The determination of whether a question is foreground or background depends upon your level of experience. The experienced clinician will have very few background questions that need to be researched. On the other hand, the novice has so many unanswered questions that most are of a background nature. The graph in Fig. 2.1 shows the relationship between foreground and background questions and the clinician's experience.

When do you want to get the most current evidence? How often is access to EBM needed each day for the average clinician? Most physician work is based upon knowledge gained by answering background questions. There are some situations where current (and best) evidence is more helpful. These include questions that are going to make a major impact for your patient. Will the disease kill them, and if so how long will it take and what will their death be like? These are typical questions that a cancer patient would want to know about. Other reasons for searching for the best current evidence include problems that recur commonly in your practice, those in which you are especially interested, or those for which answers are easily found. The case where you are confronted with a patient whose problem you cannot solve and for which there is no good background information would lead you to search for the most current (foreground) evidence.

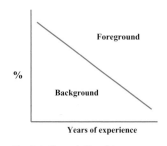

Fig. 2.1 The relationship between foreground and background questions and the clinician's experience.

The clinical question: structure of the question

The first and most critical part of the EBM process is to ask the right question. We are all familiar with the computer analogy, "garbage in, garbage out." The clinical question (or query) should have a defined structure. The **PICO** model has become the standard for stating a searchable question. A good question involves **Patient**, **Intervention**, **Comparison**, and **Outcome**. These must be clearly stated in order to search the question accurately.

　The **patient** refers to the population group to which you want to apply the information. This is the patient sitting in your office, clinic, or surgery. If you are too specific with the population, you will have trouble finding any evidence for that person. Therefore, you must initially be pretty general in your specification of this group. If your patient is a middle-aged man with hypertension, there may be many studies of the current best treatment of hypertension in this group. However, if you had a middle-aged African-American woman in front of you, you may not find studies that are limited to this population. Asking about treatment of hypertension in general will turn up the most evidence. You can then look through these studies to find those applicable to that patient.

The **intervention** is the therapy, exposure (to a potentially harmful process), or diagnostic test which you are interested in applying to your patient. This could simply be a new drug. If you are answering a question about the causes of diseases or risk factors leading to premature mortality, you will be looking for etiology. We will discuss studies of diagnostic tests in more detail in Chapters 20–26.

The **comparison** is the intervention (therapy, etiology, or diagnostic test) against which the intervention is measured. A reasonable comparison group is one that would be commonly encountered in clinical practice. Testing a new drug against one that is never used in current practice is not going to help the practitioner. The comparison group ought to be a real alternative and not just a "straw man." The use of placebo in many studies is no longer considered ethical since there are acceptable treatments for the problem being studied.

The **outcome** is the endpoint of interest to you or your patient. Not all outcomes are important to the patient. One type of outcome is the surrogate outcome. This refers to disease markers that ought to cause changes in the disease process. However, this may not always be true. Studies of heart-attack patients done in the 1960s showed that some died suddenly from irregular heart rhythms. These were identified before death by the presence of abnormal beats (premature ventricular contractions, PVCs) on the electrocardiogram. Physicians thereafter began treating all patients with heart attacks with drugs to suppress PVCs and noted that there was a lower rate of patients with PVCs. They thought this would reduce deaths in all patients with heart attacks. But a large study found that the death rate actually increased when all patients were given these drugs. While they prevented death in a small number of patients who had PVCs, they increased death rates in other (and unfortunately in a majority of) patients. The most important outcomes are the ones that matter to the patient, most often death, disability, or full recovery.

Putting EBM into context in the current practice of medicine: the science and art of medicine

Although most physicians believe that they practice EBM all the time, the observed variation in practice suggests otherwise. EBM can be viewed as an attempt to standardize the practice of medicine. At the same time, it is not "cookbook" medicine. The application of EBM may suggest the best approach to a specific clinical problem. However, it is still up to the clinician to determine whether the individual patient will benefit from that approach. If your patient is very different from those for whom there is evidence, you may be justified in taking another approach to solve the problem. This ought to be based upon sound background and pathophysiological information.

Evidence-based medicine is only one part of an ongoing process of lifelong learning for physicians. It is not a club with which you can beat your opponent senseless through the stellar application of profound pronouncements. It should be part of the everyday practice of all physicians.

It is only slightly more than 50 years since statistics was first felt to be an important part of the medical curriculum. In a 1947 commentary in the *British Medical Journal* entitled Statistics in the medical curriculum?[5] Sir Austin Bradford Hill lamented that most physicians would interpret this as "What! Statistics in the medical curriculum?" We are now in a more enlightened era. We recognize the need for physicians to be able to understand the nature of statistical processes and to be able to interpret these for their patients. This goes to the heart of the science and art of medicine.

The science is in the literature and in the ability of the clinician to interpret that literature. The art is in determining to which patients the literature will apply and then communicating the results to the patients. You learn scientific facts during the first two years of medical school that will be the building blocks for caring for your future patients. The clinical and basic sciences are the foundation of the science of medicine. Having a critical understanding of new advances in medicine through reading the medical literature is an important part of this science. You will also learn the art of medicine. This includes the ability to perform an adequate history and physical examination of your patient so that you can extract the maximum amount of evidence to use for good medical decision making. You will also need to give information to your patient about their illness and be able to empower them to act appropriately to effect a cure or control and moderate the illness. Finally, you must be able to know when to apply the results of the most current literature to your patient. When is the patient close enough in characteristics to the population group studied and when should other approaches to the patient's illness be used?

Finally, Fig. 2.2 is a reprint from the *BMJ* (the journal formerly known as the *British Medical Journal*) which is a humorous look at alternatives to evidence-based medicine.

[5] A. Bradford Hill. *Br. Med. J.* 1947; ii: 366.

Departments of Education and Medicine, New Children's Hospital, Westmead, NSW 2145, Australia
David Isaacs
clinical professor
Dominic Fitzgerald
staff physician

Correspondence to:
D Isaacs
davidi@nch.edu.au

BMJ 1999;319:1618

Clinical decisions should, as far as possible, be evidence based. So runs the current clinical dogma.[1 2] We are urged to lump all the relevant randomised controlled trials into one giant meta-analysis and come out with a combined odds ratio for all decisions. Physicians, surgeons, nurses are doing it[3-5]; soon even the lawyers will be using evidence based practice.[6] But what if there is no evidence on which to base a clinical decision?

Participants, methods, and results

We, two humble clinicians ever ready for advice and guidance, asked our colleagues what they would do if faced with a clinical problem for which there are no randomised controlled trials and no good evidence. We found ourselves faced with several personality based opinions, as would be expected in a teaching hospital. The personalities transcend the disciplines, with the exception of surgery, in which discipline transcends personality. We categorised their replies, on the basis of no evidence whatsoever, as follows.

Eminence based medicine—The more senior the colleague, the less importance he or she placed on the need for anything as mundane as evidence. Experience, it seems, is worth any amount of evidence. These colleagues have a touching faith in clinical experience, which has been defined as "making the same mistakes with increasing confidence over an impressive number of years."[7] The eminent physician's white hair and balding pate are called the "halo" effect.

Vehemence based medicine—The substitution of volume for evidence is an effective technique for brow beating your more timorous colleagues and for convincing relatives of your ability.

Eloquence based medicine—The year round suntan, carnation in the button hole, silk tie, Armani suit, and tongue should all be equally smooth. Sartorial elegance and verbal eloquence are powerful substitutes for evidence.

Providence based medicine—If the caring practitioner has no idea of what to do next, the decision may be best left in the hands of the Almighty. Too many clinicians, unfortunately, are unable to resist giving God a hand with the decision making.

Diffidence based medicine—Some doctors see a problem and look for an answer. Others merely see a problem. The diffident doctor may do nothing from a sense of despair. This, of course, may be better than doing

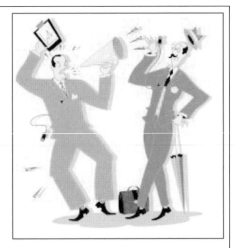

something merely because it hurts the doctor's pride to do nothing.

Nervousness based medicine—Fear of litigation is a powerful stimulus to overinvestigation and overtreatment. In an atmosphere of litigation phobia, the only bad test is the test you didn't think of ordering.

Confidence based medicine—This is restricted to surgeons (table).

Comment

There are plenty of alternatives for the practising physician in the absence of evidence. This is what makes medicine an art as well as a science.

Contributors: DI and DF each contributed half the jokes and will both act as guarantors.
   Funding: None.
   Competing interests: None declared.

1 Evidence Based Medicine Working Group. Evidence-based medicine: a new approach to teaching the practice of medicine. *JAMA* 1992;268: 2420-5.
2 Rosenberg W, Donald A. Evidence based medicine: an approach to clinical problem solving. *BMJ* 1995;310:1122-6.
3 Sackett DL, Rosenberg WM, Gray JAM, Haynes RB, Richardson WS. Evidence based medicine: what it is and what it isn't. *BMJ* 1996;312:71-2.
4 Solomon MJ, McLeod RS. Surgery and the randomised controlled trial: past, present and future. *Med J Aust* 1998;169:380-3.
5 McClarey M. Implementing clinical effectiveness. *Nursing Management* 1998;5:16-9.
6 EBM and the IMF. *J Exponential Salaries* 1999;99:1-9.
7 O'Donnell M. *A sceptic's medical dictionary.* London: BMJ Books, 1997.

Basis of clinical practice

Basis for clinical decisions	Marker	Measuring device	Unit of measurement
Evidence	Randomised controlled trial	Meta-analysis	Odds ratio
Eminence	Radiance of white hair	Luminometer	Optical density
Vehemence	Level of stridency	Audiometer	Decibels
Eloquence (or elegance)	Smoothness of tongue or nap of suit	Teflometer	Adhesin score
Providence	Level of religious fervour	Sextant to measure angle of genuflection	International units of piety
Diffidence	Level of gloom	Nihilometer	Sighs
Nervousness	Litigation phobia level	Every conceivable test	Bank balance
Confidence*	Bravado	Sweat test	No sweat

*Applies only to surgeons.

Fig. 2.2 Isaacs, D. & Fitzgerald, D. Seven alternatives to evidence based medicine. *BMJ* 1999; 319: 1618. Reprinted with permission.

3

Causation

Heavier than air flying machines are impossible.

Lord Kelvin, President of the Royal Society, 1895

Learning objectives

In this chapter you will learn:
- cause-and-effect relationships
- Koch's principles
- the concept of contributory cause
- the relationship of the clinical question to the type of study

The ultimate goal of medical research is to increase our knowledge about the interaction of a particular agent (cause) with our health or disease (effect). Causation is the relationship between an exposure and an outcome such that the exposure resulted in the outcome. However, the strength of an association may not be equivalent to proving a cause-and-effect relationship. In this chapter, we will discuss the theories of causation. By the end of this chapter you will be able to determine the type of causation in a study. The stronger the design of a study, the more likely it is to prove a relationship between cause and effect.

Cause-and-effect relationships

Most biomedical research studies try to prove a relationship between a particular cause and a specified effect. The **cause** may be a risk factor resulting in a disease, or a treatment helping alleviate suffering. The **effect** is a particular outcome that we want to measure. Not all study designs are capable of proving a cause-and-effect relationship. We will discuss these study designs in a later chapter.

The cause is also called the **independent variable**. The researcher or the environment sets this. The cause is a risk factor (or exposure), diagnostic test, or treatment. The effect is called the **dependent variable**. It is dependent upon the action of the independent variable. It can be an outcome (death, survival, etc.) or a degree of improvement on a clinical score or the detection of disease by a diagnostic test. You ought to be able to identify the cause and effect easily in the study you are evaluating. The structure of the study should obviously describe which variable is which. If not, there are problems with the study design. In some studies relating to the prognosis of disease, time is the independent variable.

Types of causation

It's not always easy to establish a link between a disease (or any effect) and its suspected cause. For example, we think that hyperlipidemia (elevated levels of lipids or fats in the blood) is a cause of cardiovascular disease. But how can we be sure that this is a cause and not just a related factor? Perhaps hyperlipidemia is caused by inactivity or a sedentary lifestyle and the lack of exercise causes both cardiovascular disease and hyperlipidemia.

This may even be true with acute infections. *Streptococcus viridans* is a bacterium that can cause infection of the heart valves. However, it takes more than the presence of the bacterium in the blood to cause the infection. We cannot say that the presence of the bacterium in the blood is sufficient to cause this infection. There must be other factors such as local deformity of the valve or immunocompromise that make the valve prone to infection.

In a more mundane example, it has been noted that the more churches a town has, the more robberies occur. Does this mean that clergy are robbing people? No – it simply means that a third variable, population, explains the number both of churches and of muggings. Likewise, we know that *Streptococcus viridans* is a cause of subacute endocarditis. But it is neither the only cause, nor does it always lead to the result of an infected heart valve. How are we to be sure?

In medical science, there are two types of cause-and-effect relationships: **Koch's postulates** and **contributory cause**. Robert Koch, a nineteenth-century microbiologist, developed his famous postulates as criteria to determine if a certain microbiologic agent was the cause of an illness. Acute infectious diseases were the scourge of mankind before the mid twentieth century. As a result of better public health measures (water treatment and sewage disposal) and antibiotics these are less of a problem today. Dr. Koch studied the anthrax bacillus as a cause of habitual abortion in cattle. He created the postulates while trying to determine the exact cause of the illness. This was an attempt to determine the relationship between the agent causing the illness and the illness itself.

Koch's postulates stated four basic steps to prove causation. First, the infectious agent must be found in all cases of the illness. Second, when found it must be able to be isolated from the diseased host and grown in a pure culture. Next, the agent from the culture when introduced into a healthy host must cause the illness. Finally, the infectious agent must again be recovered from the new host and grown in a pure culture. This entire cascade must be met in order to prove causation.

While this model may work well in the study of infectious diseases, most modern illnesses (the ones you will see as a clinician) are chronic and degenerative in nature. Illnesses such as diabetes, heart disease and cancer tend to be multifactorial in their **etiology** (cause). There are multiple factors causing or exacerbating the illness, and usually multiple factors that can alleviate the illness. It is virtually impossible to pinpoint a single cause or the effects of a single treatment, and most research studies of these diseases cannot clearly determine a single cause and effect. Stronger studies of these diseases are more likely to point to useful clinical information relating one particular cause with an effect on the illness.

Applying **contributory cause** helps prove causation in these complex and multifactorial diseases. The requirements for proof are less stringent than Koch's postulates. However, since the disease-related factors are multifactorial, it is more difficult to prove that any one factor is decisive in either causing or curing the disease. Contributory cause recognizes that there is a large gray zone in which some of the many causes and treatments of a disease overlap.

First, the cause and effect must be seen together more often than would be expected to occur by chance alone. This means that they can be linked more often than would be expected if that relationship (linkage) was untrue and any concurrence of those two factors was a random event. Second, the cause must always be noted to precede the effect. If there were situations for which the effect was noted before the occurrence of the cause, that would negate this relationship in time. Finally and ideally, it should be able to be shown that changing the cause changes the effect. This last factor is the most difficult to prove and requires an intervention study be performed. Contributory cause to prove the nature of a chronic and multifactorial illness must minimally show association and temporality. However, to strengthen the causation, the change of the effect by a changing cause must also be shown. Table 3.1 compares Koch's postulates and contributory cause.

Causation and the clinical question

The components of causation are both parts of the **clinical question**. Since this is the first step in EBM, it is useful to put the clinical question into the context of causation. The **intervention** (exposure, test, or treatment) is the **cause** that is being investigated. In most studies this is compared to another cause, named the **comparison**. The **outcome** of interest is the **effect**. You will learn to use good searching techniques to make sure that the study you find answers this query in

Table 3.1. Koch's   postulates vs. contributory cause

Koch's postulates (most stringent)

(1) **Sufficient**: if the agent (cause) is present the disease (effect) is present
(2) **Necessary**: if the agent (cause) is absent, the disease (effect) is absent
(3) **Specific**: the agent (cause) is associated with only one disease (effect)

Contributory cause (most clinically relevant)

(1) Not all patients with the particular cause will develop the effect (disease): the cause is **not sufficient**
(2) Not all patients with the specific effect (disease) were exposed to the particular cause: the cause is **not necessary**
(3) The cause may be associated with several diseases (effects) and is therefore **non-specific**

Table 3.2. Cause and effect relationship for most common types of studies

Type of study	Cause	Effect
Etiology, harm, or risk	Medication, environmental, or genetic agent	Disease, complication, or mortality
Therapy or prevention	Medication, other therapy, or preventive modality	Improvement of symptoms or mortality
Prognosis	Disease or therapy	Time to outcome
Diagnosis	Diagnostic test	Accuracy of diagnosis

the best (most powerful) manner possible. The intervention, comparison, and outcome all relate to the patent **population** being studied.

Primary clinical research studies can be roughly divided into four types. The type of study is determined by the elements of cause and effect. They are studies of **etiology** (or harm or risk), **therapy**, **prognosis**, and **diagnosis**. (There are numerous secondary study types that will be covered later in the book.) The nomenclature used for describing the cause and effect in these studies can be somewhat confusing and is shown in Table 3.2.

- Studies of etiology, harm, or risk compare groups of patients that have or don't have the outcome and look to see if they do or don't have the risk factor. They can also go in the other direction, starting from the presence or absence of the risk factor and finding out who did or didn't have the (outcome) disease. The direction of the study can be either forward or backward in time. A useful way of looking at this category is to look for **cohort**, **case–control** or **cross-sectional** studies. In the case of studies of etiology, the causative factor for a disease is the cause and the presence of disease is the outcome.

• Studies of therapy or prevention tend to be **randomized clinical trials**, in which some patients get the therapy (or prevention) being tested and the others don't. The outcome (effect) is compared between the two groups.

• Studies of prognosis look at disease progression over time. They can be either cohort studies or randomized clinical trials. We will discuss the various types of studies in later chapters.

• Studies of diagnosis are unique in that we are looking for some diagnostic maneuver or test that will separate those with a disease from those who may have a similar presentation and yet not have the disease. Usually these are cohort, case–control, or cross-sectional studies.

There is a relationship between the clinical question and the study type. In general the clinical question can be written as: among (population) patients with a particular disease, does the presence of (intervention) a therapy or risk factor (compared with no presence), change the (outcome) probability of an adverse event? For a study of risk or harm, we can write this as: among patients with **disease** or **characteristic**, does the presence of (exposure to) **risk factor**, compared with the absence of (lack of exposure to) **risk factor**, worsen the **outcome**? We can also write it as: among patients with exposure or non-exposure (population) to a risk factor (intervention and comparison), are they more likely to have the outcome of interest? For therapy, the question is: among patients with **disease** or **characteristic**, does the presence of (exposure to) **therapy**, compared with the use of placebo or **standard therapy**, improve the **outcome**? The form of the question can help you perform better searches, as we will see in the next chapter. Through regular practice, you will learn to write better questions.

4

The medical literature: an overview

It is astonishing with how little reading a doctor can practice medicine, but it is not astonishing how badly he may do it.

Sir William Osler (1849–1919)

Learning objectives

In this chapter you will learn:
- the scope and function of the articles you will find in the medical literature
- the function of the main parts of a research article

The medical literature is the source of most of our current information on the best medical practices. This literature consists of different types of articles including research studies. To be an intelligent reader of the medical literature you must understand the information that different types of article are capable of providing. In order to evaluate the results of a research study, you must understand what clinical research articles are designed to do and what they are capable of accomplishing. Each part of a study contributes to the final results of the published research.

Where is clinical research found?

In your medical career, you will read (and perhaps also write) lots of research papers. All medical specialties have at least one primary peer-reviewed journal. Most have several. There are also many general-interest medical journals. One of the things you will notice is that not all journals are created equal. Peer-reviewed journals are "better" than non peer-reviewed journals since their articles are more carefully screened and contain fewer "problems." Many of these journals have a statistician on staff to assure that the statistical tests used are correct.

The *New England Journal of Medicine* and the *Journal of the American Medical Association (JAMA)* are the most widely read and prestigious general medical journals in the United States. The *Lancet* and the *British Medical Journal (BMJ)* are the other top English-language journals in the world. However, even these excellent journals print "imperfect" studies. The consumer of this literature (you) is responsible for determining how to use the results of clinical research. You will have to interpret the results of these research studies to your patients. They will read about studies in the lay press and base their decisions about health care upon what popular magazine writers and editors say in these articles and accompanying editorials. In order to interpret the studies your patients are reading about in the media you require a healthy skepticism of the content of the medical literature as well as a working knowledge of critical appraisal. Other physicians, journal reviewers, and even editors may not be as well trained as you.

Non-peer-reviewed and minor journals may still have articles and studies that give good information. Many of the articles in these journals tend to be expert reviews or case reports. These are useful for reviewing and relearning background information. However, no matter how prestigious the journal, no study is perfect. But all studies have some degree of useful information. A partial list of common and important medical journals is included in the Bibliography.

What are the important types of article?

There are several broad types of article that you should be familiar with. Each has its own strengths and problems. These are different from clinical research studies such as epidemiological studies (case–control, cohort or cross-sectional) and randomized clinical trials. We will discuss the common types of clinical research studies in Chapter 6.

Animal or **basic science** (**bench research**) studies are usually considered pure research. They may be of questionable usefulness in humans (your patients) since people are not laboratory rats and *in vitro* does not always equal *in vivo*. Because of this, they may not pass the "so what?" test. However, they are useful preliminary studies, and they may justify and suggest human clinical studies. It is only through these types of studies that medicine will continue to push the envelope of our knowledge of physiological and biochemical mechanisms of disease.

Animal or other bench research is often used to justify certain treatments. This leap of faith may result in potentially harmful or at best not helpful treatments being given to patients. An example of potentially useful basic science research is the discovery of angiostatin, a chemical that stops the growth of blood vessels into a tumor. Publication of research done in mice showing that infusion of this chemical caused regression of tumors resulted in a sudden increase in inquiries to physicians from families of patients with cancer hoping that they would be able to obtain the drug and get a cure. Unfortunately, this was not going to happen. First the drug had to be given to patients in a clinical trial, and this showed results that were much less dramatic. Similar results happened with bone-marrow transplant therapy for breast cancer.

The discovery of two forms of the enzyme cyclo-oxygenase (COX 1 and 2) was done in animals and using basic research in humans. COX 2 is a primary enzyme in the inflammatory process, while COX 1 is the primary enzyme in the maintenance of the mucosal protection of the stomach. Inhibition of both enzymes is the primary action of most non-steroidal anti-inflammatory drugs (NSAIDs). With the discovery of these two enzymes, drugs selective for inhibition of the COX 2 enzyme were developed. These had anti-inflammatory action without causing gastric mucosal irritation and gastrointestinal bleeding. This looked like a real advance in medicine and the drugs were equivalent in anti-inflammatory action to the other NSAIDs. However, to extend the use of this class of drug to routine pain management is probably not warranted. Clinical studies have demonstrated equivalence in pain control with other NSAIDs, but only modest reductions in side effects, and these came at a very large increase in cost.

Basic science research is important to increase the content of biomedical knowledge. Recent basic science research has demonstrated the plasticity of the nervous system. When I was in medical school, it was standard teaching that nervous-system cells were permanent and not able to regenerate. Current research now shows that new brain and nerve cells can be grown. This research has been done in animals and in humans. While not clinically useful at this time, it is promising research for the treatment of degenerative nerve disorders such as Alzheimer's disease.

The results of these studies are sometimes accepted without question because of a feeling that since they measure basic physiologic processes they are more reliable. A recent study by Bogardus *et al.* found that there were significant methodological problems in many studies of molecular genetics (essentially, basic science) techniques in clinical settings (clinical studies).[1] While this book focuses on clinical studies, the principles discussed also apply to basic research studies.

Editorials are opinion pieces written by a recognized expert on a given topic. Most often they are published in response to a study in the same journal issue. Editorials are the vehicle that puts a study into perspective and shows its usefulness in clinical practice. They give "contextual commentary" on the study. Because an expert is giving an opinion, the piece incorporates their **biases**. They should be well referenced.

---

[1] S. T. Bogardus, J. Concato & A. R. Feinstein. Clinical epidemiological quality in molecular genetic research: the need for methodological standards. *JAMA* 1999; 281: 1919.

A **clinical review** article seeks to review all the important studies on a given subject to date. It is written by an expert or someone with a special interest in the topic and is more up to date than a textbook. It is subject to the authors' biases in reporting the results of the referenced studies. The strength of the review depends upon the strength of each individual study. Although useful to update one's own knowledge, it should not be accepted uncritically. It is most useful for new learners updating their background information. However, if you are familiar with the background literature and can determine the accuracy of the citations and subsequent recommendations, a review can help to put clinical problems into perspective. This type of review is different from a systematic review.

Meta-analysis or **systematic review** is a relatively new technique to provide a comprehensive and objective analysis of all clinical studies on a given topic. It attempts to combine many studies and will be more objective in reviewing these studies. The authors apply statistical techniques to quantitatively combine the results of the selected studies. We will discuss the details on evaluating these types of article in Chapter 31.

Components of a clinical research study

Clinical studies should be reported upon in a standardized manner. Most journals have now accepted the IMRAD style. This stands for Introduction, Methods, Results, and Discussion. First proposed by Day in 1989, it is now the standard for all clinical studies reported in the English-language literature.[2] Structured abstracts proposed by the SORT (Standards of Reporting Trials) group are also now being used in most medical journals. The structure of the abstract follows the structure of the full article (Table 4.1).

The **abstract** is a summary of the study. It should accurately reflect what actually happened in the study. Its purpose is to give you an overview of the research and let you decide if you want to read the article in the first place. The abstract includes a sentence or two on each of the elements of the article. These include the introduction, study design, population studied, interventions and comparisons, outcomes measured, primary or most important results, and conclusions. The abstract may not completely or accurately represent the actual findings of the article and often does not contain important information found only in the article. Therefore it should never be used as the sole source of information about the study.

---

[2] R. A. Day. The origins of the scientific paper: the IMRAD format. *AMIAJ* 1989; 4: 16–18.

Table 4.1. Components
of reported clinical
studies

(1) Abstract
(2) Introduction
(3) Methods
(4) Results
(5) Discussion
(6) Conclusion
(7) References/bibliography

The **introduction** is a brief statement of the problem to be solved and the purpose of the research. It describes the importance of the study by giving the reader a brief overview of previous research on the same or related topics or the scientific justification for doing the study. The hypotheses being tested should be *explicitly* stated. Too often, the hypothesis is only implied, potentially leaving the study open to misinterpretation. As we will learn later, only the **null hypothesis** can be directly tested. Therefore, the null hypothesis should either be explicitly stated or obvious from the statement of the expected outcome of the research (called the **alternative hypothesis**).

The **methods** section is the most important part of a research study. Unfortunately, it is also the least frequently read. It includes a detailed description of the **research design**, the population sample, and the process of the research. There should be enough details to allow anyone reading the study to replicate the experiment. Careful reading of this section will suggest potential biases and threats to the validity of the study.

(1) The **sample** is the population being studied. It should also be the population to which the study is intended to pertain. The processes of **sample selection** and/or **assignment** must be adequately described. This includes the **eligibility requirements** or **inclusion criteria** (who could be entered into the experiment) and **exclusion criteria** (who is not allowed to be in the study and why). It also includes a description of the **setting** in which the study is being done. The site of research (community outpatient clinic, specialty practice, hospital, or others) may influence the types of patient enrolled in the study.

(2) The **procedure** describes both the experimental processes and the outcome measures. It includes **data acquisition, randomization** (how were subjects allocated to different groups?), and **blinding** conditions (are the treating professionals, observers, or participants aware of the nature of the study and is it **single-, double-,** or **triple-blinded**?). The variables examined (all the outcome measures), how they are measured, and the quality of these measures

(the **instruments** and **measurements**) should all be explicitly described. In studies that depend on record review, the process by which that review was carried out should be explicitly described.

(3) The **statistical analysis section** includes types of **data** (**nominal**, **ordinal**, **interval**, **ratio**, **continuous**, or **dichotomous**), how the data are described (**measures of central tendency** and **dispersion** of data), and what **analytic** (**inferential**) statistical tests will be used to assess statistical relationships (differences, etc) between two or more variables. It should also note the levels of α **and** β **error** and the **power**.

The **results** section should summarize all the data pertinent to the purpose of the study. It should also give an explanation of the **statistical significance** of the data. This part of the article is not a place for commentary or opinions – "just the facts!"[3] All important sample and subgroup characteristics, and the results of all important research outcomes, should be included. The degree of variability in measurements (e.g., standard deviations or standard error of the mean), the **measures of central tendency** and **dispersion**, and the **p values** or **confidence intervals** should be given so that readers may determine for themselves if the results are statistically and/or clinically significant. The tables and graphs should be clearly and accurately labeled.

The **discussion** includes an interpretation of the data and a discussion of the clinical importance of the results. It should flow logically from the data shown, incorporating other research about the topic, and explaining why this study did or did not corroborate the results of those studies. Unfortunately, this section is often used to "spin" the results of a study in a particular direction and will over- or under-emphasize certain results. It should include a discussion of the statistical and clinical significance of the results.

(1) The **statistical significance** is a mathematical phenomenon depending only on the number of subjects (**sample size**), the **precision** of the data (degree of variability of the results), and the magnitude of the difference found between groups (**effect size**). As the sample size increases a smaller effect size will become statistically significant.

(2) The **clinical significance** means that the results are important and will be useful in clinical practice. If a small effect size is found it may not be clinically important. A study with enough subjects can find statistical significance if even a tiny difference in outcomes of the groups is found. This result may make no difference in the practice of medicine (i.e., for one patient). What is important is a change in status that matters for a given patient (the one sitting in front of you at the moment).

---

[3] Sargent Friday (played by Jack Webb) in the 1960s television show *Dragnet*.

(3) Interpretation of **non-significant results** (absence of evidence of an effect) must be included. The finding that no statistically significant difference was found does not conclusively mean that no relationship exists. The study may not have had adequate **power** to find the results statistically significant. This is especially true for studies with small sample sizes. Absence of evidence of an effect is not the same thing as evidence of absence of an effect.

(4) Finally, the discussion should address all **potential biases** in the study and hypothesize on their effects on the study conclusions. The directions for future research in this area should then be addressed.

The study results should be accurately reflected in the **conclusion** section, a one-paragraph summary of the final outcome. Important sources of bias should be mentioned as disclaimers. Pitfalls in the interpretations of study conclusions include the use of biased language and incorrect interpretation of results not supported by the data. Studies sponsored by drug companies or written by authors with other conflicts of interest may be more prone to these biases. All sources of conflict of interest should be listed either at the start or at the end of the article.

The **references/bibliography** section demonstrates how much the author has included or acknowledged the work of others. This includes a comprehensive reference list including all important studies of the same or similar problem. This is an area which you will be better at interpreting when you have immersed yourself in a specialty area for a while and are able to evaluate this author's use of the literature. Be wary if there are multiple citations of works by just one or two authors (especially if by the author(s) of the current study).

How can you get started?

You have to decide which journals to read. The *New England Journal of Medicine* is a great place for medical students to start. It publishes important and high quality studies and includes lots of correlation with basic sciences. There are also excellent case discussions, review articles, and basic-science articles. In general, begin by reading the abstract. This will tell you if you really want to know what this study is about in the first place. If you don't care about this topic, go on to the next article. Remember, that what you read in the abstract should not be used to apply the results of the study to a clinical scenario. You still need to read and evaluate the article, especially the methods section. *JAMA* (*Journal of the American Medical Association*) is another excellent journal with a lot of studies about medical education and the operation of the health-care system. For readers in the United Kingdom, the *Lancet* and the *BMJ* (*British Medical Journal*) are equivalent journals for the student to begin with.

The rest of this book will present a set of useful skills that will assist you in evaluating clinical research studies. Initially, we will focus on learning how to critically evaluate the most common clinical studies. Specifically, these are studies of therapy, risk, harm, and etiology. Appendix 2 is a useful outline of steps to help you to do this. Later the book will focus on studies of diagnostic tests, clinical decision making, cost analyses, survival analyses (prognosis), and meta-analyses or systematic reviews.

5

Searching the medical literature

Sandi Pirozzo, B.Sc., M.P.H.

Senior Lecturer in Epidemiology, School of Population Health, University of Queensland, Brisbane, Australia

Through seeking we may learn and know things better. But as for certain truth, no man has known it, for all is but a woven web of guesses.

Xenophanes (sixth century BC)

Learning objectives

In this chapter you will learn:
- how to use a clinical question to initiate a medical literature search
- how to formulate an effective search strategy to answer specific clinical questions
- the most appropriate database to use to answer a specific clinical question
- the use of Boolean operators in developing a search strategy
- the types and uses of various evidence-based review databases

To become a lifelong learner, the physician must be a competent searcher of the medical literature. This requires you to be able to develop an effective search strategy for a clinical question. By the end of this chapter you will understand how to write a clinical question and formulate a search of the literature. Once you have written an answerable clinical question and decided on the best study design that could answer the question, your next task is to search the literature and find the best available evidence. While this might appear an easy task, unless you know which database to use and have good searching skills, it can be time-consuming, frustrating and wholly unproductive! This chapter will take you through some common databases and provide you with information that will make your search for evidence both efficient and rewarding.

Introduction

Finding all relevant studies that have addressed a single question is not an easy task. There are currently over 22 000 journals and 10 million articles in the biomedical literature. Although increasing each year, only a small proportion of journals is indexed in databases. A systematic approach to searching this literature is essential in order to identify the best evidence available to answer a clinical question.

Use of different databases

Of all the databases that index medical and health-related literature, **MEDLINE** is probably the best known. It was developed by the National Library of Medicine at the National Institutes of Health in the USA. It is the world's largest general biomedical database and indexes approximately one-third of all biomedical articles. Since it was the first medical literature database available for electronic searching, most clinicians are familiar with its use. Due to its size and breadth, it is sometimes a challenge to get exactly what you want from it. We will look at this database first, after we discuss some basic principles of searching.

In addition to MEDLINE, there are other databases that are more specialized and may yield more clinically useful information, depending on the nature of your query. The database you select depends on the content area and the type of question being asked. The database for nursing and allied health studies is called **CINAHL** and the one for psychological studies is called **PsycINFO**. If you are searching a question of therapy or intervention, then the **Cochrane Library** can be a particularly useful resource. It provides systematic reviews of trials of health-care interventions and a registry of controlled clinical trials. A list of relevant databases and other online resources is provided in the Bibliography.

Developing effective information retrieval strategies

Having selected the most appropriate database you must develop an effective search strategy to retrieve the best available evidence on your topic. This section will give you a general searching framework to apply to any database. Databases often vary in terms of software used, internal structure, indexing terms, and amount of information that they give. However, the principles behind developing a search strategy remain the same.

The first step is to identify the key words or concepts in your study question. This starts a systematic approach to breaking down the question into its individual components. The most useful way of dividing a question into its components is to use the PICO format that we introduced in Chapter 2. To review: P stands for the population of interest; I is the intervention, whether a therapy, diagnostic test, or risk factor; C is the comparison (to the intervention); and O is the outcome of interest.

We can represent a PICO question pictorially using a Venn diagram. We will use an example of the following question: *What is the mortality reduction in colorectal*

Fig. 5.1 Venn diagram for
colorectal screening search.
Comparison is frequently
omitted in search strategies.

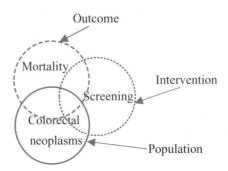

Fig. 5.1 Venn diagram for
colorectal screening search.
Comparison is frequently
omitted in search strategies.

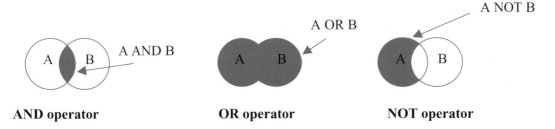

AND operator   OR operator   NOT operator

Fig. 5.2 Boolean operators (AND,
OR and NOT). Blue areas
represent the search results in
each case.

*cancer as a result of performing hemoccult of the stool (fecal occult blood test)
screening in well-appearing adults?* Using the PICO format, we recognize that
mortality is the **outcome**, screening with the hemoccult is the **intervention**, not
screening is the **comparison**, and adults who appear well but do and don't have
colorectal neoplasms is the **population**. The Venn diagram for that question is
shown in Fig. 5.1.

Once the study question has been broken into its components, they can be
combined using Boolean logic. This consists of using the terms **AND**, **OR** and
NOT as part of the search. The AND operator is used when you wish to retrieve
those records containing both terms. Using the AND operator serves to narrow
your search and reduces the number of citations recovered. The OR operator is
used when at least one of the terms must appear in the record. It broadens the
search, should be used to connect synonyms or related concepts, and will increase
the number of citations recovered. Finally, the NOT operator is used to retrieve
records containing one term and not the other. This also reduces the number of
citations recovered and is useful to eliminate potentially irrelevant documents. Be
careful using this operator as it can eliminate useful references too. It can be used
to narrow initially wide-ranging searches. The use of these operators is illustrated
in Fig. 5.2.

Let's use the example of our question about the effect of hemoccult screening
on colon-cancer mortality. The combination of the initial search terms *colorectal
neoplasms AND screening* represents the overlap between these two terms and
retrieves only articles that use both terms. This will give us more articles than if

we used all three terms in one search: *screening AND colorectal neoplasms AND mortality*. That combination represents a smaller area, the one where all three terms overlap, and will retrieve only articles with all three terms.

Although the overlap of all three parts may have the highest concentration of relevant articles, the other areas may still contain many relevant articles. We call this a high-specificity search. The set we retrieve will contain a high proportion of articles that are useful, but many others may be missed. Hence, if the *disease AND study factor* combination (*colorectal neoplasms AND screening*) yields a manageable number of citations, it is best to work with this and not further restrict the search by using the outcomes (*screening AND colorectal neoplasms AND mortality*).

Everyone searches differently! Most people will start big (most hits possible) and then begin limiting the results. Look at these results along the way to make sure you are on the right track. My preference is to start with the smallest number of search terms that gives a reasonable number of citations and then add others (in a Boolean fashion) as a means of either increasing (OR operator) or limiting (AND or NOT operators) the search. Usually, for my purposes, anything less than about 50 to 100 citations to look through by hand is reasonable. Remember that these terms are entered into the database by hand and errors of classification will occur. The more you limit your searches the more likely you will be to miss important citations. In general, both the outcome and study design terms are options usually needed only when the search results are very large and unmanageable.

You can use more complex combinations like *(mortality AND screening) OR (mortality AND colorectal neoplasms) OR (screening AND colorectal neoplasms)* to capture all the overlap areas between all three circles. This strategy will yield a higher number of hits (but less than all three terms with OR connecting them). However, it may not be appropriate if you are looking for a quick answer to a clinical question since you will then have to hand-search more citations. Whatever strategy you choose to start with, try it. You never know (a priori) what you are going to get.

Use of synonyms and wildcard symbol

When the general structure of the question is developed and only a small number of citations is recovered, it may be worthwhile to look for synonyms for each component of the search. For our question about mortality reduction in colorectal cancer from fecal occult blood screening in adults, we can use several synonyms. Screening can be *screen* or *early detection*, colorectal cancer can be *bowel cancer*, and mortality can be *death* or *survival*. Since these terms are entered into the database by coders they may vary greatly from study to study for the same events. What you miss with one synonym, you may pick up with another.

We can also use the truncation or "wildcard" symbol to find all the words with the same stem. Thus our search string can become *(screen* OR early detection) AND (colorectal cancer OR bowel cancer) AND (mortality OR death* OR survival)*. The term *screen** is shorthand for words beginning with "screen." It will turn up screen, screened, screening, etc. The wildcard is extremely useful but should be used with caution. If you were searching for information about hearing problems and you used *hear** as one of your search terms you would retrieve not only articles with the word "hear" and "hearing" but also all those articles with the word "heart!" Note that the wildcard symbol varies between systems: most commonly it is an asterisk (*) or dollar sign ($).

MEDLINE

MEDLINE is available online for free using the PubMed website at www.pubmed.gov. This provides a very user-friendly interface, and the best way to get to know it is to use it, explore its capabilities, and experiment. Rather than provide a comprehensive tutorial on searching PubMed, this chapter will focus on a few of the features that are most helpful in the context of evidence-based medicine.

PUBMED clinical queries: searching using methodological filters

Within PubMed there is a special feature called **clinical queries**, which can be found in the left-hand side bar of the PubMed page. It uses a set of built-in search filters (based on methodological search techniques developed by Haynes in 1994) for the best evidence on clinical questions in four study categories: diagnosis, therapy, etiology and prognosis. In turn each of these categories may be searched with an emphasis on **specificity** (most of the articles retrieved should be relevant, but many articles may be missed) or **sensitivity** (the proportion of relevant articles will decrease, but many more articles will be retrieved). You can also search for a systematic review of your search topic by clicking on the "systematic review" option. Fig. 5.3 shows the PubMed clinical queries page. In order to continue searching in clinical queries, you need to click on the "clinical queries" link in the left-hand side bar each time you conduct a search. If you do not do this, searches will be conducted in general PubMed. Clicking on the "filter table" option within clinical queries allows you to see how each filter is interpreted in PubMed query language.

It is best to start with the specificity emphasis when initiating your search and then add terms to the search if not enough articles are found. Once you enter your search terms in the query box and click on "go," PubMed will display your search results. Your search is then displayed with your search terms as you entered

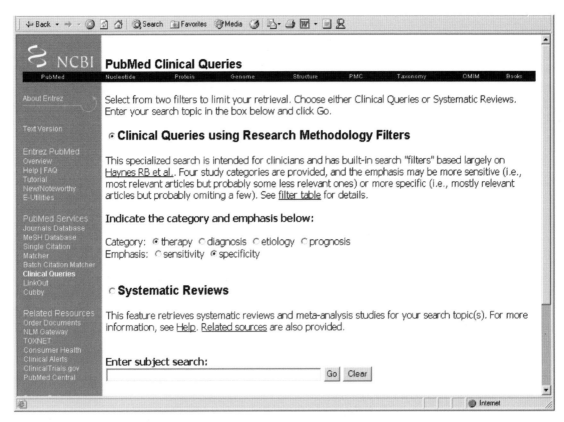

them combined with the methodological filter terms. Below the query box is the features bar, which provides access to additional search options. The PubMed query box and features bar are available from every screen except the clinical queries home page. You must return to the clinical queries homepage to enter a new clinical queries search.

You may enter one or more terms (e.g., *vitamin c AND common cold*) in the query box. The terms are searched in various fields of the record. Boolean operators AND, OR, NOT must be in upper-case (e.g., *vitamin c OR zinc*). The truncation or wildcard symbol (*) is used in the same manner as previously described. PubMed searches for the first 150 variations of a truncated term. If a truncated term (e.g., *staph**) produces more than 150 variations, PubMed displays a warning message such as "Wildcard search for 'staph*' used only the first 150 variations. Lengthen the root word to search for all endings!"

Fig. 5.3 PubMed "clinical queries." (National Library of Medicine. Used with permission.)

Limits

The features bar consists of **limits**, **preview/index**, **history**, **clipboard**, and **details**. If you want to limit your search, click "limits" from the features bar. This

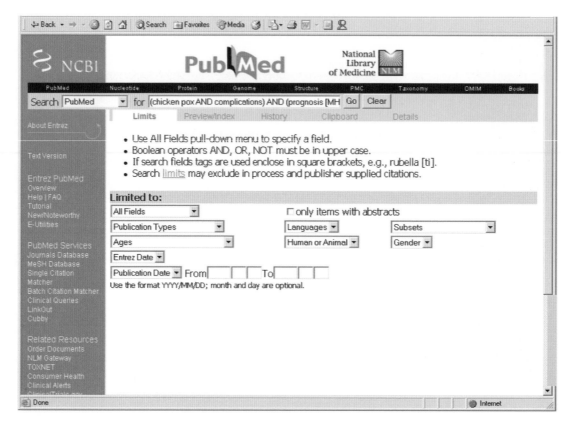

Fig. 5.4 The "limits" window in PubMed. (National Library of Medicine. Used with permission.)

opens the Limits window shown in Fig. 5.4, which offers a number of useful ways of reducing the number of retrieved articles. You can restrict your search to words in a particular field within a citation, to a specific age group or gender, to human or animal studies, to articles published with abstracts or in a specific language, or to a specific publication type (e.g., meta-analysis or RCT).

You can also limit by either Entrez date or publication date. The "Entrez date" is the date the citation was entered into the system; the publication date is the month and year it was published. And lastly, under the subset pull-down menu, you may limit your retrieval to a specific subset of citations within PubMed, such as AIDS-related or other citations. If you have applied limits to a search the check-box next to "limits" will be marked and a listing of your limit selections will be displayed. To turn off the existing limits, click on the check-box to remove the check before running your next search.

History

PubMed will retain your entire search strategy and results, which can be viewed by clicking on "history" from the features bar. This feature is only available after

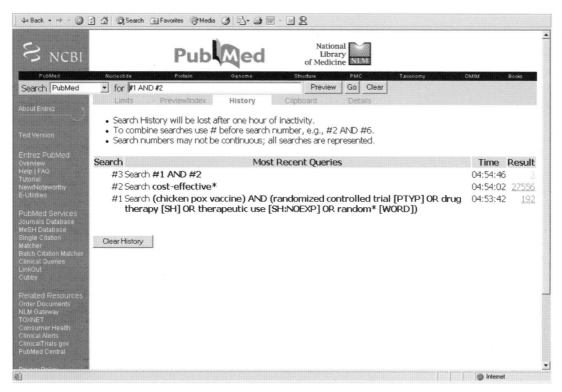

Fig. 5.5 The history of a search in PubMed. (National Library of Medicine. Used with permission.)

you run your first search and lists and numbers your searches in the order in which you ran them. As shown in Fig. 5.5, the history displays the search number, your search query, the time of search, and the number of citations in your results. You can combine searches or add additional terms to an existing search by using the number (#) sign before the search number: e.g., *#1 AND #2*, or *#1 AND (drug therapy OR diet therapy)*. Once you have entered a revised search strategy in the query box, click "go" to view the search results. Click "clear history" to remove all searches from the history screen and the preview/index screen. The maximum number of queries held in history is 100. Once the maximum number is reached, PubMed will remove the oldest search from the history to add the most recent search. The search history will be lost after one hour of inactivity on PubMed. PubMed will move a search statement number to the top of the history if the new search is the same as a previous search.

The preview/index allows you to enter your search terms one at a time using pre-selected search fields. It is useful for finding specific references.

Clipboard

The clipboard gives you a place to collect selected citations from one or several searches to print or save for future use. The maximum number of items that can be placed in the clipboard is 500. Once you have added items to the clipboard, you can click on "clipboard" from the features bar to view your selections. Citations in the clipboard are displayed in the order they were added. To place an item in the clipboard, click on the check-box to the left of the citation, go to the send menu and select "clipboard," then click "send." Once you have added a citation to the clipboard, the record-number color will change to green. If you send to the clipboard without selecting citations, PubMed will add all of your search results (up to 500 citations) to the clipboard.

Saving

When you are ready to save or print your clipboard items it is best to change them to ordinary text. This will simplify your printout and save paper as you will not print all the PubMed motifs and icons. To do this, click on "clipboard" on the features bar. You should see only the articles that you placed on the clipboard. The send menu will now read "text." Click on the send button to transfer. A new page will be displayed which resembles an ordinary text document for printing. You can also use this "send to text" option for single references if you want to omit all the graphics. To save the entire set of search results click the display pull-down menu to select the desired format and then select "send to file" from the send menu. To save specific citations click on the check-box to the left of each citation (you may move to other pages in the retrieval process) and when you have finished making your selections, select "send to file."

The maximum number of items that can be saved is 10 000. If you try to save a file with more than 10 000 citations, PubMed will display a message that instructs you to refine your search! The default file name for saving searches is query.fcgi. Consider changing the name to something more meaningful to you, and change the fcgi extension, if you wish to open the file in a text editor or word-processing package.

General searching in PubMed

If you are not finding the evidence you need in the clinical queries search, or if you find an author who has written extensively in an area of interest and you wish to search for other papers by this author, use the general search page in PubMed. Begin by clicking on the PubMed symbol in the top left-hand corner of the screen and the general search screen will be displayed (Fig. 5.6). Simply type your search terms in the query box and your search results will be displayed as before.

MeSH

In looking for synonyms to broaden or improve a search you should consider using both text words and keywords (index terms) in the database. One of

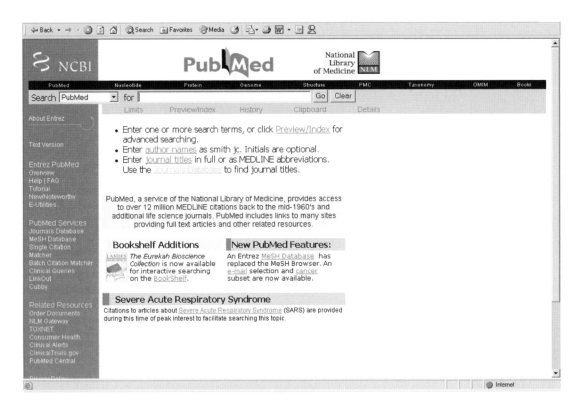

Fig. 5.6 General search screen in PubMed. (National Library of Medicine. Used with permission.)

MEDLINE's great strengths is its MeSH (Medical Subject Headings) system. By default, PubMed automatically "maps" your input to the appropriate MeSH terms, so you can take advantage of the system without even realizing you are doing so. But you can also perform a specific MeSH search by clicking on the "MeSH database" link in the left-hand side bar. If you type in "colorectal cancer" you will be led to the MeSH term *colorectal neoplasms* (Fig. 5.7). You can then refine the search by clicking on the term to bring up the detailed display (Fig. 5.8). This allows you to select subheadings (*diagnosis, etiology, therapy*, etc.) to narrow your search, and also gives you access to the MeSH tree structure.

The "explode" (exp) feature allows you to capture an entire subtree of MeSH terms within a single word. Thus, for our search term *colorectal neoplasms*, the "explode" incorporates the entire MeSH tree below *colorectal neoplasms* (Table 5.1). You can also click on any specific terms in the tree that you desire. You will then get all the descriptors for that MeSH term and all those under it.

Select the appropriate MeSH term, with or without subheadings, and with or without explosion, and use the send menu to "send to search box." Your search terms will appear in the query box at the top of the screen. Click "search PubMed" to execute the search.

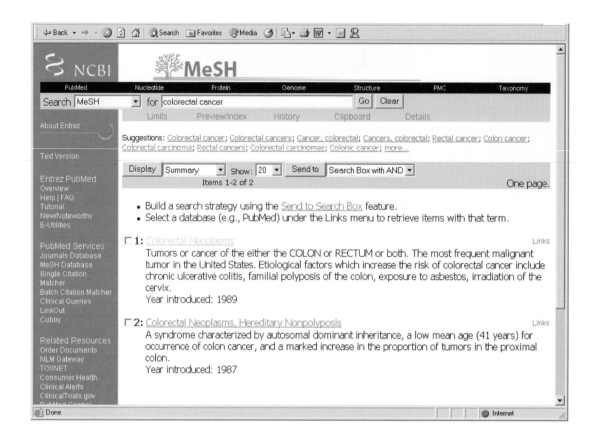

Fig. 5.7 PubMed MeSH database.
(National Library of Medicine.
Used with permission.)

The search will automatically explode your term unless you restrict by selecting the "do not explode this term" box. Each of these articles has been indexed by at least one of the MeSH keywords from the tree. To see the difference that exploding a MeSH term makes, repeat the search using the term *colorectal neoplasms* in the search window without exploding. You will probably retrieve about one-quarter of the articles you retrieved in the previous search.

A common question that novice users of PubMed often ask is "how do I find out the MeSH keywords that have been used to categorize a paper?" Knowing the relevant MeSH keywords will help to focus and/or refine the search. There is a simple way to do this. Once you have found a relevant citation, click on the author link to view the abstract. Then go to the "display" icon and open it as shown in Fig. 5.9. Select MEDLINE and click "display." The record is now displayed as it is indexed and you can scroll down and check out the MeSH terms for this paper. The initials MH precede them. MeSH terms do not appear for articles that are in process. You can also link to "related articles." This will allow you to find other relevant citations, but no limits apply here.

Table 5.1. A MeSH tree containing the term colorectal neoplasms

Neoplasms
    Neoplasms by Site
        Digestive System Neoplasms
            Gastrointestinal Neoplasms
            Intestinal Neoplasms
                Colorectal Neoplasms
                    Colonic Neoplasms
                        Colonic Polyps +
                        Sigmoid Neoplasms
                    Colorectal Neoplasms, Hereditary
                    Nonpolyposis
                    Rectal Neoplasms
                      Anus Neoplasms +

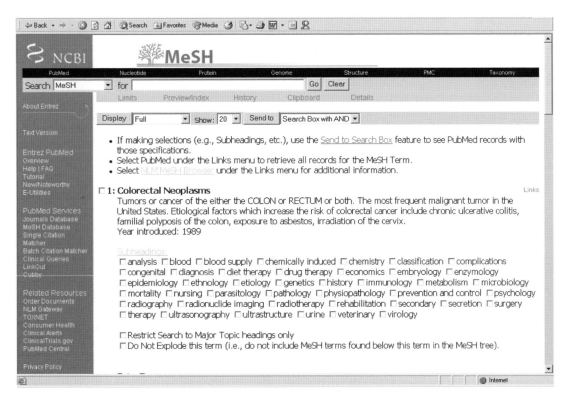

Fig. 5.8 PubMed MeSH database with subheadings. (National Library of Medicine. Used with permission.)

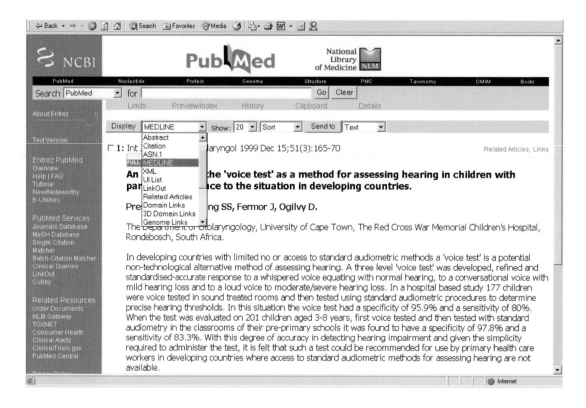

Fig. 5.9 The "display" menu in
PubMed. (National Library of
Medicine. Used with
permission.)

While the MeSH system is useful, it should supplement rather than usurp the
use of textwords so that incompletely coded articles are not missed.

Methodological terms and filters

MeSH terms cover not only subject content but also a number of useful terms
on study methodology. For example, if we are considering questions of therapy,
many randomized trials are tagged in MEDLINE by the specific methodological
term *randomized controlled trial* or *clinical trial*. You may limit your search to one
of these types in PubMed under the limit feature by using the publication types
pull-down menu.

An appropriate methodological filter may help confine the retrieved studies
to primary research. For example, if you are interested in whether screening (an
intervention) reduces mortality from colorectal cancer, then you may wish to
confine the retrieved studies to controlled trials. The idea of methodological terms
may be extended to multiple terms that attempt to identify particular study types.
Such terms are used extensively in the clinical queries search.

Note that many studies do not have the appropriate methodological tag. The
Cochrane Collaboration and the United States National Library of Medicine

(NLM) are working on correctly retagging all the controlled trials, but this is not so for other study types.

Field searching

Frequently you will want to shorten your search time by searching in a specific field. Someone may have told you about a recent article by a particular author renowned for work in the area that you are interested in searching. Or you may recall seeing a relevant study in a particular journal in the library. Knowing how to search in specific fields will prove to be invaluable in these circumstances. The field labels and the method of searching will differ slightly depending on the software you are using to access MEDLINE. In most cases software other than PubMed will either be Ovid Technologies (Ovid) or SilverPlatter Information (WebSPIRS/WinSPIRS). These are both proprietary search engines for finding medical articles. If you want to search for an article with "colorectal cancer" in the title using PubMed, select the title field in the limits option using the fields pull-down menu for your search term. Or you can simply type "colorectal cancer[ti]" in the query box. In others browsers, typing "colorectal cancer in ti" (if using WebSPIRS) or "colorectal cancer.ti" (if using Ovid) will retrieve this set of articles.

The field-label abbreviations can be found by accessing the help menu. The most commonly used field labels are abstract (ab), title (ti), source (so), journal (jn), and author (au). The difference between source and journal is that "source" is the abbreviated version of the journal title, while "journal" is the full journal title. In PubMed you can select the journal or author simply by using the journals database located on the left-hand side bar or by typing in the author's last name and initials in the query box. Remember, when you search using "text words," the program searches for your word in any of the available fields. For example, if "death" is one of your search terms then you will retrieve articles where "death" is an author's name as well as those in which it occurs in the title or abstract. Normally this isn't a problem but be careful when you use "wildcard" searches.

The process of identifying papers is an iterative one. It is best initially to devise a strategy on paper. However, this will inevitably miss useful terms and the process will need to be repeated and refined. The results of the initial search are used to retrieve relevant papers which can then be used in two ways to identify missed papers. You can search the bibliographies of the relevant papers for articles missed by the initial search. You can also perform a citation search, using the Science Citation Index database to identify papers that have cited the identified relevant studies, some of which may be subsequent primary research. These "missed" papers are invaluable and provide clues on how the search may be broadened to capture further papers by studying the MeSH terms that have been

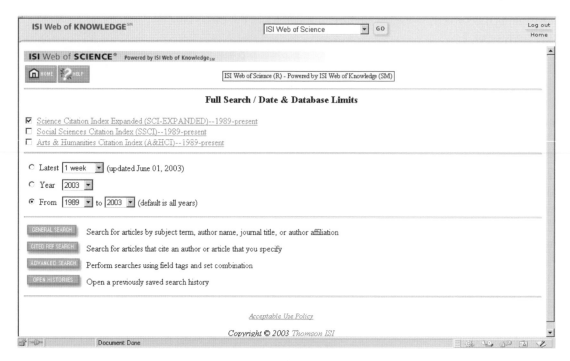

Fig. 5.10 Citation databases "full search" window. (Web of Science, Thomson ISI. Used with permission.)

used. The whole procedure may then be repeated using the new terms identified. This iterative process is sometimes referred to as "snowballing."

Using the Science Citation Index

The ISI Science Citation Index is accessed through *Web of Science* and covers approximately 5,600 of the world's leading science journals. Your library must be a subscriber in order for you to use this database. It is a compilation of all the cited references from journal articles published during a particular year and allows you to take a known, relevant paper and find other more recent papers that cite it. Go to the ISI Web of Science at isiknowledge.com and click on the "full search" icon. Fig. 5.10 displays the full search window.

Click on the box next to the Science Citation Index and, unless you specifically want references only from the last few years, you can leave the year selection on the default setting of "all years." Now click on the "cited ref search" icon. Type in the author, the journal and the year of publication of the article you want to search as shown in Fig. 5.11 and then click "lookup."

You will notice that the journal title is typed in the "cited work" window, although it is not clearly indicated that this is what is required. In fact, new users frequently make the mistake of typing the title of the article in this window and then wonder why no articles are retrieved. If you are not sure how to abbreviate the journal title, click on "list" and scroll through the alphabetical index until you find the journal

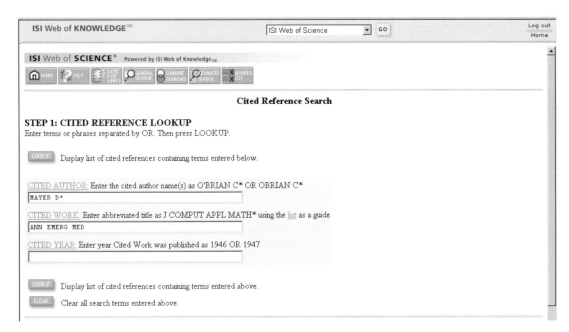

you are looking for. It is also worth noting that the journal abbreviations may be different to what you are accustomed to seeing in MEDLINE. For example, the *British Medical Journal* is abbreviated to "BMJ" in MEDLINE but in the Science Citation Index it is "Brit Med J." You will be unsuccessful in your search if you use the wrong journal abbreviation.

Fig. 5.11 An example of a cited reference search. (Web of Science, Thomson ISI. Used with permission.)

Hand-searching

If the relevant articles appear in a limited range of journals or conference proceedings, it may be feasible and desirable to search these by hand. This is obviously more important for unindexed or very recent journals, but may also pick up relevant studies not easily identified from titles or abstracts. Fortunately, the Cochrane Collaboration is systematically hand-searching a number of journals to identify controlled trials and a master list is maintained on their website (www.cochrane.org). This should be checked before undertaking your own hand-search. However, for other types of question and study there has been no such systematic search. The abstracts of Cochrane Reviews are available without charge and can be browsed or searched.

The Cochrane Library

The final database that we will cover is the Cochrane Library. Actually the Cochrane Library contains several databases, the most important of which we will look at in turn. But first some background about the Cochrane Library might prove useful. The Cochrane Library owes it genesis to an astute British epidemiologist and doctor, Archie Cochrane, who is best known for his influential book *Effectiveness and Efficiency: Random Reflections on Health Services*, published in 1971. In the book, he suggested that because resources would always be limited they should be used to provide equitably those forms of health care which had been shown in properly designed evaluations to be effective. In particular, he stressed the importance of using evidence from randomized controlled trials (RCTs) because these were likely to provide much more reliable information than other sources of evidence. Cochrane's simple propositions were soon widely recognized as seminally important – by lay people as well as by health professionals. In his 1971 book he wrote: "It is surely a great criticism of our profession that we have not organised a critical summary, by specialty or subspecialty, adapted periodically, of all relevant randomised controlled trials."[1]

His challenge led to the establishment during the 1980s of an international collaboration to develop the Oxford Database of Perinatal Trials. In 1987, the year before Cochrane died, he referred to a systematic review of randomized controlled trials (RCTs) of care during pregnancy and childbirth as "a real milestone in the history of randomized trials and in the evaluation of care" and suggested that other specialties should copy the methods used.

The Cochrane Collaboration was developed in response to Archie Cochrane's call for systematic and up-to-date reviews of all health-care-related RCTs. His suggestion that the methods used to prepare and maintain reviews of controlled trials in pregnancy and childbirth should be applied more widely was taken up by the Research and Development Programme, initiated to support the United Kingdom's National Health Service. Funds were provided to establish a "Cochrane Centre," to collaborate with others, in the UK and elsewhere, to facilitate systematic reviews of randomized controlled trials across all areas of health care. When the Cochrane Centre was opened in Oxford in October 1992, those involved expressed the hope that there would be a collaborative international response to Cochrane's agenda. This idea was outlined at a meeting organized six months later by the New York Academy of Sciences. In October 1993 – at what was to become the first in a series of annual Cochrane Colloquia – 77 people from eleven countries co-founded the **Cochrane Collaboration**. It is an international organization that aims to help people make well-informed decisions about health care by preparing, maintaining, and ensuring the accessibility of systematic reviews of the effects of health-care interventions.

Several databases are included in the Cochrane Library but the ones most pertinent to our requirements are as follows:

---

[1] A. L. Cochrane. *Effectiveness & Efficiency: Random Reflections on Health Services.* London: Royal Society of Medicine, 1971.

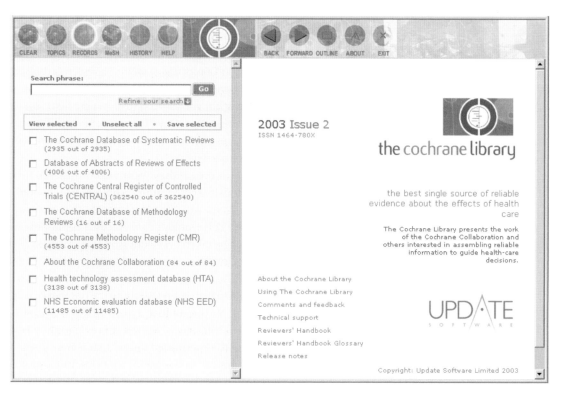

The Cochrane Database of Systematic Reviews (CDSR) contains systematic reviews of the effects of health care prepared by the Cochrane Collaboration. In addition to complete reviews, the database contains protocols for reviews currently being prepared.

The Database of Abstracts of Reviews of Effects (DARE) includes structured abstracts of systematic reviews which have been critically appraised by reviewers at the NHS Centre for Reviews and Dissemination in York and by other people.

The Cochrane Central Register of Controlled Trials (CENTRAL) is a bibliographic database of controlled trials identified by contributors to the Cochrane Collaboration and others.

Fig. 5.12 Search screen in the Cochrane Library. (Cochrane Library. Used with permission.)

Searching in the Cochrane Library

Each screen in the Cochrane Library has a "toolbar" at the top as shown in Fig. 5.12. The toolbar helps you to move between screens and within documents. Below the toolbar on the left is a "search" box in which you can enter your search term or terms, and below that is a list of the databases, with the number of records retrieved by the latest search ("hits"). The right-hand side of the screen is used for displaying selected documents.

The search strategies you have learned thus far are also applicable to the Cochrane Library, with a few exceptions. All text is searched in the default setting (e.g., titles, abstracts, authors' names, citations, keywords). Thus if you enter a search term and it is a word in one of the systematic reviews, that systematic review will be one of your hits even though it may not be directly relevant to your search. If you would like to restrict your search to a specific field you can select "refine your search" below the search window. Then click the "go" button to return to re-run the search with the restrictions. It is not necessary to use upper-case letters for your Boolean operators.

By default, records are selected as if they were joined by AND. If you enter "stroke unit" it is equivalent to "stroke AND unit". Similarly, if you enter "primary care" as a search term, the program will retrieve all records that contain the word "primary" and the word "care". This would include records containing sentences such as "Particular care should be taken in selecting primary studies." If you want to search for a phrase then enclose the search terms within quotation marks (e.g., "primary care").

There are a number of steps to use when searching the databases using MeSH terms. First, click on "MeSH" on the toolbar, type a single word in the MeSH search window, and click on the "thesaurus" button or press the enter key. Choose an initial MeSH heading from the "permuted index" that is now displayed. This is an index of all terms that appear in the MeSH tree structures, and all MeSH phrases containing the entered word are displayed. Use the scroll bar to browse the permuted index, and choose the term that most clearly defines what you want to search for by clicking on it to highlight it and open the MeSH tree(s) containing the term. Your chosen term will be displayed within the MeSH tree(s) in red.

You can now move both up and down through the tree structure to select either more general or more specific terms. The list directly below a term displayed in red shows the direct "children" of that term. To move up or down a level in a MeSH tree, click to highlight a term above or below the current one. The tree display will be re-drawn with the newly selected term now shown in red. Repeat the procedure until you are sure that you want to search either on the term shown in red only or on this term and the terms below it.

Finally, you can search the chosen term. With the term shown in red, you have two main options. Click on "single term" to search only for the term shown in red or click on "explode all trees" to search for the term in red and all of the "children" of this term.

Once you have performed a search, your results will be shown as hits against each database on the database list. Fig. 5.13 shows the results of a search for studies assessing the efficacy of low-fat diets in obesity. The search terms used were *obesity and ((low next fat) near diet*)*. Using the search string *((low next fat) near diet*)* ensures that we will retrieve studies with a variety of permutations of the same words (e.g., "low fat diet" or "diets low in fat"). Working from the top

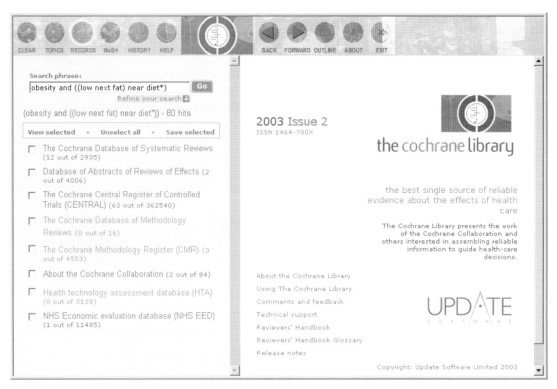

Fig. 5.13 Results of a
Cochrane search. (Cochrane
Library. Used with
permission.)

of the screen down we can see that we have retrieved 12 hits in the Cochrane
Database of Systematic Reviews. There are also 2 hits in the Database of Abstracts
of Reviews of Effects and 63 in the Cochrane Central Register of Controlled Trials.

We can view any of these results by clicking on the name of the database. For
example, if we click on "Cochrane Database of Systematic Reviews" the screen
displayed in Fig. 5.14 will appear. Note that eight of the 12 hits are complete
reviews, and four are protocols.

To view any of the hits we simply click on the title of the review in the results list,
as shown in Fig. 5.15, and the text of the document appears on the right-hand side
of the screen. Scroll down to read the review. All Cochrane reviews are presented
in the same way, with an abstract followed by the full text of the review.

To view any of the other Cochrane reviews, or any of the hits from the other
databases in the Cochrane Library, simply select another title from the results list.

The Cochrane Library can be accessed online through most medical libraries,
as long as the library has a subscription. In many countries free national provision
has been arranged.

It is of course possible to print Cochrane reviews, but it should be emphasized
that most reviews are very large documents. If you simply click on the print icon
you will be printing the entire document, and some of them are up to 90 pages

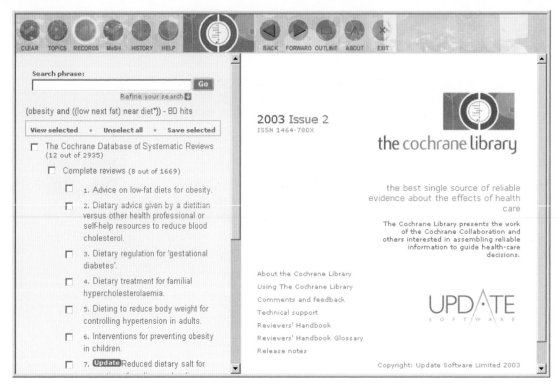

Fig. 5.14 Results of a search in the Cochrane Database of Systematic Reviews. (Cochrane Library. Used with permission.)

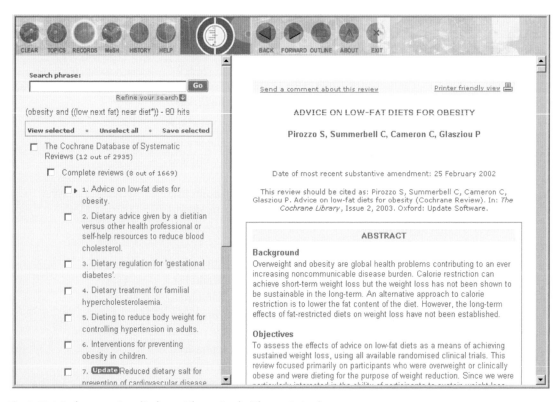

Fig. 5.15 A Cochrane review. (Cochrane Library. Used with permission.)

long. It is preferable to select the section(s) you need. In many cases, simply printing the abstract (1–2 pages) will suffice.

Other databases

Other evidence-based medicine databases are available on various search engines. Portions of the Cochrane Library and the American College of Physicians (ACP) Journal Club are available on Ovid. The ACP Journal Club is also available on the American College of Physicians website. Finally, don't forget about your helpful librarians. If you need help or run into problems searching, your local hospital medical librarians will be able to provide valuable assistance.

6

Study design and strength of evidence

Louis Pasteur's theory of germs is ridiculous fiction.

Pierre Pachet, Professor of Physiology, Toulouse University, 1872

Learning objectives

In this chapter you will learn:
- the unique characteristics, strengths, and weaknesses of common clinical research study designs
  - descriptive – cross-sectional, case reports, case series
  - timed – prospective, retrospective
  - longitudinal – observational (case-control, cohort, non-concurrent cohort), interventional (clinical trial)
- the different levels of evidence and how study design affects the strength of evidence.

There are different types of research study. Not all studies are able to show the same things since different research study designs accomplish different goals. Therefore, the first step in assessing the validity of a research study is to determine the study design. Each study design has inherent strengths and weaknesses. The ability to prove causation and expected potential biases will be determined by the design of the study.

Identify the study design

When critically appraising a research study, you must first understand what different research study designs are able to accomplish. The type of study will suggest potential biases you can expect. There are two basic categories of study that are easily recognizable. These are **descriptive** and **longitudinal** studies. We will discuss each type and its subtypes separately.

A classification commonly used to characterize longitudinal clinical research studies is by the direction of the study in time. Characterizations in this manner, or so-called timed studies, have traditionally been divided into **prospective** and **retrospective** study designs. These are terms which can easily be misapplied and should not be referred to except as generalizations. Prospective studies begin at a time in the past and subjects are followed to the present time. Retrospective studies begin at the present time and look back on the behavior or other characteristics of those subjects in the past. Since these terms are often used incorrectly, they should be abandoned.

Descriptive studies

Descriptive studies are records of events. These include studies that look at a series of cases or a cross-section of a population to look for particular characteristics. For example, a novel treatment of several patients yields promising results after several cases are reported and the authors want other physicians to try the therapy. **Case reports** describe individual cases and **case series** describe accounts of an illness or treatment in a small group of patients. In **cross-sectional studies** the interesting aspects of a group of patients (including potential causes and effects) are all observed at the same time.

Case reports and case series

Case reports or small numbers of cases are often the first description of a new disease, clinical sign, symptom, treatment, or diagnostic test. They can also be a description of a curriculum, operation, patient-care strategy, or other health-care process. Some case reports can alert physicians to a new disease that is about to become very important. For example, AIDS was initially identified when the first cases were reported in two case series in 1981. The series consisted of two groups of previously healthy homosexual men, one with a rare type of pneumonia (*Pneumocystis carinii* pneumonia) and the other with a rare cancer (Kaposi's sarcoma). These diseases had previously only been reported in immunocompromised people. This start of the AIDS epidemic, a fact that was not evident from these first two reports, quickly became evident as more clinicians noticed cases of these rare diseases.

Most case reports are descriptions of rare diseases or rare presentations of common diseases and are unlikely to occur very soon again, if ever. A recent case series reported on two cases of stroke in young people related to illicit methamphetamine use. To my knowledge, we have not been deluged with a rash of young methamphetamine users with strokes. Although it makes pathophysiological sense, the association may only be a fluke. Case reports are a useful venue to report unusual symptoms of a common illness. The individual clinician cannot use this information immediately on all patients with this symptom, but should wait and carefully observe those patients before deciding to do any further evaluation.

New treatments or tests described in a study **without any control group** also fall into this category. At best, these descriptive studies can suggest future directions for research on the treatment or test being reported, using more stringent study designs. Case studies and cross-sectional studies have certain strengths. They are cheap and relatively easy to do with existing medical records and potential clinical material is plentiful. If you see new presentations of disease or interesting cases, you can easily write a case report. However, their weaknesses outweigh their strengths. These "studies" do not provide explanations and cannot show association between cause and effect. Therefore, they do not provide much useful evidence!

Since no comparison is made to any control group, contributory cause cannot be proved. A good general rule for case studies is to "take them seriously and then ignore them." By this is meant that you should never change your practice based solely on a single case study or series (except as noted below) since the probability of seeing the same rare presentation or rare disease is quite remote.

There is one situation in which a case series may be useful. Called the "all-or-none case series," this occurs when there is a **very dramatic** change in the outcome of patients reported in a case series. There are two ways this can occur. First, **all** (or almost all) patients died before the treatment became available and **some** (or many more) in the case series survive. Second, **some** (or most or many) patients died before the treatment became available, but **none** (or almost none) in the case series die. This is roughly what happened when penicillin was first introduced. Prior to this time, most patients with pneumonia died of their illness. When penicillin was first given to patients with pneumonia, most of them lived. The credibility of these case reports depends on the numbers of cases reported, the relative severity of the illness, and the accuracy and detail of the case descriptions given in the report.

The case series can be abused. It can be likened to a popular commercial for Life cereal from the 1970s. In the scene two children are unsure if they will like Life, the new cereal, so they ask their little brother, Mikey, to try it. He likes it and they both say "Mikey liked it!" Too often, a series of cases is presented showing apparent improvement in the condition of several patients that is attributed to a particular therapy. The authors conclude that this means it should be used as the new standard of care. The fact that everyone got better is not proof that the therapy (or other intervention) in question is causative. This is called the "Mikey liked it" phenomenon.[1]

---

[1] This construct is attributed to J. Hoffman, *Emergency Medical Abstracts*, 2000.

Cross-sectional studies

Cross-sectional studies are descriptive studies that look at a sample of a population to see how many people (in that population) are afflicted with a particular disease (effect) and how many have a particular risk factor (cause). Cross-sectional studies record events and observations – diseases or other outcomes (effect) and risk factors (cause) – in this population at a single instant in time.

The strengths of cross-sectional studies are that they are relatively cheap, easy, and quick to do. The data are usually available through medical records or statistical databases. They are useful **initial exploratory studies** especially to screen or classify aspects of disease. They are capable of demonstrating an **association** between the cause and effect. Several patients with a rare disorder can be compared to suitable controls. In order to draw conclusions from this study, patient exposure to the risk factor being studied must continue until the outcome occurs. If the exposure began long before the outcome occurs and is intermittent, it will be more difficult to associate the two. If done properly, cross-sectional studies are capable of calculating the **prevalence** of disease in the population. Prevalence is the percentage of people in the population with the outcome of interest at any point in time. Since all the cases are looked at in one instant of time, cross-sectional studies cannot calculate **incidence**, the rate of appearance of new cases over time.

There are more disadvantages to these types of study. The rules of cause and effect for contributory cause cannot be fulfilled. Since the risk and outcome are measured at the same time, you cannot be certain which is the cause and which the effect. A cross-sectional study found that teenagers who smoked early in life were more likely to become anxious and depressed as adults than those who began smoking at a later age. Does teenage smoking cause anxiety and depression in later years, or are those who have subclinical anxiety or depression more likely to smoke at an early age? It is impossible to tell if the cause preceded the effect, the effect was responsible for the cause, or both are related to an unknown (**confounding** or **surrogate**) third factor. This is more likely to be true if the time from the cause to the effect is short. For example, it is very common for people to visit their doctor just before their death. The visit to the doctor is not a risk factor for death but is a "surrogate" marker for severe (and potentially life-threatening) illness. These patients visit their doctors for symptoms associated with their impending deaths.

Cross-sectional studies are subject to **prevalence–incidence bias**. This occurs because the risk factor appears to cause the disease (occurrence) when in reality it simply affects the duration or prognosis of the disease. An association was noted between HLA-A2 antigen and the presence of acute lymphocytic leukemia in children in a cross-sectional study. It was assumed to be a risk factor for occurrence of the disease. Subsequent studies found that long-term survivors had the HLA-A2

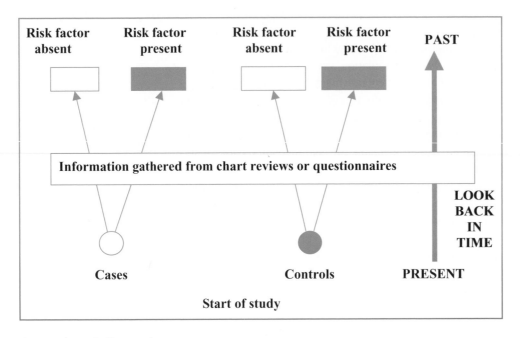

Fig. 6.1 Schematic diagram of a
case-control study.
antigen and its absence was associated with early mortality. HLA-A2 antigen was not a risk factor for the disease but an indicator of good prognosis.

Longitudinal studies

This is a catchall term describing either observations or interventions made over a given period of time. There are three basic longitudinal study designs. These are **case–control** studies, **cohort** studies (and the related **non-concurrent cohort**), and **clinical trials**. These are **analytic (inferential)** studies. They look for a statistical association between risk factors (cause) and outcomes (effect).

Case-control studies

These were previously called retrospective studies. There is a unique feature that should be used to identify a case-control study. The subjects are initially selected because they either have (**cases**) or do not have (**controls**) the outcome of interest. They are grouped by the absence or presence of the outcome. Fig. 6.1 is a schematic description of a case-control study. The purpose of the study is to find out the odds of exposure to the risk factor among the cases and compare this to the odds of exposure among the controls. You can do this by reviewing elements that occurred in the past, looking for suspected risk factors. This type of study is good to screen for potential risk factors of disease.

The strengths of case-control studies are that they are relatively easy, cheap, and quick to do from previously available data. They can be done using current patients and asking them about events that occurred in the past. They are well suited for studying rare diseases since the study begins with subjects who already have the outcome. Each case patient may then be matched up with one or more suitable control patients. Ideally the controls are as similar to the cases as possible, other than in the outcome and exposure to the risk factor being compared. Fewer diseased subjects can detect significant differences in exposures between them and the controls. They are good exploratory studies and can look at many risk factors for one outcome. The results can then be used to suggest new hypotheses for a stronger study (cohort or clinical trial) to be done later.

Unfortunately, there are many serious weaknesses in case-control studies, making them only fair sources of evidence in general. Since the data are collected retrospectively, data quality may be poor. Data often come from a careful search of the medical records of the cases and controls. The advantage is that these records are usually easily available. They may be of questionable reliability since you are relying on descriptions (often subjective) to determine exposure and outcome. Record reviewers use subjective standards to determine the presence of the cause and effect. This type of **implicit review** of charts introduces the researcher's bias in interpreting the measurements or outcomes. Stronger case-control studies will use **explicit reviews**. They are better but are more difficult to perform. Only clearly objective measures are reviewed or the chart material is reviewed in a blinded manner using previously determined outcome descriptors.

When a patient is asked to remember something about a medical condition that occurred in the past, their memory is subject to **recall bias** or **reporting bias**. Those with the disease are more likely to recall exposure to many risk factors simply because they have the disease. Similarly, subjects in the sample may not be representative of all patients with the outcome since they have been specially sought out. This is called **sampling bias** or **referral bias** and commonly occurs in studies done at specialized referral centers. The referred patients may be different from those seen in a primary-care practice. In referral centers, only the most severe cases of a given disorder will be seen, thus limiting the generalizability of the findings.

When determining many potential risk factors for an outcome using a case-control study a **derivation set** is developed. The results of this study should be used cautiously since any association discovered may have turned up by chance alone. The study can then be repeated using a cohort study design to look at those factors that have the highest correlation with the outcome in question to see if the association still holds (called a **validation set**).

Case-control studies can only study one disease (outcome) at a given time. Prevalence or incidence cannot be calculated since the ratio of cases to controls is preselected by the researchers. They cannot prove contributory cause since

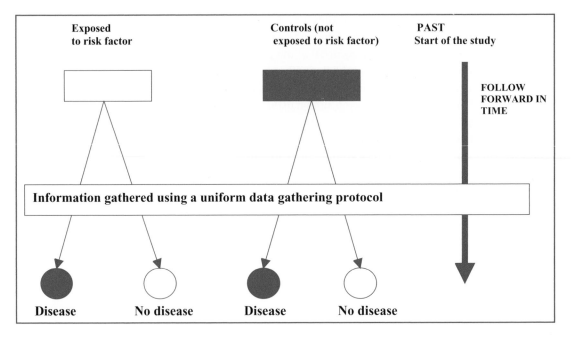

Fig. 6.2 Schematic diagram of a cohort study.

they cannot show that the cause preceded the effect. Finally, they cannot alter the cause to change the effect.

Cohort studies

These were previously called **prospective studies** since they are usually done prospectively in time. The name comes from the Latin *cohors*, meaning a tenth of a legion marching together in time. However, they can be and are now as frequently done retrospectively (**non-concurrent cohort study**). The cohort is a group of patients who are selected based on the presence or absence of the risk factor (Fig. 6.2). They are followed in time to determine which of them will develop the outcome (disease). The **probability** (incidence or risk) of developing the outcome can be calculated for each group. The degree of risk is then compared between the two groups.

The cohort study is one of the strongest research study designs. They are powerful studies that can determine the incidence of disease. They are able to show that the cause is associated with the effect more often than by chance alone. Since they are done prospectively, they can show that the cause preceded the effect. They do not attempt to manipulate the cause and cannot prove that altering the cause alters the effect. This is an ideal study design for answering questions of etiology, harm, or prognosis. It is easier to collect the data in an objective and uniform fashion. There is usually no recall bias, except possibly in non-concurrent cohort studies. If the study is done in the present, the investigators can predetermine the entry criteria, what measurements are to be made, and how they are best made.

Their main weakness is that they are expensive in time and money. The startup and ongoing monitoring costs may be prohibitive. This is a greater problem when studying rare or uncommon diseases. It may be difficult to get enough patients to find clinically or statistically significant differences between the patients who are exposed and those not exposed to the risk factor. Since the cohort must be set up prospectively by the presence or absence of the risk factor, they are not good studies to uncover new risk factors.

Confounding variables are those affecting the risk factor and the outcome. They may affect the exposed and unexposed groups differently and bias the conclusions. Patients who leave the study (**patient attrition**) can cause loss of data about the outcomes. The cause of their attrition from the study may be directly related to some conditions of the study. Therefore, it is imperative for researchers to account for all patients. In practice an acceptable level of attrition is less than 20%. However, this should be used as a guide rather than an absolute value. A lower rate of attrition may bias the study if the reason patients were lost from the study is related to the risk factor. If patients change some aspect of their behavior or exposure to the risk factor after the initial grouping of subjects, **misclassification bias** can occur. Safeguards to prevent these issues should be clearly outlined in the methods section of the study.

A special case of the cohort study, the **non-concurrent cohort study** is also called a **database study**. It is essentially a cohort study that begins in the present and utilizes data on events that took place in the past. The cohort is still separated by the presence or absence of the risk factor. This is usually not the original reason that patients were entered into the study. Non-concurrent prospective studies are not retrospective studies, but have been called "retrospective cohort studies". They have essentially the same strengths and weaknesses as cohort studies.

In a typical non-concurrent cohort study design, the cohort is put together in the past and many baseline measurements are made. The follow-up measurements and determination of outcomes are made when the data are finally analyzed. The data will have been collected incidentally for another study and analyzed later for a new risk factor. This is a risk factor other than that for which the original study was done. For example, a cohort of motor-vehicle-accident trauma patients is collected to look at the relationship of wearing seat belts to death. After the data are collected, the same group of patients is looked at to see if there is any relationship between severe head injury and the wearing of seat belts.

The data are available from databases that have already been set up, and should be gathered in an objective manner or at least without regard for the association which is being sought (data gatherers are ideally blinded to the outcomes). Non-concurrent cohort studies rely on historical data and may suffer some of the

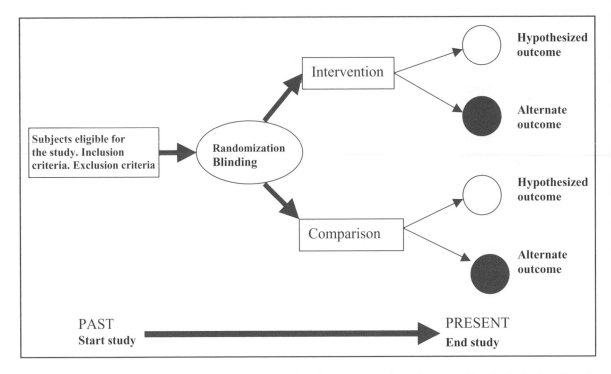

Fig. 6.3 Schematic diagram of a randomized clinical trial.

weaknesses associated with case-control studies regarding the lack of uniformity of data recorded in the data base and subjective interpretation of records.

To review

> Subjects in **cohort studies** are initially grouped according to the presence or absence of **risk factors** regardless of whether the group was assembled in the past or the present
>
> Subjects in **case-control studies** are initially grouped according to the presence or absence of the **outcome**

Clinical trials

A **clinical trial** is a cohort study in which the investigator intervenes by manipulating the presence or absence of the risk factor (usually a therapeutic maneuver). Clinical trials are human experiments (**interventional studies**). Cohort and case-control studies are **observational studies** in which there is no intervention. An example of a clinical trial is a study in which a high-soy-protein diet and a normal diet were given to middle-aged male smokers to determine if it reduced their risk of developing diabetes. Fig. 6.3 is a schematic diagram of a randomized clinical trial.

Clini[...] [...]terized by the presence of a control group identical to the [...] [...]very way except for their exposure to the intervent[...] [...]g controlled clinical trials should be **randor**[...] [...]ve an equal chance of being placed[...] [...]placebo, or standardized therapy[...] [...] being tested). Subjects and experimenters should be [...] [...] group assignment during the study.

Clinical trials are the only study design that can fulfill all the rules of contributory cause. They can show that the cause precedes the effect and that altering the cause alters the effect. When properly carried out they will have fewer methodological biases than any other study designs.

However, they are far from perfect. The most common weakness of controlled clinical trials is that they are very expensive. Because of the high costs, multi-center trials that utilize cooperation between many research centers and are funded by industry or government are becoming more common. Unfortunately, the high cost of these studies has resulted in more of them being paid for by large biomedical (pharmaceutical or technology) companies. This could represent a conflict of interest for the researcher, whose salary and research support is dependent on the largess of the company providing the money. Patient attrition and compliance may also compromise the results. There may be ethical problems when the study involves giving potentially harmful, or withholding potentially beneficial, therapy. The Institutional Review Boards (IRB) of the institutions doing the research should address these. A poorly designed study should not be considered ethical by the IRB. However, it is still your responsibility to determine how ethical a study is based upon the methodology. The fact that a study is a randomized controlled trial (RCT) does not in itself guarantee validity, and there can still be serious methodological problems that will bias the results.

7

Instruments and measurements: precision and validity

Not everything that can be counted counts, and not everything that counts can be counted.

Albert Einstein (1879–1955)

Learning objectives

In this chapter you will learn:
- different types of data as basic elements of descriptive statistics
- instrumentation and measurement
- precision, accuracy, reliability, and validity
- how researchers should optimize these factors

All clinical research studies involve observations and measurements of the phenomena of interest. Observations and measurements are the desired output of a study. The instruments used to make them are subject to error, which may bias the results of a study. The first thing we will discuss is the type of data that can be generated from clinical research. This chapter will then introduce concepts related to instruments and measurements.

Types of data and variables

There are several different ways of classifying data. They can be classified by their function (**independent** or **dependent**), nature (**nominal**, **ordinal**, **interval**, or **ratio**), and whether they are **continuous**, **discrete**, or **dichotomous**.

When classifying variables by function we want to know what the variable does to the experiment. Is it the effect or the cause? In most clinical trials one variable is held constant relative to the other. The **independent** variable is under the control of or can be manipulated by the investigator. Generally this is the cause of interest such as a drug, other treatment, or diagnostic test. The **dependent** variable changes as a result (or an effect) of the action of the independent variable. It is usually the outcome of the treatment or the presence of a particular diagnosis. We want to find out if a change in the independent variable will produce a change in the dependent variable. The nature of each variable should be evident from the study design.

When classifying variables by their nature, we mean the "mathematical" characteristics of the number generated for that variable. **Nominal** data are named categories. One can assign a number to each of these categories, but it would have no intrinsic significance and cannot be used to compare one piece of the data-set to another. Changing the number assignment has no effect on the interpretation of the data. Examples of nominal data are classification of physicians by specialty or of patients by the type of cancer from which they suffer.

Ordinal data is nominal data for which the order of the variables has importance and intrinsic meaning. But there is no mathematical relationship between data points. Typically, certain pain scores (the so-called Likert scales), opinion scales, severity of injury scores (as reflected in a score such as the Trauma Score where lower numbers are predictive of worse survival than higher ones), or the grading and staging of a tumor (higher numbers are worse in these cases) are examples of ordinal data. Common questionnaires asking the participant to state whether they agree, are neutral, or disagree with a statement are also examples of an ordinal scale. Although there is a "directional value" to each of these answers, there is no numerical mathematical relationship between them.

Interval data is ordinal data for which the interval between each number is also a meaningful real number. However, interval data has an arbitrary zero point. Therefore, there is no ratio relationship between two points and they are not directly proportional. One example is temperature in Celsius where $64\,°C$ is $32\,°C$ hotter than $32\,°C$ but not twice as hot. Another example is the common IQ score where 100 is average, but 200 is not twice as smart (although it is super-genius, and less than 0.01% the population have a score this high).

Ratio data is interval data that has an absolute zero value. This results in a meaning for both absolute and ratio, or relative, changes in the variable. Examples of ratio variables are the temperature in degrees Kelvin ($100\,°$Kelvin is $50\,°K$ hotter than $50\,°K$ and is twice as hot), age (a 10-year-old is twice as old as a 5-year-old), and common biological measurements such as pulse, blood pressure, respiratory rate, blood chemistry measurements, and weight.

Data can be described as either having or lacking continuity. **Continuous** data may take any value within a defined range. For most purposes we choose to round off to an easily usable number of digits. This is called the number of significant places. (Do you remember this from high school and college?) Height is an example of a continuous measure since a person can be 172 cm or 173 cm or 172.58763248... cm tall. The practical useful value would be 172.6 or 173 cm.

Values for **discrete** data can only be whole numbers. For example, a piano is an instrument with only discrete values (i.e., there are only 88 keys, therefore only 88 possible notes). Scoring systems like the Glasgow Coma Score (measuring neurological deficits) and other ordinal scales contain only discrete variables and (mathematically) can have only integer values.

We commonly use **dichotomous** data to describe binomial outcomes, those variables that can have only two possible values. Obvious examples are alive or dead, yes or no, normal or abnormal, and better or worse (or not better). Sometimes researchers convert continuous variables to dichotomous ones. Selecting a single cutoff as the division between two states does this. For example, serum sodium is defined as normal if between 135 and 145 mEq/dl. Values over 145 define hypernatremia, and values below this don't. This has the effect of dichotomizing the value of the serum sodium into either hypernatremic or not hypernatremic.

Measurement in clinical research

All natural phenomena can be measured. Errors may occur in that process. These can be classified into two categories: random and systematic. **Random error** is characteristically unpredictable in direction or amount. Random error leads to a lack of precision due to the innate variability of the biological or sociological system being studied. This biological variation occurs in most bodily functions. For example, in a given population, there will be a more or less random variation in the pulse or blood pressure. Many of these random events can be described by the normal distribution. Random error can also be due to the lack of precision of the measuring instrument. An imprecise instrument will get slightly different results each time the same event is measured. Certain measurements are inherently more precise than others. Serum sodium measured inside rat muscle cells will show less random error than the degree of depression in humans. There can also be innate variability in the way that different researchers (or physicians) interpret the data on certain patients.

Systematic error represents a consistent distortion in direction or magnitude of the results. For example, researchers could consistently use a blood-pressure cuff that always reads high by 10 mm Hg. More commonly, the measurement can be influenced by knowledge of other aspects of the patient's situation. Researchers may respond differently to some patients in the study. In a study of asthma, the researcher may consistently coach some research subjects differently in performing the peak expiratory flow rate (PEFR), an effort-dependent test. Non-random assignment of subjects can result in bias. Researchers could preferentially assign patients with bronchitis (almost always gets better on its own) to the placebo group when studying the effect of antibiotics on bronchitis and pneumonia (sometimes gets better on its own, but more slowly). If the patients assigned to placebo get better as often as those taking antibiotics, this may have occurred because the placebo patients were going to get better more quickly anyway. Systematic (or systemic) error is a function of the person making the measurement or the calibration of the instrument.

Both types of errors may lead to incorrect results. The researcher's job is to minimize bias in the study. We are usually more successful at reducing systematic error. However, it is the reader's job to determine if bias exists, and if so to what extent and in what direction that bias can change the study results.

Instruments and how they are chosen

Common **instruments** include physical "machines" like the thermometer or sphygmomanometer (blood-pressure cuff and manometer) and survey items such as questionnaires or pain scales. By their nature, objective measurements made by physical instruments such as automated blood-cell counters may be very precise. They may also be affected by random variations in the body. An example of this is hemodynamic pressure measurement (arterial or venous pressure, oxygen saturation, airway pressures) taken by transducers. The actual measurement may be very precise, but there can be lots of random variation around the true measurement. Subjective instruments include questions that must be answered either yes or no or with an ordinal scale (0, 1, 2, 3, 4, or 5) or by placing an x on a pre-measured line. Measures of pain or anxiety are common examples.

Measurements, the data that instruments give us, are the final goals of research. They are the result of applying an instrument to the process of systematically collecting data. For the instruments mentioned above, the measurements are temperature (thermometer), blood pressure (sphygmomanometer), number of yes or no answers (on a survey), and level of pain (location of x on a line as a percentage of the total length of the line). The quality of the measurements is only as good as the quality of the instrument used to make them.

Good instrument selection is a vital part of the research study design. The researcher must select instruments that will measure the phenomena of interest. If you wish to measure blood pressure accurately and precisely, a standard blood-pressure cuff would be a reasonable tool. You could also measure blood pressure using an intra-arterial catheter attached to a pressure transducer. This will give a more precise result, but the additional precision may not help in the ultimate care of the patient. If survival is the desired outcome, a simple record of the presence or absence of death is the best measure. For measuring the cause of death, the death certificate can also be the instrument of choice, but has been shown to be inaccurate.

When subjective outcomes (pain, anxiety, quality of life, or patient satisfaction) are measured, the selection of an instrument becomes more difficult. Pain, a very subjective measure, is appreciated differently by different people. Some patients will react more strongly and show more emotion than others in response to the same levels of pain. There are standardized pain scores available that have been validated in research trials. The most commonly used pain scale is the Visual Analog Scale (VAS). A 10-cm line is placed on the paper with one end labeled "no pain at all," and the other end "worst pain ever." The patient puts a mark on the scale corresponding to the pain level. This can be repeated using the same level of pain as a validation of the scale. The best outcome measure when using this scale is the change in the pain score, not the absolute score. Since pain is quantitated differently, it is only the difference in scores that is likely to be similar. In fact, when this was studied, it was found that patients would use consistently similar differences for the same degree of pain.[1]

Another type of pain score is the Likert Scale. This is a five- or six-point ordinal scale in which each of the points represents a different level of pain. A sample Likert Scale begins with 0 = no pain, continues with 1 = minimal pain, and ends with 5 = worst pain ever. The reader must be careful when interpreting studies using this type of scoring system. Personal differences in the quantification may result in large differences in the score. A patient who puts a 3 for their pain is counted very differently from a patient who puts a 4 for the same level of pain. The differences in pain level have not been quantitated and as it is an ordinal scale the results may not be used the same way as a VAS score, which behaves like a continuous variable. Likert scales are very useful for measuring opinions about a given question. For example, when evaluating a course, you are given several graded choices such as strongly agree, agree, neutral, disagree or strongly disagree.

Similar problems will result with other questionnaires and scales. The reader must become familiar with the commonly used survey instruments in their specialty. Commonly used scores in studies of depression are the Beck Depression Inventory or the Hamilton Depression Scale. In the study of alcoholism, the commonly used scores are the CAGE score, Michigan Alcohol Screening Test (MAST), and the Alcohol Use Disorders Identification Test (AUDIT). The reader is responsible for understanding the limitations of each of these scores when reviewing the literature. This will require you to look further into the use of these tests when you first start to review the medical literature. Sometimes scores are developed specifically for a study. In that case, they must be independently validated before use.

A common problem in selecting instruments is the practice of measuring **surrogate markers**. These may or may not be related to the outcome of interest and may not be predictive of it. For example, the degree of blood flow through a coronary artery (as measured by "TIMI grade") is a good measure of the flow

---

[1] K. H. Todd & J. P. Funk. The minimum clinically important difference in physician-assigned visual analog pain scores. *Acad. Emerg. Med.* 1996; 3: 142–146; and K. H. Todd, K. G. Funk, J. P. Funk & R. Bonacci. Clinical significance of reported changes in pain severity. *Ann. Emerg. Med.* 1996; 27: 485–489.

of blood through the artery. But it may not predict the ultimate survival of a patient. The first measure (TIMI grade flow) is a **disease-oriented outcome** while survival is a **patient-oriented outcome**. **Composite outcomes** will more often achieve statistical significance when each individual outcome is too infrequent to demonstrate statistical significance. Only consider using these if all the outcomes are important to your patient. An example is the use of death and recurrent transient ischemic attack (TIA or "mini-stroke") as an outcome. Death is important to all patients, but recurrent TIA (transient by definition) may not have the same level of importance, and should not be considered equal when measuring outcome events.

Attributes of measurements

Measurements should be precise, accurate, reliable, and valid. **Precision** simply means that the measurement is nearly the same value each time it is measured. This is a measure of random variation or error. Statistically it states that there is a small amount of variation around the true value of the variable being measured. In statistical terminology this is equivalent to a small standard deviation or range around the middle value (mean or median) of multiple measurements. For example, if each time a physician takes a blood pressure, the same measurement is obtained, we can say that the measurement is precise. The same measurement can become imprecise if not repeated the same way, for example if different blood-pressure cuffs are used. **Reliability** is often used loosely as a synonym of precision and incorporates durability or reproducibility of the measurement. It tells you that no matter how often you repeat the measurement you will get the same result. We are looking for instruments that will give precise, consistent, reproducible, and dependable data.

   Accuracy is a measure of the trueness of the result. This tells you how close the measured value is to the true (or actual) value. Statistically, it is equivalent to saying that the mean (arithmetic average) of all measurements taken is the actual value of the thing being measured. For example, indirect blood-pressure measurements using a manometer and blood-pressure cuff correlate closely to direct intra-arterial measurements in healthy, young volunteers using a pressure transducer. This means that the blood pressure measured using the manometer and blood-pressure cuff is accurate. The measurement will be inaccurate if the manometer is not calibrated properly or if an incorrect cuff size is used.

   Precision and accuracy are direct functions of the instruments chosen to make the measurements. **Validity** tells us that the measurement actually represents what we want to measure. We may have accurate and precise measurements that are not valid. For example, weight is a less valid measure for obesity than skin fold thickness or body mass index. Blood pressure measured with a standard blood-pressure cuff is a valid measure of the intra-arterial pressure. A single blood-sugar measurement is not a valid measure of **overall** diabetic control. A test called glycosylated hemoglobin is a valid measure of this.

Types of validity

There are several definitions of validity. The first set defines validity by the process in which it is determined. This includes **criterion-based, predictive**, and **face validity**. The second definition determines where validity is found in a clinical study. This includes **internal** and **external validity**.

Criterion-based or **construct validity** is a description of how close the measurement of the phenomenon of interest is to other measurements of the same thing using different instruments. This means that there is a study showing that the measurement of interest agrees with other accepted measures of the same thing. For example, the score of patients on the CAGE (alcoholism screening) questionnaire correlates with the results on the more complex and previously validated Michigan Alcohol Screening Test (MAST) for the diagnosis of alcoholism. Similarly, blood-pressure cuff readings correlate with intra-arterial blood pressure as recorded by an electrical pressure transducer.

Predictive validity is a type of criterion-based validity that describes how well the measurement predicts an event. This could be the result of another measurement or a particular outcome. For example, lack of fever in an elderly patient with pneumonia predicts a higher mortality than in the same group of patients with fever. This was determined from studies of factors related to a specific outcome, mortality, in elderly patients with pneumonia.

Finally, **face validity** is how much common sense the measurement makes. It is a statement of the fact that the instrument measures the phenomenon of interest and makes sense. For example, the measured performance of a student on one multiple-choice examination should predict that student's performance on another multiple-choice examination. Performance on an observed examination of a standardized patient accurately measures the student's ability to accurately perform a history and physical examination on any patient (face validity). However, this must be validated since in the testing situation some students may freeze up, which they wouldn't do when face-to-face with a real patient.

Validity can also be classified by the potential effect of bias on a study. Internal and external validity are the terms used to describe this and are the most common ways to classify validity. You should use this schema to assess all research studies. **Internal validity** exists when precision and accuracy are not distorted by bias introduced into a study. An internally valid study precisely and accurately measures what is intended. Internal validity is threatened by problems in the way a study is designed or carried out, or with the instruments used to make the measurements.

External validity exists when the measurement can be generalized and the results extrapolated to other (clinical) situations or populations. External validity is threatened when the population studied is too restricted to be able to apply the results to another (usually larger) population.

Schematically, truth in the study is a function of internal validity. The results of an internally valid study are true and there is no serious source of bias that can produce a fatal flaw and invalidate the study. Truth in the universe (all other patients with this problem) is only present if the study is externally valid. The process by which this occurs will be discussed in a later chapter.

Improving precision and accuracy

In the process of designing a study, the researcher should maximize precision, accuracy, and validity. The **methods section** detailing the protocol used in the study should enable the reader to determine if enough safeguards have been taken to assure a valid study. The protocol should be explicit and given in enough detail to be reproduced easily by anyone reading the study.

There are four possible error patterns that can occur in the process of measuring data. (1) Both precision and accuracy can be good: the result is equal to the true value and there is only a small degree of variation around that value (the standard deviation is small). (2) The results may be precise but not accurate: the result is not equal to the true value, but there is only a small degree of variation around that value; this pattern is characteristic of systematic error. (3) Results that are accurate but not precise are typical of random error: the result is equal to the true value but there is a large amount of variation around that value (the standard deviation is large). (4) The result may be neither accurate nor precise: this is due to both random and systematic error; in this case the result of the study is not equal to the true value and there is a large amount of variability around that value. Look for these patterns of error (or potential error) when reviewing a study.

Using exactly reproducible and objective measures can increase precision. Standardizing the performance of the measurements and training of observers will also increase precision. Automated instruments can give more reliable measurements, assuming that they are regularly calibrated. The number of trained observers should be kept to a minimum. More observers increase the likelihood that one will make a serious error.

Making **unobtrusive** measurements reduces subject bias. Unobtrusive measurements are those which cannot be detected by the patient. For example, taking a blood pressure is obtrusive while simply observing a patient for an outcome (death or living) is (usually) non-obtrusive. Watching someone work and recording his or her efficiency is obtrusive since it could result in a change in behavior (the **Hawthorne effect**). Unobtrusive measurements are made in a **blinded** manner. If the observer is unaware of the group to which the patient is assigned, there is less risk that the measurement will be biased. Blinding creates the climate for consistency and fairness in the measurements, and results in reduced systematic error. Non-blinded measurements can lead to differential treatment being given to one of the groups. This can lead to **contamination** or **confounding** of the results. In **single blinding**, either the researcher or the patient doesn't know who is in each group. In **double blinding**, neither the researchers nor subjects know who is in each group. **Triple blinding** occurs if the patient, person treating, and researcher measuring are all blind to the treatment being rendered.

Tests of inter- and intra-rater reliability

Different observers can obtain different results when they measure the temperature of a child using a thermometer because they use slightly different techniques (e.g., the time the thermometer is left in the patient) or different ways to read the mercury level.

Improve precision by minimizing inter- and intra-observer variation. The researcher should account for variability between observers and between measurements made by the same observer. Variability between two observers or between multiple observations by a single observer can introduce bias into the results. Therefore at least a subset of all the measurements should be repeated and the variability of the results measured. This is called **inter-observer** and **intra-observer** variability. Tests for inter-observer and intra-observer variability should be done before the study is completed. Inter-observer variability occurs when two or more observers obtain different results when measuring the same phenomenon. Intra-observer variability occurs when the same observer obtains different results when measuring the same phenomenon on two or more occasions. Both of these are measured by the kappa statistic.

The **kappa statistic** measures the degree of agreement beyond chance between two observers (the inter-rater agreement) or for multiple measurements made by a single observer (the intra-rater agreement). It is a quantitative measure of the degree of agreement between measurements.

We often assume that all diagnostic tests are precise. Many studies have demonstrated that most non-automated tests have a degree of subjectivity in their interpretation. This has been seen in commonly used x-ray tests such as CT scan, mammography, and angiography. It is also present in tests commonly considered to be the Gold Standard such as the interpretation of tissue samples from biopsies or surgery.

We will show how to do this using a clinical example. One morning, two radiology residents were reading mammograms. The first resident (no. 1) had

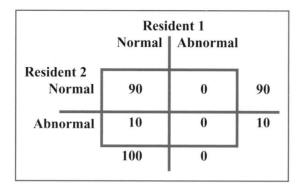

Fig. 7.1 Observed agreement between two residents when one (no. 1) reads them all as normal and the other (no. 2) reads 90 as normal and 10 as abnormal.

	Resident 1		
	Normal	**Abnormal**	
Resident 2			
Normal	90	0	90
Abnormal	10	0	10
	100	0	

Fig. 7.2 Observed agreement between two residents when both (no. 1 and no. 2) read 90 as normal and 10 as abnormal, but there is no relationship between their readings. The 90% read normal by no. 1 are not the same as the 90% read as normal by no. 2.

	Resident 1		
	Normal	**Abnormal**	
Resident 2			
Normal	81	9	90
Abnormal	9	1	10
	90	10	

been on night call and was pretty tired. He didn't really feel like reading these, knowing that in any case his readings would be reviewed by the attending. He also reasoned that since this was a screening clinic for young women (average age 32) there would be very few positives. This particular radiology department had a computerized reading system. The resident pushed either the "normal" or the "cancer" button on a console and that reading would be entered in the file. After reading the first three as negative, he fell asleep on the "negative" button.

The second resident (no. 2) was really interested in mammography and had slept all night (since she was not on call). She carefully read each study and pushed the appropriate button. She read 90 films as normal and 10 as suspicious for early breast cancer. The two residents' readings are tabulated in the 2 × 2 table in Fig. 7.1.

Observed agreement = 90/100 = 90%. Is an agreement of 90% very good? What would the agreement be if they read the mammograms by chance alone? We know that there are 90% normals and 10% abnormals. So let's assume that each read the films with that proportion of each result and do the same 2 × 2 table (Fig. 7.2). Agreement by chance = (81 + 1)/100 = 82%.

	Resident 1 Normal	Resident 1 Abnormal	
Resident 2 Normal	25	25	50
Abnormal	25	25	50
	50	50	A

	Resident 1 Normal	Resident 1 Abnormal	
Resident 2 Normal	50	0	50
Abnormal	0	50	50
	50	50	B

Fig. 7.3 Kappa for chance agreement only (A, $\kappa = 0.0$) and for perfect agreement (B, $\kappa = 1.0$).

Kappa is the ratio of the actual agreement beyond chance and the potential agreement beyond chance. The actual agreement beyond chance is the difference between the actual agreement found and that expected by chance. In our example it is $90 - 82 = 8\%$ (0.08). The potential agreement beyond chance is the difference between the highest possible agreement (100%) and that expected by chance alone. In our example, $100 - 82 = 18\%$ (0.18).

$$\text{Kappa} = (0.90 - 0.82)/(1.00 - 0.82) = 0.08/0.18 = 0.44$$

Overview of kappa statistic

You should use the kappa statistic when you want to know the **precision** of a measurement or the **inter-observer consistency** (or indeed intra-observer consistency). This gives a reasonable estimate of how "easily" the measurement is made. The "easier" to make, the more likely that two different observers will agree on the result.

Kappa ranges from 0 to 1 where 0 means that there is no agreement and 1 means there is complete agreement beyond that expected by chance alone. You can see from making a 2×2 table that if there is an equal number in each cell the agreement occurs purely by chance (Fig. 7.3). Similarly if there is perfect agreement the agreement is very unlikely to be completely by chance. However, it is still possible: if there are only a few readings in each cell, the agreement could have occurred by chance, and there was a chance (even though it is small) that there was 100% agreement. Confidence intervals (which we will discuss later in the book) should be calculated to determine the range within which (statistically) 95% of possible kappa values will be found.

The value of kappa is as a measure of the significance of the agreement in making a measurement of the data. Some experts have related the value of kappa to qualitative descriptors, and these are shown in Table 7.1. In general, look for a kappa higher than 0.6 before you consider the agreement to be reasonably acceptable.

Table 7.1. Interpretation of the kappa statistic

$$
\text{Kappa} = \frac{\text{actual agreement between measurements beyond chance}}{\text{potential agreement between measurements beyond chance}}
$$

Range: 0–1 (0 = no agreement; 1 = complete agreement)

Numerical level of kappa	Qualitative significance
0.0–0.2	slight
0.2–0.4	fair
0.4–0.6	moderate
0.6–0.8	substantial
0.8–1.0	almost perfect

There are other statistics that (more or less) measure the same thing. These are the standard deviation on repeated measurements, coefficient of variation, correlation coefficient of paired measurements, and Cronbach's alpha.[2]

---

[2] A more detailed discussion of kappa can be found in D. L. Sackett, R. B. Haynes, G. H. Guyatt & P. Tugwell *Clinical Epidemiology: a Basic Science for Clinical Medicine.* (2nd edn.) Boston: Little Brown, 1991.

8

Sources of bias

Of all the causes which conspire to blind
Man's erring judgment, and misguide the mind;
What the weak head with strongest bias rules, –
Is pride, the never-failing vice of fools.

Alexander Pope (1688–1744): Essay on Criticism

Learning objectives

In this chapter you will learn:
- sources of bias
- threats to internal and external validity
- how to tell when bias threatens the conclusions of a study

All studies involve observations and measurement of the phenomena of interest. The observations and instruments used to make these measurements are subject to error. Bias introduced into a study can result in systematic error. These errors may then affect the results of the study and could invalidate the conclusions. Since there is no such thing as a perfect study, in reading the medical literature you should be familiar with common sources of bias in clinical studies. By understanding how these biases could effect the results of the study, it is possible to detect bias and predict the potential effect on the conclusions. You can then determine if this will invalidate the study conclusions enough to deter you from using the results in your patients' care. This chapter will give you a schema for looking for bias, and present some common sources of bias.

Overview of bias in clinical studies

Bias was a semilegendary Greek statesman who tried to make peace between two city-states by lying about the warlike intention of the enemy state. His ploy failed and ultimately he told the truth, allowing his city to win the war. His name became forever associated with slanting the truth as a means to accomplish an end.

Bias is defined as the systematic introduction of error into a study that can distort the results in a non-random way. It is almost impossible to eliminate all sources of bias even in the most carefully designed study. It is the job of the researcher to attempt to remove as much bias as possible. It is the job of the reader to find any possible bias and assess the importance and potential effects of this bias on the results of the study. Virtually no study is 100% bias-free and not all bias will result in an invalid study.

After identifying a source of bias, you must determine the likely effect of that bias on the results of the study. If this is likely to be great, internal validity and the conclusions of the study are threatened; if it could completely change the results of the study, it is called a "fatal" flaw. The results of a study with a fatal flaw should generally not be applied to your current patients. Results of studies with only small potential effects of bias can be accepted and used with caution. Bias can be broken down into three areas according to its source: the population being studied, the measurement of the outcome, and miscellaneous sources.

Bias in the population being studied

Selection bias

Selection or sampling bias occurs when patients are selected in a manner that will systematically influence the outcome of the study. There are several ways that this type of bias can occur. Subjects who are volunteers or paid to be in the study may have different characteristics than the "average person" with the disease in question. Another form of selection bias occurs when patients are chosen for a study based upon certain characteristics. These characteristics may then change the outcome of the study. A few examples will help demonstrate the effects of this bias.

An investigator offered free psychiatric counseling to women who had just had an abortion if they took a free psychological test. He found the incidence of depression was higher in these women than in the general population. He concluded that having an abortion caused depression. It is more likely that women who had an abortion and were depressed (therefore needing counseling) would sign up for the study. Women who had an abortion and were not depressed would be less likely to sign up for the study and take the "free" psychological test. This is a potentially fatal flaw of this study, and therefore the conclusion is biased.

Patients with suspected pulmonary embolism (PE, blood clot in the lung), were studied with angiograms (x-ray of the blood vessels in the lung capable of showing a blood clot) and other tests, to find the correlates of this diagnosis. It was found that those patients with a positive angiogram (showing a PE) were less likely to have a blood clot in the leg (DVT, deep venous thrombosis, which can break off and migrate to the lung) than patients with a negative angiogram (showing no blood clot, or no PE). The authors concluded that DVT was not a risk factor for PE. The study did not include all patients in the universe with possible PE, but only those with a high enough "clinical" suspicion of a PE to be referred for an angiogram. This is a form of selection bias. The presence of a DVT is a risk factor for a PE and could lead to treatment rather than angiogram. Therefore, patients suspected of having PE and who didn't have DVT were more likely to be selected for angiogram. Similarly, DVT patients with no signs or symptoms of PE who were entered into the study only because they had a DVT wouldn't have a PE. Again, this is a fatal flaw and should not change your approach to these patients.

Referral bias

Referral bias is a special form of selection bias. Studies performed in tertiary care or referral centers often use only patients referred for specialty care as subjects. This eliminates cases that are milder and more easily treated, and those diagnosed at an earlier stage, who are more likely to be seen in a primary care provider's office. Obviously the subjects in the study are not like those patients with similar complaints seen in a primary care office, who will be much less likely to have unusual causes for their symptoms. This limits external validity and the results should not be generalized to all patients with the same complaint or problem.

Patients presenting to a neurology clinic with headaches occurring days to weeks after apparently minor head traumas were given a battery of tests: CT scan (computerized tomogram) of the head, EEG (electroencephalogram or "brain waves"), MRI (magnetic resonance imaging) scan of the brain, and various psychological tests. Most of these tests were normal, but some of the MRIs showed minor abnormalities. None of these required any special additional treatment. Most of the patients with the abnormalities on the MRI had a brief loss of consciousness at the time of injury. The authors concluded that all patients with any loss of consciousness after minor head trauma should have immediate MRI scans done. The study patients reflected only those who were referred to the neurologist and who therefore had persistent problems from their head injury. They did not measure the percentage of all patients with head injuries who had loss of consciousness for a brief period of time and who had the reported MRI abnormalities. The results, even if significant in this selected population, would not apply to the general population of all head-injured patients.

Spectrum bias

Spectrum bias occurs when only patients with classical or severe symptoms are selected for a study. This makes the expected outcomes more or less likely than for the population as a whole. For example, patients with definite subarachnoid hemorrhages (bleeding in or around the brain) who have the worst headache of their life and present with coma or a severe alteration of their mental status will almost all have a positive CT of their head showing the bleed. Those patients who have similar headaches but no neurological symptoms are much less likely to have a positive CT of the head. Selecting only those patients with severe symptoms will bias the study and make the results inapplicable to those with less severe symptoms.

Detection bias

Detection bias is a form of selection bias that preferentially includes patients in a study if they have been exposed to a particular risk factor. In these cases, exposure causes a sign or symptom that precipitates a search for the disease and then is blamed for causing the disease. Estrogen therapy was thought to be a risk factor for the development of endometrial (uterine) cancer. Patients who had cancer and were in a tumor registry were compared to a similar group of women who were referred for D&C (diagnostic scraping of the uterine lining) or hysterectomy (removal of the uterus). The proportion of women taking estrogen was the same in both groups, suggesting no relationship between estrogen use and cancer of the uterus.

Of the women in the D&C or hysterectomy group who were taking estrogen (the risk factor), many turned out to have uterine cancer. Did estrogen cause cancer? Estrogen caused the bleeding, which led to a search for a cause (by D&C), and this found cancers. This and subsequent studies showed that there was a relationship between postmenopausal estrogen therapy and the development of this cancer.

Recall bias

Recall or reporting bias occurs most often in a retrospective (case–control or non–concurrent cohort) study. When asked about certain exposures, cases are more likely than controls to recall that they were exposed. It is human nature to search for a reason for an illness. This is a potential problem whenever subjective information determines exposure and is less likely to occur when objective information is used. A study was performed looking for the connection of childhood leukemia to living under high-tension wires. Mothers of children with leukemia were more likely to remember living anywhere near a high-tension power line than were mothers without a leukemic child. **Exposure suspicion bias** is a type of recall bias that occurs on the part of the researcher. When asking subject patients about exposure, researchers might phrase the question in ways that encourage recall bias. The control subjects similarly might be asked in subtly different ways that could make them less likely to recall the exposure.

Non-respondent bias

Non-respondent bias occurs because those people who don't respond to a survey may be different in some fundamental way from those who respond. The reason for not responding may be related to the study. Past studies have noted that smokers are less likely to respond to a survey than non-smokers when it contains questions about smoking. This makes the results of such a survey biased. It is also true that healthy people are more likely to participate in these surveys than unhealthy ones. This will underestimate the apparent ill effects of smoking, as the bias of having more healthy people in the study group.

Membership bias

Membership bias occurs because the health of some group members differs in a systematic way from the general population. This is obvious when one group of subjects is from health clubs, has higher average education, or is from other groups that might intrinsically be more health-conscious than the average person. It is a problem with studies that look at nurses or physicians and attempt to extrapolate the results to the general population. Socioeconomic factors may distinguish these groups and limit generalizability when analyzing a study.

A recent review of all studies of thrombolytic (clot-dissolving) therapy for acute myocardial infarction (AMI, heart attacks) was conducted. The reviewers found that, on average, patients who were eligible for the study were younger and healthier than patients who were ineligible for inclusion in the study or patients not enrolled (invited to participate as a subject) in the study but treated with these drugs anyway. Overall, study patients got more intensive therapy for their AMI in many other ways. The mortality for study patients was less than half that of ineligible patients and about two thirds that of non-study patients.

Berkerson's bias is a specific bias that occurs when patients in a selected ward of a hospital are the control subjects. These patients may share characteristics that (as a group) separate them from the cases. This difference in baseline characteristics will affect the outcome of the study.

Bias in the measurements of the outcome

Subject bias

Subject bias is a constant distortion of the measurement by the subject. In general, patients try to please their doctors and will tell them what they think the doctor wants to hear. They also may consciously change their behavior or responses in order to please their physicians. They may not report some side effects and may overestimate the amount of medications taken. They may report more improvement if they know they were given a therapy approved of by their doctor rather than the placebo or control therapy. Only effective blinding of subjects (and ideally, also of observers) can prevent this.

Observer bias

Observer bias is the conscious or unconscious distortion in perception of reporting the measurement by an observer. It also occurs when physicians treat patients differently because of the group to which they are assigned. Physicians in a study may give more intensive treatment to their patients who are assigned to the intervention group rather than to the placebo or comparison group. They may interpret the answers to questions on a survey differently in patients known to be in the active treatment rather than control group. An observer not blinded to patient selection may report the results of one group of patients differently from those of the other group. One form of this bias is the situation in which patients who are the sickest may be either preferentially included or excluded from the sample because of bias on the part of the observer making the assignment to each group. This is known as **filtering** and is a form of **selection bias**.

Data collected retrospectively by reviewing the medical records may have poor data quality. The records used to collect data may contain inadequate detail and possess questionable reliability. They may also use varying standards to judge symptoms, signs of disease severity, or outcomes. This is a common occurrence in chart review or retrospective (case–control or non-concurrent cohort) studies. The **implicit review** of charts introduces the researchers bias in interpreting both measurements and outcomes. If there are no objective and explicit criteria for evaluating the medical records (patient charts), the information contained in them is open to misinterpretation from observer bias. It has been shown to occur that researchers subconsciously fit the response to best match their hypothesis. Researchers came up with different results if they performed a blinded chart review as opposed to an unblinded review. **Explicit reviews** are better and can occur when only clearly objective outcome measures are reviewed. Even better is to have the chart material reviewed in a blinded manner. The **Hawthorne effect** occurs because being observed during the process of making measurements changes the behavior of the subject. In the physical sciences, this is known as the Heisenberg Uncertainty Principle. If subjects change their behavior, the outcome will be biased. In one study, physicians knew they were being studied to see which antibiotic they ordered for strep throat. The study was done to see if they would use less expensive antibiotics more often than expensive new ones. They acted differently and changed their clinical practices during the course of the study, prescribing many more of the low-price antibiotics during the course of the study. After the study was over, their behavior went back to baseline. This bias can be prevented through the use of unobtrusive, blinded, or objective measurements.

Misclassification bias

Misclassification bias occurs when the status of patients or their outcomes is incorrectly classified. When the subject patient is given an inaccurate diagnosis (possibly due to lack of comparison to a "gold standard" diagnosis), they will be counted with the wrong group. In some situations, the diagnosis is not appropriate for the treatment. For instance, in a study of antibiotic treatment of pneumonia, patients with bronchitis can be misclassified as having pneumonia. Those patients would all get better with or without antibiotics, making it harder to find a difference in the outcomes of the two treatment groups. Patients may also change their behaviors or risk factors after the initial grouping of subjects, resulting in misclassification bias on the basis of exposure. This is a common bias in cohort studies.

Misclassification of outcomes (distinguishing cases from controls) is a source of bias in case–control studies, and you must know how accurately the cases and controls are being identified. If the disorder (outcome) is relatively common some of the control patients may be affected. One way of compensating for this bias is to "dilute" the control group with extra patients. This will reduce the extent to which misclassification of cases (incorrectly counted as controls) will affect the data. Let's say that you wanted to find out if people who killed themselves by playing Russian Roulette were more likely to have used alcohol than those who committed suicide by shooting themselves in the head. You would look at death investigations and find those that were classified as suicides and those that were classified as Russian Roulette. However, you suspect that some of the Russian Roulette cases may have been misclassified as suicides to "protect the victim." To compensate for this, or dilute the effect of the bias, you decide that your control group will include three suicide deaths for every one Russian Roulette death. Obviously if Russian Roulette deaths are routinely misclassified, this strategy will not result in any change in the bias. This is called **outcome misclassification**. Outcome classification based upon subjective data (including death certificates) is more likely to exhibit this misclassification. This bias can be prevented with objective standards for classification of patients, which should be clearly outlined in the methods section of the study.

Miscellaneous sources of bias

Confounding

Confounding refers to the presence of several variables that could explain the apparent connection between the cause and effect. If a particular variable is present more often in one group of patients than in another, it may be responsible for causing a significant effect. For example, a study was done to look for the effect of antioxidant vitamin E intake on the outcome of cardiovascular disease. It turned out that the group with high vitamin E intake also had a lower rate of smoking and a higher socioeconomic status and educational level than the groups with lower vitamin E intake. It is much more likely that those other variables are responsible for a difference in outcome (decrease in observed cases of cardiovascular disease) than the intake of vitamin E. There are statistical ways of dealing with confounding variables called **multivariate analyses**. The rules governing the application of these types of analyses are somewhat complex and will be discussed in greater detail in a later chapter. When looking at studies always look for the potential presence of confounding variables and at least make certain that the authors have **adjusted** for those variables.

Contamination and cointervention

These are more commonly seen in randomized clinical trials but can also exist in observational studies. Contamination occurs when both groups receive the same therapy as the experimental group or are exposed to the same risk as the "exposed" group. This happens less often in observational studies since we specifically separate out those people exposed to the risk factor and those who are not exposed to the risk factor. However, there may be an environmental situation by which those classified as not exposed to the risk factor are actually exposed. For example, a study is done to look at the effect of living near high-tension wires on the incidence of leukemia. Those patients who live within 30 m of a high-tension wire are considered the exposed group and those who live more than 30 m away are considered the control group. Those people who live within 3 or 5 m of that 30-m line could be misclassified and have a similar degree of exposure to those people on the other side of the line. In fact, families living 60 m from the wires may be equally affected by the electrical field if the wires they live under have four times the strength.

Cointervention occurs when one group or the other receives different medical care based partly or totally upon their group assignment. This also occurs mostly in randomized trials, but could be present in an observational study when the group exposed to one risk factor or one particular treatment also receives different therapy, or other exposure, not received by the unexposed group. This can easily occur in studies with historical controls. Historical controls require different rules to deal with them. The patients in the past may not have had access to the same advances in medical care as the patients who are currently being treated or exposed. The end results would be different if both groups received the same degree of medical care.

Patient attrition

There may be loss of valuable information due to patient attrition. Patients may drop out of the study or be lost to follow-up for many reasons, some directly related to the study. Patients who drop out may do so because a treatment or placebo is ineffective or there are too many unwanted side effects. Therefore, it is imperative for researchers to account for all patients. Studies of placebo use have demonstrated that patients who are compliant, whether given the active intervention or inert placebo, will do better than those who are non-compliant. In practice a drop-out rate less than 20% is an acceptable level of attrition. However, even a lower rate of attrition may bias the study if the reason patients were lost from the study is directly related to the study variables. This is even more important if there are differential rates of attrition between the intervention and comparison groups.

How the authors dealt with outcome measurements of subjects who dropped out, were lost to follow-up, or crossed from one group to another is extremely important. They cannot be ignored and just left out of final data calculations since this will certainly introduce bias into the final results. The data can be analyzed using a **best case / worst case** strategy, assuming that missing patients all had a poor outcome in one analysis and a good outcome in the other. The researcher can then compare the results obtained from each group and see if the loss of patients could have made a big difference.

For subjects who switch groups or don't complete therapy, an **intention-to-treat** strategy should be used. The final outcome of those patients who changed groups is analyzed with the group to which they were originally assigned even though they didn't finish the study or switched groups. We will discuss the issues of attrition and intention to treat further in the chapter on the randomized clinical trial (Chapter 15).

External validity

External validity refers to all problems in applying the study results to a larger or different population. This can occur because the subjects of a study are from only one group in the population. Age, gender, ethnic or racial groups, socioeconomic groups, and cultural groups are examples of variables that can affect external validity. Simply having only one clearly identified group of patients does not automatically mean there will be lack of external validity. There ought to be an a-priori reason that the results could be different in other groups. For example, we know that women respond differently than men to various drugs. Therefore, a study of a particular drug performed only on men could lack external validity when it comes to recommending the drug to women. However, each case must be looked at separately and the reader must determine whether external validity exists.

The result of poor external validity is **inappropriate extrapolation** or generalization of the results of a study to groups to which they do not apply. In a study of patients with heart attacks (myocardial infarction or MI), those who had frequent irregular heart beats (premature ventricular contractions or PVCs) had increased mortality. This led to the recommendation that antiarrhythmic drugs (to suppress the PVCs) be given to all patients with MI. Later studies found an increased number of deaths among patients on long-term antiarrhythmic drug therapy. Subsequent recommendations were that these drugs only be used to treat immediately life-threatening PVCs. The original study patients all had acute ischemia (lack of oxygen going to the heart muscle) while the long-term patients did not, making extrapolation to that population incorrect.

The outcome chosen should be one that matters to the patient. Ideally it is a measure of faster resolution of the problem such as reduction of pain or death rate due to the illness. In these cases, all patients would agree that the particular outcome is important. However, there are also studies that look at other outcomes. These may be important in the overall increase in medical knowledge, but not immediately important to the patient. In fact, these results called **surrogate endpoints** may not translate into improved health at all.

Suppose that I wanted to see if there was any relationship between the timing of students' taking of Step I of the USMLE and their final score. I look at all the scores and correlate them with the date the test is taken. I find that there is a strong association between board scores and date, with the higher scores occurring among students taking the boards at earlier dates. I conclude that medical students should be taking the boards as early as possible in the cycle. What I am missing is that the timing of taking the exam and the score are both dependent on another factor, class rank (or some other marker of all-around smartness). Therefore the two variables, although related, are not of importance to medical students.

Early studies of drugs for the reduction of cholesterol showed that many of the new drugs had a significant effect on lowering cholesterol. These drugs were then used in large populations as a promise to reduce the incidence of heart disease. When these drugs were tested in these populations it was found that the death rate among patients who were on the drug actually increased. Subsequently, newer drugs for this indication have been tested in large populations and found to actually reduce overall death rate. Some of the even newer drugs for this indication have not been tested for the endpoint of reduced mortality and are trying to cash in on the success of those drugs with proven reduction of death rates.

A recent study measured performance on a driving simulator. Volunteers were given a non-sedating antihistamine, a standard sedating antihistamine, or a measured amount of alcohol. The investigators found some impairment in driving performance with the sedating antihistamine and alcohol but very little with the non-sedating antihistamine. This contradicts several large case–control studies, which found increased numbers of accidents with alcohol but not with the sedating antihistamine. The conclusion that non-sedating antihistamines are safer than other antihistamines is not warranted based upon the measurement of driving simulation. If there were significant (and clinically important) impairment with sedating antihistamines, it would have been somewhat apparent in the case–control studies.

Final concerns

Chance can also lead to errors in the study conclusions. The action of chance error causes distortion of the study results in a random way. We can account for this problem with the appropriate use of statistical tests, which will be addressed in the next chapter.

There are a few more miscellaneous concerns for validity when evaluating outcome measurements. Are the measured outcomes those that are important to patients? Were all of the important outcomes included and reported upon or were only certain "main" outcomes of the research project included? If certain outcomes were measured to the exclusion of others, suspect foul play. A study may find a significant improvement in one outcome (for instance disease-free survival) while the outcome of interest for patients, and therefore the outcome of importance, is overall survival, which shows no improvement. The problems associated with subgroup analysis and composite endpoints will be discussed in the chapter on Type I errors (Chapter 11).

There is a definite **publication bias** towards the publication of studies that show a positive result. Studies that show no effect or a negative result are more difficult to get published or may never be submitted for publication. Authors are aware of this bias and as a result it also takes longer for negative studies to get written.

There is a prejudice that all studies supported or run by drug companies or other proprietary interests are inherently biased. Since these companies want their products to do well in clinical trials, it may be that the methods used to bias the studies can be quite subtle. Take the studies of antihistamines and thrombolytics mentioned earlier in this chapter. Drug-company sponsorship should be a "red flag" to look more carefully for sources of bias in the study. In general, all potential conflicts of interest should be clearly stated in any medical study article. Many journals now have mandatory requirements that this be included and prominently displayed. However, as the examples below illustrate, there are still some problems with this policy.

You must evaluate each study on its own merits. If you think bias exists, you must be able to demonstrate where it is and how it could affect the study. The medical industry is funding more and more research. These companies have a lot of power when it comes to deciding what research gets done and what gets published. There were two recent cases showing abuse of this power.

Table 8.1. Looking for sources of bias: a checklist

Check the methods section for the following

(1) The methods for making all the measurements were fully described with a clearly defined protocol for making these measurements.
(2) The observers were trained to make the measurements and this training was adequately described and standardized.
(3) All measurements were made unobtrusively, the subjects were blinded to the measurement being made, and the observers (either the ones providing care or the ones making the measurements or interpreting the results) were blinded.
(4) Paired measurements were made (test–retest reliability) or averaged and intra-observer or inter-observer reliability of repeated measurements was measured.
(5) The measurements were checked against a known "gold standard (the measurement accepted as being the truth) and checked for their validity either through citations from the literature or by a demonstration project in the current study. Readers may have to decide for themselves if a measurement has face validity. You will know more about this as you learn more background material about the subject.
(6) The reasons for inclusion and exclusion must be spelled out and appropriate.
(7) Patients who drop out or cross over must be clearly identified and the results appropriately adjusted for this behavior.
(8) The most appropriate outcome measure should be selected. Be suspicious of composite or surrogate outcome measures.

In one case, Boots Pharmaceuticals, the maker of Synthroid (a brand of levothyroxine, a thyroid hormone commonly taken to replace low thyroid levels) sponsored a study of their drug against generic thyroid replacement medication. The study was done at Harvard and when the researchers found that the two drugs were equivalent, they submitted their findings to *JAMA*. The company notified both Harvard and *JAMA* that they would sue in court if the study were printed. Harvard and *JAMA* both stepped down and pulled the article. That news was leaked to the *Wall Street Journal*, which published the account, and Boots relented, allowing the study to be published in *JAMA*.

In the second case, a researcher at the Hospital for Sick Children in Toronto was the principal investigator in a study of a new drug to prevent the side effect of iron accumulation in children with a disease requiring them to get multiple transfusions. The drug appeared to be associated with severe side effects. When she attempted to make this information known to authorities at the university, the company threatened legal action and she was removed from the project. When other scientists at the university stood up to support her, she was removed from her job. When the situation became public and the government stepped in, she was rehired by the university, but in a lower position. The issues of conflict of interest in clinical research will be discussed in more detail in Chapter 16.

This chapter was an introduction to common sources of bias. There are many other sources of bias that have been named. There is an excellent article by Dr. David Sackett on sources of bias.[1] The accompanying checklist (Table 8.1) will help the novice reader identify potential sources of bias.

[1] D. L. Sackett. Bias in analytic research. *J. Chronic Dis.* 1979; 32: 51–63.

9

Review of basic statistics

There are three kinds of lies: lies, damned lies, and statistics.

Benjamin Disraeli, Earl of Beaconsfield (1804–1881)

Learning objectives

In this chapter you will learn:
- evaluation of graphing techniques
- measures of central tendency and dispersion
- populations and samples
- the normal distribution
- use and abuse of percentages
- simple and conditional probabilities
- basic epidemiological definitions

Clinical decisions ought to be based on valid scientific research from the medical literature. These studies consist of both epidemiological and clinical research. The competent interpreter (consumer) of these studies must understand basic epidemiological and statistical concepts. Critical appraisal of the literature and good medical decision making require an understanding of the tools of basic probability.

What are statistics and why are they useful in medicine?

Nature is a random process. The world is full of variation especially when it comes to complex biological systems. It is virtually impossible to describe the operations of a given biological system with a single and simple formula or fact. Since we cannot measure all the parameters of every biological system we are interested in, we make approximations and deduce how often they are true. Because of the innate variation in biological systems or organisms it is hard to tell real differences in a system from random variation or "noise." Statistics seeks to describe this randomness by telling us how much "noise" there is in the measurements we make of a system or organism. By "filtering" out this noise, statistics allows us to approach a correct value of the underlying facts of interest.

Descriptive and inferential statistics

Descriptive statistics is concerned with the presentation, summarization, and utilization of data. These include techniques for graphically displaying the results of a study and mathematical indices that summarize the data with a few key numbers. These are **measures of central tendency** (**mean**, **median**, and **mode**) and **measures of dispersion** (**standard deviation**, **standard error of the mean**, **range**, **percentile**, and **quartiles**). In medicine, we usually study a small number of patients with a given disease, a **sample**. What we are actually interested in finding out is how all patients with that disease (the entire **population**) will respond. **Inferential statistics** can tell us whether or not we can generalize the data gathered from the sample to a larger group of subjects or the entire population.

Visual display (graphing) of data

The purpose of a graph is visually to display the data in a form that allows the observer to draw conclusions about the data. Graphs can be deceptive. The reader is responsible for being able to evaluate the accuracy and truthfulness of graphic representations of the data. There are several common deceptions to watch for when evaluating and reading graphs.

There must be a well-defined zero point. Lack of zero point (Fig. 9.1) is always illegal (inappropriate or improper). This technique makes small differences look bigger by emphasizing only the upper portion of the scale. It is legal to start at zero, break the line up with two diagonal hash marks just above the zero point, and then continue from a higher value (as in Fig. 9.2). This still exaggerates the changes in the graph, but now the reader is warned and will consider the results accordingly.

The axes of the graph should be relatively equally proportioned. **Lack of proportionality**, a much more subtle technique, is still illegal. It serves to emphasize the drawn-out axis relative to the other (less drawn-out) axis. This visually exaggerates smaller changes in the axis that is drawn to the larger scale. (Fig. 9.3) Both axes should have their variables drawn to roughly the same scale (Fig. 9.4).

Another deceptive graphing technique can be seen in some pharmaceutical advertisements. This consists of the use of three-dimensional shapes to demonstrate the difference between two groups (usually the effect of a drug on a patient outcome). One example uses cones of different heights to demonstrate the difference between the end point of therapy for the drug produced by the company and its closest competitor. The height of each cone is the percentage of patients

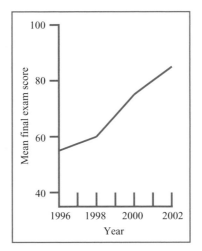

Fig. 9.1 Illegal graph due to the lack of a defined zero point. This makes the change in mean final exam scores appear to be much greater (relatively) than they truly are.

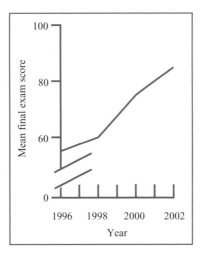

Fig. 9.2 Legal version of the graph in Figure 9.1 created by putting in a defined zero point. Although the change in mean final exam scores still appears to be relatively greater than they truly are, the reader is notified that this distortion is occurring.

responding in each group. Visually, the cones represent a larger volume than simple bars or even triangles, making the drug being advertised look like it caused a much larger effect. For more information on deceptive graphing techniques, the reader is referred to E.R. Tufte's classic book on graphing.[1]

Types of graph

Stem-and-leaf plots

Stem-and-leaf plots are shortcuts used as preliminary plots for graphs called simple histograms. The stem is made up of the digits on the left side of each

[1] E. R. Tufte. *The Visual Display of Quantitative Data*. Cheshire, CT: Graphics Press, 1983.

Fig. 9.3 Illegal graph due to the lack of proportionality of the x and y axes. This makes it appear as if the change in mean final exam scores occurred over a much shorter time period than in reality.

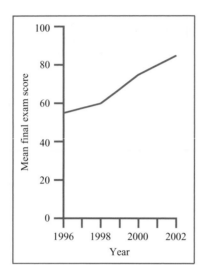

Fig. 9.4 Legal graph with proportioned x and y axes, giving a true representation of the rise in exam scores gradually over time.

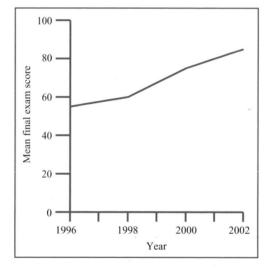

value (tens, hundreds, or higher) and the leaves are the digits on the right side (units, or lower) of each number. Let's take, for example, the following grades on a hypothetical statistics exam:

96 93 84 75 75 71 65 74 58 87 66 90 76 68 65 78 78 66 76 88 99 88 78

90 86 98 67 66 87 57 89 84 78

In this example, the first digit (the tens) forms the stem and the second digit (the units), the leaves. In creating the stem-and-leaf plot, first list the tens digits, and then next to them all the units digits which have that tens digit in common. Our example becomes the stem-and-leaf plot in Fig. 9.5.

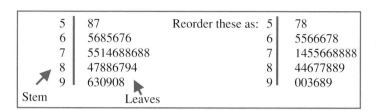

Fig. 9.5 Stem-and-leaf plot of grades in a hypothetical statistics exam.

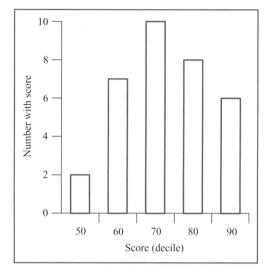

Fig. 9.6 Bar graph of the data in Fig. 9.5.

This can be rotated 90° counterclockwise and redrawn as a bar graph (bar chart) or histogram. The y-axis shows the number of observations in each category. It can also show the percentages of the total in each category. The categories (tens digits in our example) appear as the x-axis. This shows the relationship between the independent variable (exam scores) and the dependent variable (number of students with a score in each 10% increment of grades).

Bar graphs, histograms and frequency polygons

The most common types of graphs used in the medical articles are bar graphs, histograms, and frequency polygons. A bar graph (Fig. 9.6) can be simply drawn by turning the stem-and-leaf plot counterclockwise 90° and replacing the numbers with bars. A histogram is a bar graph in which the bars touch each other (Fig. 9.7). As a rule, the author should attempt to make the contrast between bars on a histogram as clear as possible. A frequency polygon shows how often each observation occurs (Fig. 9.8 is a frequency polygon of the data in Fig. 9.5). A cumulative frequency polygon (Fig. 9.9) shows how the number of accumulated events is distributed. Here the y-axis is usually the percentage of the total events.

Fig. 9.7 Histogram of the data in
Fig. 9.5.

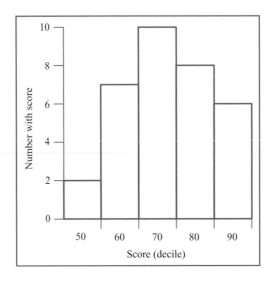

Fig. 9.8 Frequency polygon of
the data in Fig. 9.5.

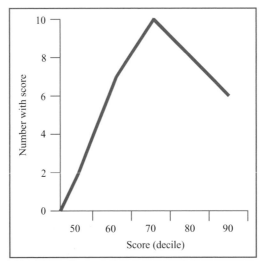

Box-and-whisker plots

Box-and-whisker plots (as in Fig. 9.10) are common ways to represent the range of values for a single variable. The central line in the box is the median. The box edges are the 25th and 75th percentile values and the lines on either side represent the limits of 95% of the data. The stars represent extreme outliers.

Measures of central tendency and dispersion

There are two numerical measures that describe a data-set. They are central tendency and dispersion. There are three measures of central tendency, describing the center of a set of variables: the mean, median and mode.

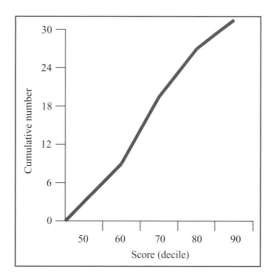

Fig. 9.9 Cumulative frequency polygon of the data in Fig. 9.5.

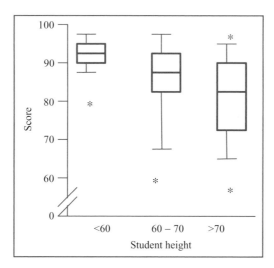

Fig. 9.10 Box-and-whisker plot of scores on the statistics test by student height.

The **mean** (μ or $\bar{x}$) is the arithmetical center, commonly called the arithmetic average. It is the sum of all measurements divided by the number of measurements. Mathematically, $\mu = (\Sigma x_i)/n$. In this equation, x_i is the numerical value of the i th data point and n is the total number of data points. The mean is strongly effected by **outliers**. These are extreme numbers on either the high or low end of the distribution (producing a high degree of **skew**). Therefore, it will not be a representative central value if the data are highly skewed. The mean should not be used for ordinal data and is meaningless in that setting unless the ordinal data has been shown to behave like continuous data in a symmetrical distribution. This is a common error and may invalidate the results of the experiment.

The **median** (M) is the middle value of a set of data points. There are the same numbers of data points above and below M. For an even number of data points, M is the average of the two middle values. The median is less affected by outliers and by data that are highly skewed. It should be used when dealing with ordinal variables or when the data are highly skewed. There are special statistical tests for dealing with these types of data.

The **mode** is the most common value or the one value with the largest number of data points. It is used for describing nominal and ordinal data and is rarely used in clinical studies.

There are several ways to describe the degree of dispersion of the data. The common ones are the range, percentiles, variance, and standard deviation. The standard error of the mean is a measure that describes the dispersion of a group of samples.

The **range** is simply the highest value to the lowest value. It gives an overview of the data spread around a central value. It should be given whenever there is either a large spread of data values or when the range is asymmetrical about the value of central tendency.

Quartiles divide the data into fourths, and **percentiles** into hundredths. The lowest quarter of values lie below the lower quartile (or 25th percentile), the lower half below the 50th percentile, and the lowest three-quarters below the upper quartile (or 75th percentile). The **interquartile range** is the difference between the 25th and 75th percentile values.

The **variance** (σ^2 or s^2) is a statistical measure of variation. It is the average of the squares (more or less) of the differences between each value and the mean. This is the sum of the squares of the differences between each value and the mean divided by n (the number of data points in the sample). It is often divided by $n - 1$, and either method is correct. This assumes a normal distribution of the variables (see below). Mathematically, $s^2 = (\Sigma(x_i - \mu)^2)/(n - 1)$. The **standard deviation** (SD, s, or σ) is simply the square root of the variance.

The **standard error of the mean** (SEM) is the standard deviation of the means of multiple samples that are all drawn from the same population. If the population size is greater than 30 and the distribution is normal, the SEM is estimated by the equation $\mathbf{SEM} = \mathbf{SD}/\sqrt{n}$ (where n is sample size).

Populations and samples

A **population** is the set of all possible members of the group being studied. The members of the population have various attributes in common. The more things they have in common, the more homogeneous and therefore restrictive the population. An example would be all white males between 40 and 65 years of age. **Generalizability** of the population is often a problem. The less they have in

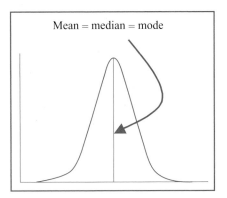

Fig. 9.11 Symmetrical curve. Mean, median and mode are the same.

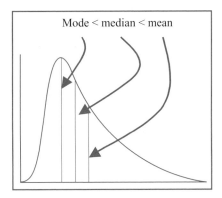

Fig. 9.12 Skewed curve (to the right). Mode < median < mean.

common, the more generalizable the results of data gathered for that population. For example, a population that included all males is more generalizable than one that only includes men under age 25. The population size is symbolized by capital **N**.

A **sample** is a subset of the population chosen for a specific reason. An example could be all white males available to the researcher on a given day for a study on attitudes about health care. Reasons to use a sample rather than the entire population include **convenience**, **time**, **cost**, and **logistics**. The sample may or may not be representative of the entire population, an issue which has been discussed in the chapter on sources of bias (Chapter 8). The sample size is symbolized by lower-case n.

Histograms or frequency polygons show how many subjects in a sample or population (the y-axis) have a certain characteristic value (the x-axis). When plotted in this manner, we call the graph a distribution of values for the given sample. Distributions can be **symmetrical** or **skewed**. By definition, a symmetrical distribution is one for which the mean, median and mode are identical. Many curves (distributions of variables) are asymmetrical. **Skew** describes the degree to which the curve is asymmetrical. Figs. 9.11 and 9.12 show symmetrical and skewed distributions. They are said to be skewed to the right (positive skew, Figure 9.13) when

Fig. 9.13 Curve with skew to the right (positive skew).

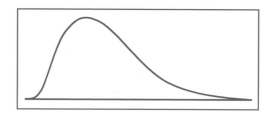

Fig. 9.14 Curve with skew to the left (negative skew).

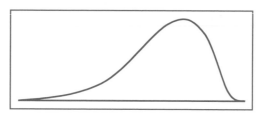

the extreme (or outlier) values are to the right side or positive side of the bulk of the data. Those skewed left (negative skew, Fig. 9.14) have the extreme values to the left of, or negative relative to, the majority of the data points. Skew should be discussed when presenting and evaluating data. The mathematical measures used to describe data are different for skewed distributions than for symmetrical ones.

The normal distribution

The Gaussian or normal distribution (Fig. 9.15) is also called the bell-shaped curve. It is named after Carl Frederick Gauss, a German mathematician. However, he did not discover the bell-shaped curve. Abraham de Moivre (a French mathematician) discovered it about 50 years earlier. It is a special case of a symmetrical distribution, and it describes the frequency of occurrence of many naturally occurring phenomena. For the purposes of most statistical tests, we assume normality in the distribution of a variable. It is better defined by giving its properties:

(1) The mean, median and mode are equal (i.e., the curve is **symmetric** around the mean – not skewed or skew = 0)

(2) The tails of the curve get closer and closer to the x-axis as you move away from the mean and they never quite reach it no matter how far you go (i.e., they approach the x-axis asymptotically)

There are specific numerical equivalents to various standard deviations of the normal distribution, as shown in Table 9.1. For all practical purposes **68%** of the population are within one standard deviation of the mean (± 1 SD), **95%** are within two standard deviations of the mean (± 2 SD), and **99%** are within three standard deviations of the mean (± 3 SD). The 95% interval (± 2 SD) is a range commonly referred to as the normal range or the Gaussian definition of the normal range.

Table 9.1. Properties of the normal distribution

(1) One standard deviation (± 1 SD) on either side of the mean encompasses 68.2% of the population
(2) Two standard deviations (± 2 SD) is an additional 27.2% (95.4% of total)
(3) Three (± 3 SD) is an additional 4.4% (99.8% of total)
(4) Four (± 4 SD) is an additional 0.2% (99.99% of total)
(5) Five (± 5 SD) includes (essentially) everyone (99.9999% of total)

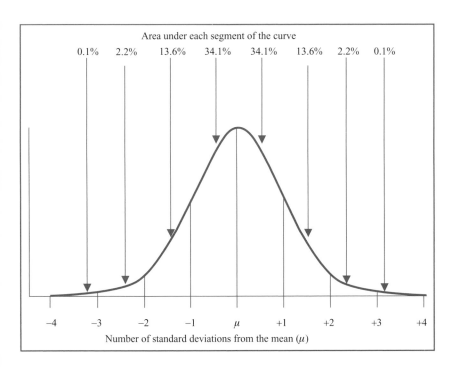

Fig. 9.15 The normal distribution.

The normal distribution is the basis of most statistical tests and concepts we will use in critical evaluation of the medical literature.

Percentages

Percentages are commonly used in reporting results in the medical literature. Percentage improvement or percentage of patients who achieve one of two dichotomous end points are the preferred method of reporting the results. These are commonly called **event rates**. A percentage is a ratio or fraction (**numerator** divided by **denominator**) multiplied by 100 to create a whole number. Obviously, inaccuracies in either the numerator or denominator will result in inaccuracy of the percentage. Percentages can be **misleading** in two important ways.

Percent of a percent will usually show a very large result, even when there is only a small absolute change in the variables. Consider two drugs (we'll call them t-PA and SK) which have different mortality rates. In a particular study, the mortality rate for patients given t-PA was 7% (experimental event rate, EER) while that for SK was 8% (control event rate, CER). The absolute difference (absolute risk reduction, ARR = |EER − CER|) is 1%, a small number, but the relative improvement in mortality (relative risk reduction, RRR = |EER − CER|/CER) is ($1/8 \times 100\% = 12.5\%$, a much larger (and more impressive) number. Using the latter without prominently acknowledging the former is misleading. It is a commonly used technique in pharmaceutical advertisements.

Percentages of small numbers can be misleading in a more subtle way. In this case, the percentage is likely simply to be inaccurate. Twenty percent of ten subjects seems like a large number, yet represents only two subjects. The fact that these two had (for example) an adverse reaction to a drug could have occurred simply by chance and the percentage could be much lower ($< 1\%$) or higher ($> 50\%$) when the same intervention is studied in a larger population sample. When there are only a small number of subjects or results in a study, the percentage may be given as long as the overall numbers are also given with equal prominence. The best way to deal with this is through the use of confidence intervals (which will be discussed in the next chapter).

Probability

Probability tells you the **likelihood** that a certain event will or will not occur relative to all possible related events or series of events of interest. Mathematically it is expressed as the number of times the event of interest occurs divided by the number of times all possible related events occur. This can be written as $P(x) = n_x/N$ where $P(x)$ is the probability of an event x occurring in a total of N possible outcome events. In this equation, n_x is the number of times x occurs. The letter P (or p) symbolizes probability. For flipping a coin once, the probability of a head is $P(\textbf{head})$. This is calculated as $P(\textbf{head}) = 1(\textbf{head})/2(\textbf{head or tail})$. The outcome of interest (one head) is divided by the total number of possible outcomes of the coin toss (one head plus one tail).

Two events are said to be **independent** (not to be confused with the independent variable) when the occurrence of one of the events does not depend on the occurrence the other event. The two events occur by independent mechanisms. The toss of a coin is a perfect example. Each toss is an independent event. The previous toss has no influence on the next one. Since the probability of a head on one toss is 1/2, if the same coin is tossed again, the probability of flipping a head does not change. It is still 1/2, and will continue to be 1/2 no matter how many heads or tails are thrown (unless of course, the coin is rigged).

Similarly, events are said to be **dependent** (not to be confused with the dependent variable) if the probability of one event affects the outcome of the other. An example would be the probability of first drawing a red ball and then a yellow ball from a jar of colored balls, without replacing the one you drew out first.

Events are said to be **mutually exclusive** if the occurrence of one absolutely precludes the occurrence of the other. Gender in humans is a mutually exclusive property. Usually! If someone is a biological male they cannot also be a biological female. Rarely they may be a hermaphrodite (having characteristics of each gender), a biological state equivalent to a flipped coin landing on its edge.

Conditional probability allows us to calculate complex probabilities, such as the probability that one event occurs given that another event has occurred. If the two events are a and b, the notation for this is $P(a \mid b)$. This is read as "the probability of event a if event b occurs." The vertical line means "**conditional upon**." This construct can be used to calculate otherwise complex probabilities in a very simple manner.

If two events are mutually exclusive (independent) the probability that either event occurs can be easily calculated. The probability that **event a or event b** occurs is simply the sum of the two probabilities. $P(a \text{ or } b) = P(a) + P(b)$. The probability of a head or a tail occurring when a coin is flipped is $P(\text{head}) + P(\text{tail})$, which is $1/2 + 1/2 = 1$, or a certain event. Similarly, the probability that **event a and event b** occurs is the product (multiply) of the two probabilities. $P(a \text{ and } b) = P(a) \times P(b)$. The probability of getting two heads on two flips of a coin is $P(\text{head on 1st flip}) \times P(\text{head on 2nd flip})$ which is $1/2 \times 1/2 = 1/4$.

Determining the probability that at least one of several mutually exclusive events will occur is a bit more complex, but the above rules allow us to make this a simple calculation. $P(\text{at least one event will occur}) = 1 - P(\text{none of the events will occur})$. We can calculate $P(\text{none of the events occurring}) = P(\text{not } a) \times P(\text{not } b) \times P(\text{not } c) \times \cdots$ For example, if we want to know the probability of getting at least one head in three flips of a coin, we could calculate the probability of getting one head, two heads and three heads and add them up, then subtract the probabilities of events that overlap (getting two heads and one tail can be done three ways with three coins). Using the above rule, the probability of at least one head is $1 - P(\text{no heads})$. The probability of no heads is the probability of three tails $(1/2)^3 = 1/2 \times 1/2 \times 1/2 = 1/8$), thus making the probability of at least one head $1 - 1/8 = 7/8$. This is an important concept in the evaluation of the statistical significance of the results of studies and the interpretation of simple lab tests.

For many lab tests we use the Gaussian distribution to define the normal values. This considers ± 2 SD as the cutoff point for normal vs. abnormal results. This means that 95% of the population will have a normal result and 5% will have an

Table 9.2. Commonly used probabilities in epidemiology

Prevalence	Probability of the presence of disease: number of existing cases of a disease/total population
Incidence	Probability of the occurrence of new disease: number of new cases of a disease/total population
Attack rate	A specialized form of incidence relating to a particular epidemic, expressed as a percentage: the number of new cases of a disease/number of persons exposed in the outbreak under surveillance
Crude mortality rate	Number of deaths for a given time period and place/mid-period population during the same time period and at the same place
Age-specific mortality rate	Number of deaths in a particular age group/total population of the same age group in the same period of time, using the mid-period population
Infant mortality rate	Deaths in infants under 1 year of age/total number of live births
Neonatal mortality rate	Deaths in infants under 28 days of age/total number of live births
Perinatal mortality rate	(Stillbirths + deaths in infants under 7 days of age)/(total number of live births + total number of stillbirths)
Maternal mortality rate	All pregnancy related deaths/total number of live births.

abnormal result. In some cases we routinely do 20 tests at once (Profile II, SMA-C, or SMA-20). What is the significance of one positive (abnormal) result? We want to know the probability that a normal person will have at least one abnormal lab test in a panel of 20 tests by chance alone. The probability that each test will be normal is 95%. Therefore, the probability that **all the tests are normal** is $(0.95)^{20} = 0.36$. Then, the probability that **at least one test is abnormal** becomes $1 - 0.36 = 0.64$. This means that there is a 64% chance that a normal person will have at least one abnormal test result that occurred purely by chance alone, when in reality that person is normal.

Basic epidemiology

Epidemiology is the study of epidemics or of disease in populations. Many of the studies that you will learn how to evaluate are epidemiological studies. On a very simplistic level, epidemiology describes the probability of certain events occurring in a population. These probabilities are described in terms of rates. This could be a rate of exposure to a toxin, disease, disability, death, or any other important outcome. In medicine, rates are usually expressed as number of cases per unit of population. The unit of population most commonly used is 100 000, although other numbers can be used (rates per 100, 1000, etc.). The rates can also be expressed as percentages.

The **prevalence** of disease is the percentage of the population that has existing cases of the disease at a given time. It is the probability that a given person in this population has the disease of interest. It is calculated as the number of cases of a disease divided by the total population at risk for the disease. The number of new cases and the resolution of existing cases affect prevalence. Prevalence increases as the number of new cases (incidence) increases and as the death (mortality) rate or cure rate decreases.

The **incidence** of a disease is the number of new cases of the disease for a given unit of population in a given unit of time. It is the probability of the occurrence of new disease. It is the number of new cases in a given time period divided by the total population. Incidence is only affected by the occurrence of new cases of disease. The occurrence of new cases can be influenced by other factors such as mass exposure to a new toxin or infectious agent, or a change in the diet of the society.

The **mortality rate** is the incidence of death. It is also the probability of death. It is the number of people who die (within a certain time) divided by the entire population (at risk of death).

An excellent resource for learning more statistics is a CD-ROM called *ActivStats*,[2] a review of basic statistics and probability. There is also an electronic textbook called StatSoft,[3] which includes some good summaries of basic statistical information.

[2] P. Velleman. *ActivStats*. Reading, MA: Addison-Wesley, 1999.
[3] StatSoft. www.statsoftinc.com/textbook/stathome.html.

10

Hypothesis testing

Medicine is the science of uncertainty and the art of probability.

Sir William Osler (1849–1919)

Learning objectives

In this chapter you will learn:
- steps in hypothesis testing
- potential errors of hypothesis testing
- how to calculate and describe the usage of control event rates (CER), experimental event rates (EER), relative rate reduction (RRR) and absolute rate reduction (ARR)
- the concepts underlying statistical testing

Interpretation of the results of clinical trials requires an understanding of the statistical processes used to analyze data. The intelligent readers of the medical literature must be able to interpret these results and determine for themselves if they are important enough to use for their patients.

Introduction

Hypothesis testing is the foundation of the scientific method. Roger Bacon suggested the beginnings of this process in the fourteenth century. Sir Francis Bacon further defined it in the seventeenth century, and it was first regularly used in scientific research in the eighteenth and nineteenth centuries. It is a process by which new scientific information is added to previously discovered facts and processes. Previously held beliefs can be tested to determine their validity. Expected outcomes of a proposed new intervention can be tested against a previously used comparison intervention. If the result of the experiment shows that the newly thought-up hypothesis is true, we have gained knowledge and can design a new experiment to further increase our knowledge. If the hypothesis being tested is false, it is "back to the drawing board" to come up with a new hypothesis (Table 10.1).

Table 10.1. Steps in hypothesis testing

(1) Gather background information
(2) State hypothesis
(3) Formulate null hypothesis (H_0)
(4) Design a study
(5) Decide on a significance level (α)
(6) Collect data on a sample
(7) Calculate the sample statistic (P)
(8) Reject or accept the null hypothesis (by comparing P to α)
(9) Begin all over again, step 1

The hypothesis

A **hypothesis** is a statement about how the study will relate the predictors (cause) and outcomes (effect). For example, a study is done to see if taking aspirin reduces the rate of death among patients with heart attacks (myocardial infarction, MI). The hypothesis is that there is a relationship between daily intake of aspirin and a reduction in the risk of death caused by MI. Another way to state this hypothesis is that there is a reduced death rate among MI patients who are taking aspirin. This is a statement of what is called the **alternative hypothesis** (H_a or H_1). The alternative hypothesis states that a difference does exist between two groups or there is an association between the predictor and outcome variables. The alternative hypothesis cannot be tested directly using statistical methods.

The **null hypothesis** (H_0) states that no difference exists between groups or there is no association between predictor and outcome variables. In our example, the null hypothesis states that there is no difference in death rate due to myocardial infarction between MI patients who took aspirin daily and those who did not.

This is the basis for formal testing of statistical significance. By starting with the proposition that there is no association, statistical tests estimate the probability that an observed association occurred due to chance alone. The customary scientific approach is to accept or reject the null hypothesis. Rejecting the null hypothesis is a vote in favor of the alternative hypothesis, which we then accept by default.

All we can know from statistical testing is the probability that the null hypothesis was falsely rejected. Therefore the validity of the alternative hypothesis is accepted by exclusion if the test of statistical significance rejects the null hypothesis. Sorry for the double talk, but this is the way statisticians talk. We want to know the probability that we reject the null hypothesis when in fact it is true (and there truly is no difference between groups). We are happy if this occurs less than 5% of the time ($P < 0.05$). This leads to our usual definition of statistical significance, $P < 0.05$. The letter P stands for the probability of obtaining the observed difference or effect size between groups by chance if in reality the null hypothesis is true and there is no difference between the groups.

Where did this 5% notion come from and what does it mean statistically? Sir Ronald Fisher (a twentieth-century British mathematician and founder of modern statistics) one day said it, and since he was the expert it stuck. He reasoned that "if the probability of such an event (falsely rejecting the null hypothesis) were sufficiently small – say, 1 chance in 20, then one might regard the result as significant." Prior to this, a level of $P = 0.0047$ (or one chance in 212) had been accepted as the level of significance.

His reasoning was pretty sound, as this thought experiment shows. How much would you bet on the toss of a coin? You pay \$1.00 (it was £1.00 in Sir Ronnie's experiment, in those days almost \$3.00) if tails come up and you get paid the same amount if it's heads. How many tails in a row would you tolerate before beginning to suspect that the coin is rigged? Sir Fisher reasoned that in most cases the answer would be about four or five tosses.

The probability of four tails in a row is $(1/2)^4$ or 1 in 16, and for five tails in a row $(1/2)^5$ or 1 in 32. One in 20 (5%) is about halfway between.[1] Is it coincidental that 95% of the population corresponds (almost exactly) to ± 2 SD of the normal distribution (actually ± 1.96 SD to be exact)? It is sobering to realize that in experimental physics, the usual P value is 0.0001 (or some such small number). They want to be really sure where a particular subatomic particle is or what it's mass or momentum are before telling the press. There is always talk (usually by pharmaceutical or biotech companies) that the level of significance of 0.05 is too low and should be increased to 0.1. This means that we will accept one chance in ten that the difference found was not true and only occurred by chance! I think this would be a poor decision, and hope that you will agree with me by the time you have finished this book.

Errors in hypothesis testing

The results of a clinical study are tested by application of a statistical test to the experimental results. The researcher asks the question "what is the probability (likelihood) that the difference between groups that I found was obtained purely by chance, and that the two groups (i.e., the results) are really the same?" Statistical tests are able to calculate this probability.

In general there are four possible outcomes of a study. These are shown in Fig. 10.1. They compare the result found in the study with the "truth in the

[1] From G. Norman & D. Streiner. *Biostatistics: the Bare Essentials*. St Louis: Mosby, 1994.

	Is the study actually valid?	
	Actually is a positive result (absolute truth)– H_0 actually false	Actually is a negative result (absolute truth)– H_0 actually true
Experiment found positive results – H_0 found to be false	Correct conclusion (Power = $1 - \beta$)	Type I error α
Experiment found negative results – H_0 found to be true	Type II error β	Correct conclusion

Fig. 10.1 Possible outcomes of a study.

universe" or the actual state of things. We cannot always determine what this is. This is called **clinical uncertainty**. We can only determine how closely we are approaching this universal truth by using statistical tests.

A **Type I error** occurs when the null hypothesis is rejected even though it is really true. In other words, concluding that there is a difference when there isn't. This is also called a **false positive** study result. There are many ways in which a Type I error can occur in a study. The reader must be wary since the writer will rarely point these out. Often they will "spin" the results. Manipulation of variables using techniques such as data dredging (or snooping or mining), one-tailed testing, subgroup analysis (especially *post hoc*), and composite-outcome endpoints may result in the occurrence of this type of error.

A **Type II error** occurs when the null hypothesis is not rejected even though it is really false. In other words, concluding there isn't a difference when in reality there is. This is also called a **false negative** study result. An example would be concluding there is no relationship between hyperlipidemia and coronary artery disease when there truly is a relationship. **Power** represents the ability of the study to detect a difference when it exists. By convention the power of a study should be greater than 80% to be considered adequate. Think of an analogy to the microscope. As the power of the microscope increases, the difference between cells that can be detected becomes smaller.

A Type II error can only be made in negative clinical trials, that is, trials reporting no statistically significant difference between groups. Therefore, when reading negative clinical trials, one needs to assess the chance that a Type II error occurred. This is important because a negative result may not be due to the lack of an effect but simply because of low power or the inability to detect the effect. From an interpretation perspective, the question one asks is "for a given β level and an effect difference that I consider clinically important, did the researcher use a large enough sample size"? Both of these concepts will be discussed in more detail in the next two chapters.

Type III and IV errors are not usually found in biostatistical or epidemiological textbooks and yet are extremely common. **Type III** errors are those that compare the intervention to the wrong drug or incorrect dose of a drug. This is fairly common in the literature and includes studies of new drugs against placebo instead of older drugs. Studies of drugs for acute treatment of migraine headaches may be done against drugs that are useful for that indication, but in doses that are inadequate for the management of the pain. The reader must have a working knowledge of the standard therapy and determine if the new intervention is being tried against the best current therapy. Studies of new antibiotics are often done against an older antibiotic that is no longer used as standard therapy.

Type IV errors are those in which the wrong study was done. For example, a new antiviral drug for influenza is tested against placebo. The drug should at least have been tested against an old antiviral drug previously shown to be effective, and not against placebo, a Type III error. But, since the current standard is prevention in the form of influenza vaccine, the correct study should in fact have been comparing the new drug against the strategy of prevention with vaccine. This is a much more complex study, but would really answer the question we have about the drugs. Any study of a new treatment should be compared to the effect of both currently available standard therapies and prevention programs.

Effect size

The actual results of the measurements showing a difference between groups are given in the results section of a scientific paper. There are many different ways to express the results of a study. The effect size is the magnitude of the outcome or association (difference between groups) that one observes. This result (δ or **effect size**) can be given either as an absolute or as a relative number (percentage or **event rate**).

The expression of the results will be different for different types of data. The effect size for outcomes that are dichotomous can be expressed as percentages. When continuous outcomes are evaluated, the mean of two (or more) groups can be compared. The standard deviations and/or range should be given with the mean. A statistical test will then calculate the P value for the difference between the two mean values. This is the probability that this difference occurred by chance alone. If the measure is an ordinal number the median is the measure that is compared. In that case, special statistical methods should be used.

The **clinically significant** effect size is the difference that is estimated to be clinically important. Since it is easier to detect a large effect (i.e., representing a 90% change) than a small one (i.e., representing a 2% change), it should be easier to detect a difference which is likely to be clinically important. However, if the sample size is large enough even a small effect size may be statistically detected. This effect size may not be clinically important even though it is **statistically significant**. We will return to this in more detail later.

Fig. 10.2 Event rates.

	Events of interest	Other events	Totals
Control or placebo group	A	B	CE = Control group events
Experimental group	C	D	EE = Experimental group events

Formulas

CER = control patients with outcome of interest / total control patients = A/CE

EER = experimental patients with outcome of interest / total experimental patients = C/EE

ARR = |CER − EER| RRR = |CER − EER|/CER

Event rate

An event is an outcome. In any study we are interested in how many events of interest happen within each of two treatment or risk groups. The outcome of interest must be a dichotomous variable for this set of calculations. The most common ones are survival, admission to the hospital, patients who had relief of pain, patients who were cured of infection, etc. Usually a positive outcome (such as survival or cure) is used. However, a negative outcome (such as death) can also be used. These are expressed as percentages. The **control group** consists of those subjects treated with placebo, comparison, or the current standard therapy. The **experimental group** consists of those subjects treated with the experimental therapy. For studies of risk, the control group is those not exposed to the risk factor, while the experimental group is those exposed to the risk factor being studied.

The rate of success (or failure) can be calculated for each group. The **control event rate** (**CER**) is the percentage of control patients who have the outcome of interest. Similarly, the **experimental event rate** (**EER**) is the percentage of experimental patients who have the outcome of interest. The (absolute) difference between the two is the **absolute rate reduction** (**ARR**). Similarly, the **relative rate reduction** (**RRR**) is the percentage of the difference between the groups. This is the difference between the two outcome rates as a percentage of the CER. Yes, this is a percentage of a percentage and you must be careful when interpreting this result. The RRR always overestimates the effect of therapy when compared with the ARR (Fig. 10.2).

Signal-to-noise ratio

Nearly all commonly used statistical tests are based on the concept of the signal-to-noise ratio. The **signal** is the relationship you are interested in and the **noise**

Fig. 10.3 Confidence and
standard error of the mean
(SEM).

Confidence = $\sqrt{n} \times$ (signal / noise)

Where the signal is the event rate, the noise is the standard deviation, and n is the sample size

SEM = $\sigma/\sqrt{n}$

where n is the sample size and σ is the standard deviation

represents random error (or variation). Statistical tests determine how much of the difference between two groups is due to random noise and how much is due to systematic or real differences in the results of interest. The statistical measure of noise is the standard deviation or standard error of the mean (Fig. 10.3).

The confidence of a statistic (result of a study) can be expressed as equal to the signal times the square root of the sample size (n) divided by the noise. Confidence is analogous to the power of a study. The signal is the effect size and the noise is the standard deviation of the effect size. Confidence in a particular result increases when the strength of the signal (effect size) increases. It also increases as the noise level (standard deviation) decreases. Finally, it increases as the sample size increases, but only in proportion to the square root of the sample size. To double the confidence, you must quadruple the sample size. Remember this relationship when evaluating study results.

Standard deviation tells you how close individual scores cluster around their mean value. A related number, the standard error of the mean (SEM) tells you how close the mean scores from repeated samples will be to the true (or expected) population mean. This is the basis for many statistical tests.

There are some limitations on the use of SEM. It should not be used to describe the dispersion of data in a sample. The standard deviation does this and using SEM is dishonest since it under-represents differences between groups. The SEM is a measure of the variability of the sample means if the study were repeated. For all practical purposes, the SEM is the standard deviation of the means of all the possible samples taken from the population. Showing one SEM with the data allows the reader to figure out the standard deviation. However, the unwary reader may not do this. A more detailed explanation of standard deviation and SEM can be found in an excellent article by David Streiner.[2] The Confidence Interval (95%) may be calculated from the SEM and the clearest way to report variation (noise) in a study would be simply to show the confidence intervals.

---

[2] D. L. Streiner. Maintaining standards: differences between the standard deviation and standard error, and when to use each. *Can. J. Psychiatry* 1996; 41: 498–502.

$$95\% \text{ CI} = \mu \pm Z_{95\%} (\sigma/\sqrt{n})$$

Where $Z_{95\%} = 1.96$ (the number of standard deviations which defines 95% of the data), $\sigma/\sqrt{n} = \text{SEM}$, and $\mu = \text{mean}$

Therefore, $95\% \text{ CI} = \mu \pm 1.96(\text{SEM})$

Fig. 10.4 95% confidence intervals (95% CI).

Confidence intervals

Confidence intervals (CI) are another way to represent the level of significance. The actual definition is that 95% of such intervals (calculated from the same experiment repeated multiple times) contain the true value of the variable for that population. For all practical purposes, the 95% CI means (in plain English) that 95% of the time we expect the true mean to be between the upper and lower limits of the confidence interval. This means that if we were to repeat the experiment 20 times, in 19 of those repeated experiments the value of the effect size would lie within the stated CI range. This gives more information than a simple P value, since one can see a range of potentially likely values. If the data assume a normal distribution and we are measuring independent events, the SEM can be used to calculate 95% confidence intervals (Fig. 10.4).

Statistical tests

The **central limit theorem** is the theoretical basis for most statistical tests. It states that if we select equally sized samples of a variable from a population with a non-normal distribution the distribution of the means of these samples will be a normal distribution. This is true as long as the samples are large enough. For most statistical tests, the sample size considered "large enough" is 30. For smaller sample sizes, other (and more complex) statistical approximations can be used.

Statistical tests calculate the probability that a difference between two groups obtained in a study occurred by chance. It is easier to visualize how statistical tests work if we assume that the distribution of each of two sample variables is two normal distributions graphed on the same axis. Very simplistically and for visual effectiveness, we can represent two sample means with their 95% confidence intervals as bell-shaped curves. There are two "tails" at the ends of the curves, each representing half of the remaining 5% of the confidence interval. If there is only some overlap of the areas on the "tails" or if the two curves are totally separate (no overlapping), the results are statistically significant. If there is more overlap

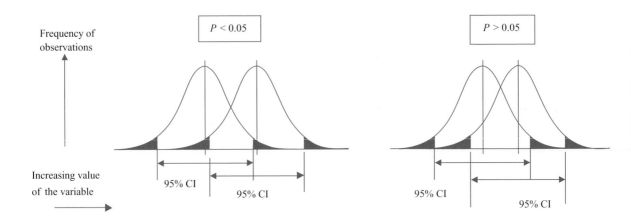

Fig. 10.5 The relationship between the overlap of 95% of possible variable values and the level of statistical significance.

such that the middle value of one distribution is inside the 95% confidence interval of the other, the results are not statistically significant (Fig. 10.5). This cannot be translated into simple overlap of the two 95% confidence intervals as statistical significance depends on multiple other factors.

Statistical tests are based upon the principle that there is an expected outcome (E) that can be compared to the actual (or observed) outcome (O). Determining the value of E is problematic since we don't actually know what value to expect in most cases. One estimate of the expected value is that found in the control group. Actually, there are complex calculations for determining the expected value that are part of the statistical test. Statistical tests calculate the probability that O is different from E – or that the (absolute) difference between O and E is greater than zero – by chance. This is done using a variety of formulas, is the meat of statistics, and is what statisticians get paid for. Actually they also get paid to help researchers decide what to measure and how to assure that the measure of interest is what is actually being measured. To quote Sir Ronnie (Fisher) again: "To call in the statistician after the experiment is done may be no more than asking him to perform a postmortem examination: he may be able to say what the experiment died of."[3]

One does not need to be a trained statistician to know which statistical test to use, but it helps. What is the average physician to do? The list in Appendix 4 is one place to start. It is an abbreviated list of the specific statistical tests that you should look for in evaluating the statistics of a study. As you become more familiar with the literature you will be able to identify the correct statistical tests more often. If the test your article uses is not on this list, you ought to be a bit suspicious. Maybe the authors found a statistician who could save the study and generate statistically significant results, but only by using an obscure test.

[3] Indian Statistical Congress, Sankhya, 1938. Sir Ronald Fisher, 1890–1962.

The placebo effect

There is an "urban myth" that the placebo effect occurs at an average rate of 35% in any study. The apparent placebo effect is more complex and made up of several other effects. Other effects, which can be confused with the true placebo effect, are the **natural course** of the illness, **regression to the mean**, other timed effects and unidentified parallel interventions. The true placebo effect is the total perceived placebo effect minus these other effects.

The natural course of the disease may result in some patients getting better regardless of the treatment given while others get worse. It will appear that they got better because of the treatment. This is true with almost all illnesses including serious infections and advanced cancers.

Regression to the mean is a natural tendency for a variable to change with time and return towards the population mean. If endpoints are re-measured they are likely to be closer to the mean than an initial extreme value. This is a commonly seen phenomenon with blood pressure values. Many people initially found to have an elevated blood pressure will have a reduction in their blood pressure over time. This is partly due to their relaxing after the initial pressure reading and partly to regression to the mean.

Other time effects that may affect the outcome measurements include the learning curve. A person gets better at a task each time it is performed. Similarly, a patient becomes more relaxed as the clinical encounter progresses. This explains the effect known as "white coat hypertension," the phenomenon by which a person's blood pressure will be higher when the doctor takes it and lower when taken later by a machine, a non-physician, or repeatedly by their own physician. Some of this effect is due to the stress engendered by the presence of the doctor; as a patient becomes more used to having the doctor take their blood pressure, the pressure decreases.

Unidentified parallel interventions may occur on the part of the physician or health-care giver (investigator) or the patient (subject), such as unconscious or conscious changes in lifestyle instituted as a result of the patient's medical problem. For example, patients who are diagnosed with elevated cholesterol may increase their exercise while they also began taking a new drug to help lower their cholesterol. This can result in a greater-than-expected rate of improvement in outcomes both in those assigned to the drug and in the controls (the placebo group).

The converse is to differentiate the true treatment effect from the perceived treatment effect. The true treatment effect is the difference between the perceived treatment effect and the various types of "placebo effect" as described above. Studies should be able to differentiate the true treatment effect from the perceived effect by the appropriate use of a control group. The control group is essentially given the placebo or standard therapy, which is equivalent to the placebo since it is the therapy that would have been given regardless of the patients' participation in the study.

A recent meta-analysis combined the results of multiple studies that had placebo and no-treatment arms and compared the results obtained by all the patients in these groups. They found that the overall effect size for the two groups was the same. The only exception was in studies for pain. In those studies, there was an overall positive effect favoring the placebo in the amount of 6.5 mm on a 100-mm scale.[4] As demonstrated by previous pain studies, this difference is not clinically significant.

[4] A. Hrobjartsson & P. C. Gotzsche. Is the placebo powerless? An analysis of clinical trials comparing placebo with no treatment *N. Engl. J. Med.* 2001; 344: 1594–1602.

11

Type I errors and number needed to treat

If this be error, and upon me prov'd,
I never writ, nor no man ever lov'd.

William Shakespeare (1564–1616): Sonnet 116.

Learning objectives

In this chapter you will learn:
- how to recognize Type I errors in a study
- the concept of data dredging or data snooping
- the meaning of number needed to treat (NNT) and number needed to harm (NNH)
- how to differentiate statistical from clinical significance
- other sources of Type I errors (subgroup analysis and composite endpoints)

Interpreting the results of a clinical trial requires an understanding of the statistical processes that are used to analyze these results. Studies that suffer from a Type I error may show apparently statistical significance when the groups are not actually different. The intelligent readers of the medical literature must be able to interpret these results and determine for themselves if these results are important enough to use for their patients.

Type I error

This occurs when the null hypothesis is rejected even though it is really true. In other words, studies that have a Type I error conclude that there is a positive effect size or difference between groups when in reality there isn't. This is a **false positive** study result. Alpha (α), known as the level of significance, is defined as the maximum probability of making a Type I error that we are willing to accept. This is the probability of rejecting the null hypothesis when it is really true and is predetermined before conducting a statistical test. The probability of obtaining the observed result, difference, or effect size by chance if the null

Fig. 11.1 One- and two-tailed
tests for the same effect size δ.

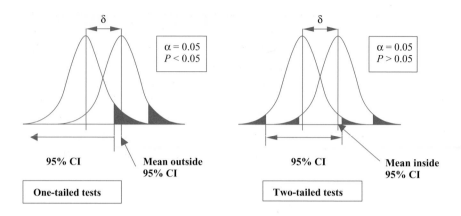

Fig. 11.1 One- and two-tailed tests for the same effect size δ.

hypothesis is true is P. This is calculated as the result of performing a statistical test.

The researcher minimizes the risk of a Type I error by setting the level of significance (α) very low. By convention, the alpha level is usually set at 0.05 or 0.01. In other words, with $\alpha = 0.05$ the researcher expects to make a Type I error in one of twenty trials. The researcher then calculates P using a statistical test. He or she compares P to α. If $\alpha = 0.05$, P must be less than 0.05 ($P < 0.05$) to show statistical significance. There are two situations for which this must be modified: two-tailed testing and multiple variables.

One-tailed vs. two-tailed tests

If we have an a-priori reason to believe that one group is clearly going to be different from the other and we know the direction of that difference, we can use a one-tailed test. The researcher must hypothesize either an increase or a decrease in the effect, not just a difference. This means that the normal distribution of one result is only likely to overlap the normal distribution of the other result on one side or in one direction. This is demonstrated in Fig. 11.1.

One-tailed tests specify the direction that you think the result will be. When asking the question "is drug A better than drug B?" the alternative hypothesis H_a is that drug A is better than drug B. The null hypothesis H_0 is that either there is no difference or drug A is worse than drug B. This automatically removes from scrutiny the possibility that drug A may actually be worse that drug B. It states that we are only interested in drug A if it is better and we have good a-priori reason to think that it really is better.

We recommend doing a two-tailed test in most circumstances. The use of a one-tailed test can only be justified if previous research demonstrated that drug A actually appears to be better and certainly is no worse than drug B. When doing a two-tailed test, we don't make any a-priori assumption about the direction of the result. A **two-tailed test** asks the question "is there any difference between groups?" In this case, the alternative hypothesis H_a is that drug A is different from drug B. This can mean that it is either better or worse, but not equivalent. The null hypothesis H_O states that there is no difference between the two drugs.

For $\alpha = 0.05$, P must be < 0.05 for statistical significance with the one-tailed test. It must be < 0.025 for the two-tailed test. Conceptually this means that the total probability of a chance (randomly occurring) error is 0.05 and that each "tail" contributes 0.025 of alpha. The requirement for $\alpha = 0.05$ is less stringent if a one-tailed test is used. In this situation, P must only be less than 0.05 rather than less than 0.025.

Multiple outcomes

The probability of making a Type I error is α for each outcome being measured. If two variables are measured, the probability of a Type I error (false positive result) is α for each variable. The probability that at least one of these two variables is a false positive is one minus the probability that neither of them is a false positive. The probability that neither is a false positive is the probability that the first variable is not a false positive $(1 - \alpha)$ and that the second variable is not a false positive $(1 - \alpha)$. The probability that neither variable is a false positive is therefore $(1 - \alpha) \times (1 - \alpha)$, or $(1 - \alpha)^2$. The probability that at least one of the two is (falsely) positive by chance then becomes $1 - (1 - \alpha)^2$. Therefore, the probability that one positive and incorrect outcome will occur only by chance if n variables are tested is $1 - (1 - \alpha)^n$.

This becomes sizable as n gets very large. **Data dredging** (or **mining** or **snooping**) is a technique by which the researcher looks at multiple variables in the hope that some or at least one will show statistical significance. This result is then reported or emphasized as the most important positive result in the study. This does a disservice as it is an example of a **Type I error**. Suspect this when there are many variables being tested, but only a few of them show statistical significance.

For example, if a researcher does a study that looks at 20 clinical signs of a given disease, it is possible that any one of them will be statistically significantly associated with the disease. For one variable, the probability that this association occurred by chance only is 0.05. Therefore the probability that no association occurred by chance is $1 - 0.05$ or 0.95. The probability that at least one of the 20 variables tested will be positively associated with the disease by chance alone is 1 minus the probability of no association. Since this is 0.95 for each variable, the probability that at least one occurred by chance becomes $1 - 0.95^{20}$ or $1 - 0.36$ or 0.64. Therefore, there is a 64% likelihood of coming up with one association that is falsely positive and occurred only by chance. If there are two abnormal values, you cannot know if both are false (occurred by chance alone) or if one is correct and which one is the correct value.

One way to get around this is by applying the **Bonferroni correction**. First we must create a new level of α, which we will call α'. The new α' will be α/n: the previous α is divided by n, the number of variables not the sample size. Therefore, P must be $< \alpha/n$ (or $\alpha/2n$ if using a two-tailed test) for the result to be statistically significant. The Bonferroni correction is used when the variables being tested are independent of each other and there are only a few (< 10) variables. This is not a true assumption in most cases and other means of estimating α' must be used.

Data dredging is a "legal" device if the study is a **derivation set**. The variables that came up positive (statistically significant) will be measured in another study using only those variables and a new sample (the **validation set**) to see if this relationship still holds. One clue to data dredging is the absence of an explicit hypothesis. This allows the researcher to find a statistically significant relationship that exists only by chance and claim it as the reason for the study. This is only legitimate if the variable that comes up positive and statistically significant in the derivation set can then become the explicit hypothesis of a validation set.

Confidence intervals (CI)

These are used more frequently now to represent the level of significance. As mentioned earlier, the true definition of the 95% CI is that 95% of such intervals (calculated by repeating the same experiment) contain the true value of the variable for that population. For all practical purposes the 95% CI is a range of values within which we would expect the true value to lie 95% of the time, or with 95% certainty. If you repeat the experiment 20 times, 19 of those times the true value will be within the stated CI range. This gives more information than a simple $p < 0.05$ value since one can see a statistically plausible range of values.

The limits of the 95% CI show how **precise** the results are. If the CI is very wide, the results are not very precise. This means that there is a great deal of random variation in the result and a very large or small value could be the true effect size. Similarly if the CI is very narrow, the results are very precise and we are more certain of the true result.

If the 95% confidence interval around the difference between two groups in studies of the effect of therapy includes the zero point, $P > 0.05$. The zero point is the point at which there is no difference between the two groups or the null hypothesis is true. If one limit of the CI is just near, and the interval does not cross the zero point, the result may only be slightly statistically significant. The addition of a few more subjects could make the result more statistically significant. However, the true effect may be very small and not clinically important.

Table 11.1. Rules of thumb for 95% confidence intervals

(1) If the point value for one (experimental) group is within the 95% CI for the other (control) group, there is likely to be no statistical significance for the difference between values
(2) If the point value for one (experimental) group is outside the 95% CI for the other (control) group, there is likely to be statistical significance for the difference between values
(3) If the 95% CI for a difference includes 0, the difference found is not statistically significant
(4) If the 95% CI for a ratio includes 1, the ratio is not statistically significant

Statistical significance vs. clinical significance

A study of a population with a very large sample size can show **statistical significance** (at the $\alpha = 0.05$ level) when the actual clinical difference between the two groups is very small. For example, if a study measuring the level of pain perception using a visual analog scale showed a statistically significant difference in pain scores of 6.5 points (on a scale 0–100) one might think this was important. Another study found that patients could not actually discriminate a difference on this scale of less than 13 points. Therefore, although statistically significant, a difference of 6.5 points would not be clinically important.

Clinicians must decide for themselves whether a result has reasonable **clinical significance**. They must then help their patients decide how much benefit will accrue from the therapy and how much risk they are willing to accept as a result of potential side effects or failure of the treatment. If a difference in effect size of the magnitude found in the study will not change the clinical situation of a given patient, that is not an important result. You must look at the overall impact of this small an effect size on patient care. This may include issues of ultimate survival, potential side effects and toxicities, quality of life, adverse outcomes and costs to the patient and society. We will cover formal cost-effectiveness analysis in Chapter 29.

Number needed to treat

A useful numerical measure of clinical significance is the **number needed to treat** (**NNT**). The NNT is the number of patients that must be treated with the proposed therapy in order to have one additional successful result. To calculate NNT you must first calculate the absolute risk reduction (ARR). This requires that the study

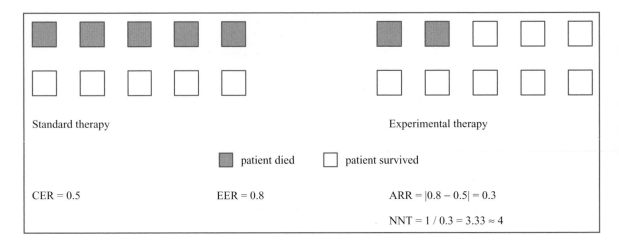

Fig. 11.2 Number needed to treat. For every 10 patients treated with the experimental treatment, there are three additional survivors. The number needed to treat is $10/3 = 3.33 \approx$ (rounded up to) 4. Therefore we must treat four patients to get one additional survivor.

outcomes are dichotomous and you can calculate the experimental (EER) and control (CER) event rates. The ARR is the absolute difference of the event rates of the two groups being compared (|EER – CER|). The NNT is one divided by the ARR (**NNT = 1/ARR**). By convention, NNT is given as 1/ARR rounded up to the nearest integer. Fig. 11.2 is a description of NNT.

We would like to see small NNTs in studies of treatment as this means that the new (experimental) treatment is a lot better than the old (standard, control, or placebo) treatment. You can compare the NNT to the risk of untreated disease and the risks of side effects of treatment. The related concept, the number needed to harm (NNH), is the number of patients that you would need to treat before an additional one is harmed (by side effects of the treatment). These two concepts (NNT and NNH) help you balance the benefit and risk of therapy. The NNH is usually calculated from studies of etiology or risk, and will be discussed in the chapter on risk assessment (Chapter 13).

For studies of prevention, NNT tends to be larger. This is fine if the intervention is relatively cheap. For example, one aspirin taken daily can prevent death after a heart attack. The NNT to prevent one death in the first five weeks after a heart attack is 40. Since aspirin is very cheap and has relatively few side effects, this is a reasonable number. The following two examples will demonstrate the use of NNT.

(1) A study of treatment for migraine headache tested a new drug sumatriptan against placebo. In the sumatriptan group, 1067 out of 1854 patients had mild or no pain at two hours. In the placebo group, 256 out of 1036 patients had mild or no pain at two hours. First the event rates are calculated, then the ARR and RRR, and finally the NNT:

EER $= 1067/1854 = 58\% = 0.58$ and CER$= 256/1036 = 25\% = 0.25$.

ARR $= 0.58 - 0.25 = 0.33$. In this case we ought to say ARI or absolute rate increase since this is the absolute increase in well-being due to the drug.

This means that 33% more patients taking sumatriptan for headache will have clinical improvement compared to patients taking placebo.

RRR = 0.33/0.25 = 1.33. This is the relative risk reduction (or in this case RRI or relative rate increase) and means that patients treated with sumatriptan are one-and-a-third times more likely to show improvement in their headache compared with patients treated with placebo therapy. The RRR (or RRI) always makes the improvement look better than the ARR (or ARI).

NNT = 1/0.33 = 3. You must treat three patients with sumatriptan to reduce pain of migraine headaches in one additional patient. This looks like a very reasonable number for NNT. However, we would never recommend placebo, and it is likely that the NNT would not be nearly this low if sumatriptan were compared against other migraine medications.

(2) Streptokinase (SK) and tissue plasminogen activator (t-PA) are two drugs that can dissolve blood clots in the arteries leading to the heart muscle and can treat a heart attack (myocardial infarction, MI). A recent study called GUSTO compared them to each other in the treatment of this disorder. In the most positive study comparing the use of these in treating MI, the SK group had a mortality of 7% (CER) and the t-PA group had a mortality of 6% (EER). This difference was statistically significant ($P < 0.05$).

ARR = |6% − 7%| or 1%. This means that there is a 1% absolute improvement in survival when t-PA is used rather than STK.

RRR = (|6 − 7|)/6 or 16%. This means that there is a relative increase in survival of 16% when t-PA is used rather than SK. This is the figure that was used in advertisements for the drug that were sent out to physicians (cardiologists, family-medicine, emergency-medicine and critical-care physicians).

NNT= 1/1% = 1/0.01 = 100. This means that you must treat 100 patients with the experimental therapy to save one additional life. This may not be reasonable especially if there is a large cost difference or significantly more side effects. In this case, STK costs $200 per dose while t-PA costs $2000 per dose. There was also an increase in the number of symptomatic intracranial bleeds with t-PA. The ARR was about 0.3%, giving an NNH of about 300. That means for every 300 patients who get t-PA, one additional patient will have a symptomatic intracranial bleed.

The number needed to screen (NNS) is a related concept that looks at how many people need to be screened for a disease in order to prevent one additional death (or other bad outcome). For example, to prevent one additional death from breast cancer you must screen 1200 women beginning at age 50. Since the potential outcome is very bad and the screening test is not invasive or intrusive (except that it is uncomfortable and may cause a very tiny number of cancers due to radiation exposure), it is a reasonable screening test. We will discuss screening tests in Chapter 26.

The NNT with surgery for clogged carotid arteries when there is 70–99% blockage to prevent one additional stroke or death at two years is 6. This is an expensive surgical intervention but with a low NNT. Therefore, assuming no or very little harm from the surgery, it would be useful to recommend it to our patients with this degree of blockage.

The NNE (number needed to expose) to secondhand smoke from a spouse to cause one additional case of lung cancer in a non-smoking spouse after 14 years of exposure is 1300. The NNE is very high, meaning that few of the people who are at risk will develop the outcome, but the baseline exposure rate is high (25% of people smoke, exposing their relatives to secondhand smoke) and the cost of intervention is very low (in dollars), making reduction of secondhand smoke very desirable.

For all values of NNT (and other similar numbers needed), confidence intervals should be given in studies that calculate these statistics. The formulas for these are very complex and are given in Appendix 3. There are several convenient NNT calculators on the web. Two sites which I recommend are those of the University of British Columbia[1] and the Centre for Evidence-Based Medicine at Oxford University.[2] In addition to the CER and EER for the groups, you also need the group size to get these confidence intervals.

Other sources of Type I error

There are two other common sources of Type I error that are seen in research studies and may be difficult to spot. Authors with a particular bias will do many things to make their preferred treatment seem better than the comparison treatment. This may not be because of conflict of interest on the part of the researcher, but simply because they are zealous in defense of their original hypothesis (belief).

An increasingly common device for reporting results uses **composite endpoints**. These are most commonly seen when a single important endpoint such as a difference in death rates shows results that are small and not statistically significant. The researcher then looks at other endpoints such as reduction in recurrence of adverse clinical events that do not cause death. The combination of both events may be reduced enough to make the study results statistically significant. A recent study looked at low-molecular-weight heparin (LMWH, an anticoagulant) for the prevention of death in certain types of cardiac event (unstable angina and

---

[1] www.healthcare.ubc.ca.
[2] www.cebm.net.

non-Q-wave infarctions). The final results were that death, heart attack or urgent surgery or angioplasty (revascularization) occurred in fewer of the LMWH group than in the standard heparin group. There was no difference between groups for death. It was only when all the outcomes were put together that the difference achieved statistical significance. In addition, the LMWH group had more intracranial bleeds and the NNT for the composite endpoint was almost equal to the NNH for the bleeds.

Sometimes a study will show a very small or non-significant difference between the intervention and comparison treatment for the overall sample group being studied. In some cases, the authors will then look at subgroups of the study population to find one that demonstrates a statistically significant association. This **post-hoc subgroup analysis** is not an appropriate way to look for significance and is a form of data dredging. The more subgroups are examined, the more likely it is that a statistically significant outcome will be found – and that it will have occurred by chance. This can determine a hypothesis for the next study of the same intervention. In that subsequent study, that subgroup will be the selected population at the start of the study and improvement looked for in that group only. A lot of time and effort is needed to get a large enough subgroup together to have a statistically significant result. In most cases, that study is unlikely to get done and the results of a subgroup analysis must be used, but with caution.

A recent study of stroke found that patients treated with thrombolytic therapy (clot-buster drugs) within three hours did better than those treated later than three hours. The authors concluded that this was the optimal time to begin treatment and the manufacturer began marketing the drugs (which are very expensive and could lead to bleeding in the brain) very heavily. Subsequent studies of patients within this time frame have not found the same reduction in neurological deficit found in the original study. The determination of the three-hour mark was a post-hoc subgroup analysis performed after the data was obtained. The authors looked for some statistically significant time period in which the drug was effective. It is possible that the drug will actually work during this time window and not during other time windows. However, a new study explicitly looking at this time window should be done to determine if the results are reproducible or if the noted association occurred by chance alone.

12

Negative studies and Type II errors

If I had thought about it, I wouldn't have done the experiment. The literature was full of examples that said you can't do this.

Spencer Silver on the work that led to the unique adhesives for 3M Post-It ® Notepads

Learning objectives

In this chapter you will learn:
- how to recognize Type II errors in a study
- how to interpret negative clinical trials using 95% confidence intervals
- how to use a nomogram to determine the appropriate sample size and interpret a Type II error

Interpretation of the results of negative clinical trials requires an understanding of the statistical processes that can account for these results. Intelligent readers of the medical literature must be able to interpret these results and determine for themselves if they are important enough to ignore in clinical practice.

The problem with evaluating negative studies

Negative studies are those that conclude that there is no statistically significant association between the cause and effect variables and no difference between the two groups being compared. This may occur because there really is no association or difference (**true negative** result) between groups. However, it can also occur because the study was unable to determine that the difference or association found was statistically significant. This is a **false negative** result and is not a trivial problem in medical research.

In a college psychology class, an interesting experiment was done. There were two sections of students in the lab portion of the class. Each section did the same experiment. On separate days, each student was given a cup of coffee. One day they got real Java and the next day decaf. After drinking the coffee, they were given a simple test of math problems that had to be completed in a specified time. Each of the students' scores was calculated. For both groups, the scores under the influence of caffeine were highest. However, when a statistical test was applied to the results, they were not statistically significant. The results could have occurred by chance greater than 5% of the time. Does caffeine improve scores on a simple math test? Are the results really no different or was the study falsely negative?

Type II error

This type of error occurs when the null hypothesis is not rejected (H_0 is accepted and no difference is found) even though it is really false (and the groups are different). The researcher concludes that there isn't a difference, when in fact there is. An example would be concluding there is no relationship between familial hyperlipidemia and the occurrence of coronary artery disease when there truly is a relationship. Another would be concluding that caffeine intake does not increase the math scores of college psychology students when in fact it does. This is called a β or **Type II error**.

We define β (beta) as the maximum probability of making a Type II error or failing to reject the null hypothesis when it is actually false. This is a convoluted way of saying that it finds the alternative hypothesis to be false, "when it ain't!" Beta is the probability of the occurrence of this wrong conclusion that an investigator must be willing to accept. The researcher does not set β directly. It can be calculated from the projected or expected study results before a study is done. The value of β is estimated from conditions of the experiment.

Power is the ability to detect a statistically significant difference when it actually exists. The researcher can reduce β and thereby increase this thing called **power**, by selecting a sufficiently large sample size (n) or making other changes in the study. Increasing the difference one wants to detect (**effect size**), using a one-tailed rather than a two-tailed test, and increasing the level of α (from 0.025 to 0.05 or higher) all **lower** the probability of making a Type II or β error.

Determining power

In statistical terminology power means that the study will reject the null hypothesis when it really is false. This is one minus the probability that a type II error is made, or $1 - \beta$. By convention we set up the experiment so that β is no greater than **0.20**. Equivalently, power should be more than **0.80** to be considered adequate for most studies. A microscope with greater power will be able to detect smaller differences between cells.

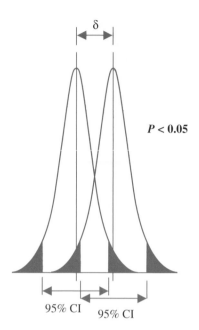

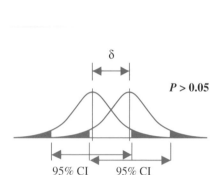

Fig. 12.1 Effect of changing sample size. Two variables with different sample sizes and the same effect size (δ). The area under the curves is proportional to the sample size (n). The samples on the left with a small sample size are not statistically significantly different ($P > 0.05$). The ones on the right with a larger sample size have an effect size that is statistically significant ($P < 0.05$).

Power depends on several factors. These include the **type of variable** (dichotomous, ordinal, or continuous – continuous is best), **statistical test** (one-tailed has more power than two-tailed), **degree of variability** (standard deviation – generally the lower, or smaller, the greater the power), **effect size** (the larger the better), and the **sample size** (the bigger the better).

These concepts are directly related to the concept of confidence discussed in Chapter 10. The confidence formula (confidence = (signal/noise) $\times \sqrt{n}$) can be written as confidence = (effect size/standard deviation) $\times \sqrt{n}$. As effect size or n increases, confidence increases. As the standard deviation increases, confidence decreases and so does power.

Effect of sample size on power

Sample size (n) has the most obvious effect on the power of a study although it is related through the square root and not directly. If the sample size is very large, a statistical test is more likely to show a level of significance for even a small effect size. This is a purely mathematical issue. The smaller the sample size, the harder it is to find statistical significance even with a large effect size. Remember the two groups of college psychology students at the start of this chapter. When the scores for the two groups were combined, the results turned out to be statistically significant. Fig. 12.1 demonstrates the effect of increasing sample size to obtain a statistically significant result.

For example we do a study to find out if ibuprofen (Motrin and others) is good for relieving the pain of osteoarthritis and find that patients taking ibuprofen

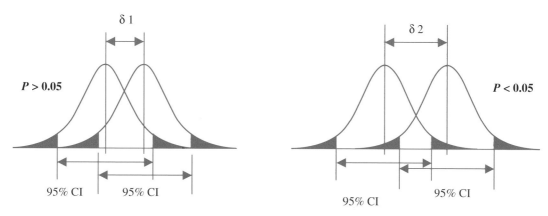

Fig. 12.2 Effect of changing effect size. Two variables with different effect sizes and the same sample size. The results of the group on the left with a small effect size are not statistically significantly different ($P > 0.05$). The ones on the right with a larger effect size have a result that is statistically significant ($P < 0.05$).

had 50% less pain than those taking placebo. There were only five patients in each group and the result (although very large in terms of effect size) was not statistically significant. We repeat the study and get exactly the same results. But this time we do it with 25 patients in each group. This time the result turns out to be statistically significant. This occurred because of an increase in power.

In the extreme, studies of tens of thousands of patients will often find very tiny effect sizes (1% or less) to be statistically significant. This is the most important reason to use the **number needed to treat** (NNT) instead of $P < 0.05$ as the best indicator of the clinical significance of a study. In terms of confidence intervals, a larger sample size will lead to narrower confidence intervals.

Effect of effect size on power

Before the experiment is done, **effect size** is estimated as the difference between groups that will be **clinically** important. The sample size needed to detect an effect size this large or larger can be calculated. It is easier to detect a large effect (e.g., 90% change) than a small one (e.g., 2% change) (Fig. 12.2). However, as we discussed above, if the sample size is large enough, even a small effect size may be statistically significant. That effect size may not be clinically important even though it is statistically significant. The conditions of the experiment can be manipulated to show a large effect size, but usually at the cost of making a Type III or IV error (as discussed in Chapter 10).

Effect of level of significance on power

The magnitude of **level of significance** (alpha, α) is how willing we are to have a result that occurred only by chance. If alpha is very small, we are willing to accept only a tiny likelihood that the effect size found occurred by chance alone. As the level of α increases, we are willing to have a greater likelihood that the effect size found occurred by chance and was not due to actual truth in the universe

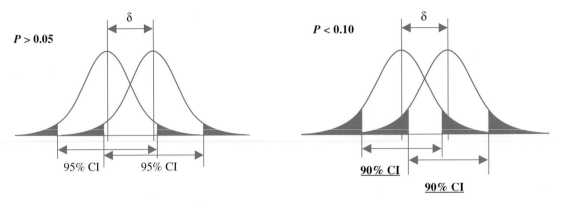

Fig. 12.3 Effect of changing alpha. Two variables with different levels of α. The samples on the left with a small $\alpha(= 0.05)$ are not statistically significantly different ($P > 0.05$). The ones on the right with a larger $\alpha(= 0.1)$ have an effect size that is statistically significant ($P < 0.10$).

(Fig. 12.3). In medicine we generally set α at 0.05, while in physics α may be set at 0.0001 or lower, since we want to be more certain that the result did not occur by chance. Those in medicine today who believe that 0.05 is too stringent and we should go to an α level of 0.1 might not be comfortable knowing that the treatment they were receiving was better than something cheaper, less toxic, or more commonly used by a chance factor of 10%.

Effect of standard deviation on power

The smaller the **standard deviation** of the data-sets the better the power of the study. If two samples each have small standard deviations, a statistical test is more likely to find them different than if they have large standard deviations. Think of the standard deviation as defining the width of a normal distribution around the mean value found in the study. When the two normal distributions are compared, the one with the smallest spread will have the most likelihood of being found statistically significant (Fig. 12.4).

Negative studies

A Type II error can only be made in a negative clinical trial. These are trials reporting no statistically significant difference or association. Therefore, when reading negative clinical trials, one needs to assess the chance that a Type II error occurred. This is important because a negative result may not be due to the lack of an important effect but simply because of the inability to detect that effect statistically. This is called a study with **low power**. From an interpretation perspective, the question one asks is, "For a given β level and a difference that I consider clinically important, did the researcher use a large enough sample size?"

Since the possibility of a Type II error is a non-trivial problem, you must perform your own interpretation of a negative clinical trial. There are three common ways of doing this. They are through the interpretation of the **confidence intervals**, by

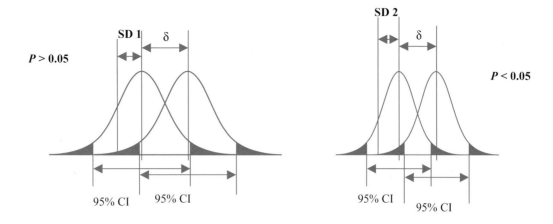

Fig. 12.4 Effect of changing precision (standard deviation). Two variables with the same sample size and effect size. In the case on the left there is a large standard deviation, while on the right there is a small standard deviation. The situation on the right will be statistically significant ($P < 0.05$) while the one on the left will not ($P > 0.05$).

using sample size **nomograms**, and with published **power tables**. We will discuss the first two methods since they can be done most simply without specialized references.

Using confidence intervals to determine significance of a negative study

Confidence intervals (CI) can be used to represent the level of significance. There are several rules of thumb that must be remembered before using CIs to determine the potential of a Type II error. If the point estimate value of one variable is within the 95% CI range of the other variable, there is no statistical significance to the difference between the two groups. If the 95% CI for a difference includes 0, the difference found is not statistically significant. If the 95% CI for a ratio includes 1, the ratio found is not statistically significant.

Unlike P values, which are only a single number, 95% CIs allow the reader actually to see a range of possible values that includes the true value with 95% certainty. For the difference between two groups, it gives the range of the most likely difference between the two groups under consideration. For a given effect size, you can look at the relationship between the limits of the CI and the **null point** (at which there is no difference or association.) A 95% CI that is skewed in one direction near the null point can be caused by low power. In that case, a larger sample size might show a statistically significant effect.

For example, in a study of the effect of two drugs on pain, the change in the visual analog score (VAS) was found to be 25 mm with a 95% CI from −5 mm to 55 mm. This suggests that a larger study would most likely find a difference that was statistically significant, although maybe not as large as 25 mm. Only a few more patients and the CI would be narrower and would "most likely" not include the null point (0). In that case, if there were no other evidence available it might be

| Begin with the sample size that was used in the study | | Use the nomogram to determine the effect size (δ) that could be found with this sample | | Potential δ < clinically important δ Ignore results (lacks power) |
| | | | | Potential δ > clinically important δ Accept results |

Fig. 12.5 Sequence of events for analyzing negative studies using sample size.

reasonable to use the "better" drug until either a more powerful study or a well-done meta-analysis showed a statistically significant or clear-cut superiority of one over the other, or equivalence of the two drugs. On the other hand, if the 95% CI were −15 mm to 60 mm, it would be unlikely that adding even a lot more patients would change the results. In this case, consider the study to be negative, at least until another and much larger study comes along.

The 95% CI can also be used to evaluate positive studies. If the absolute risk reduction (ARR) for an intervention is 0.05 with a 95% CI of 0.01 to 0.08, the intervention is better statistically, but barely significant clinically. If the intervention is extremely expensive or dangerous, its use should be strongly debated based upon that small an effect size.

Evaluating negative studies using a nomogram

There are two ways to analyze the results of a negative study using published nomograms from an article by Young and others.[1] These begin either with the sample size or with the effect size. Either method will tell you, for a study with sufficient power, what sample size was necessary, or what effect size could be found, to produce statistical significance.

In the first method, use the nomogram to determine the **effect size** that the study had the **power** to find. Begin with the sample size and work backward to find the effect size that the sample in this study had the power to find. If the effect size that could potentially have been found with this sample size was larger than the effect size you (or more correctly, your patient) would consider "clinically important," accept the study as a negative one. The clinically important difference could have been found and wasn't. On the other hand, if the clinically important effect size could not have been found with the sample size in this study, the study was too small. "Ignore" the study and consider the result a Type II error. Wait for confirmatory studies before using the information (Fig. 12.5).

[1] J. J. Young, E. A. Bresnitz & B. L. Strom. Sample size nomograms for interpreting negative clinical studies. *Ann. Intern. Med.* 1983; 99: 248–251.

| Decide on a clinically important difference | | Use the nomogram to determine the sample size (*n*) needed to find this difference | | Actual n < required n Ignore results (lacks power) |
| | | | | Actual n > required n Accept results |

The second way of analyzing a negative study is to determine the **sample size** needed to get a **clinically important effect size**. Use the nomograms starting from the effect size that you consider clinically important and determine the sample size needed to find this effect size. This effect size will most likely be bigger than the actual difference found in the study. If the actual sample size is greater than the sample size required to find a clinically important difference, accept the results as a negative trial. The study had the power to find a clinically important effect size and didn't. If the actual study sample size is less than the required sample size to find a clinically important difference, "ignore" the results with the caveats listed below. The study didn't have the power to find a difference that is clinically important (Fig. 12.6).

There are some caveats which must be considered in using this method. If the needed sample size is huge, it is unlikely that a group that large can ever be studied, so accept the results as a negative study. If the needed sample size is within about one order of magnitude greater than the actual sample size, wait for the bigger study to come along before using the information. This process is illustrated in Fig. 12.7 (dichotomos variables) and Fig. 12.8. (continuous variables). The CD-ROM has some sample problems that will help you understand this process.

Fig. 12.6 Schematic of sequence of events for analyzing negative studies using effect size.

Using a nomogram for dichotomous variables

Dichotomous variables – only two possible values (e.g., cured or not cured).
(1) Identify one group as the control group and the other as the experimental group (this should be evident from the study design)
(2) Decide what RRR (relative rate reduction) would be clinically important.
(3) RRR = (CER − EER) / CER (CER = control event rate and EER = experimental event rate)
(4) Locate this % change on the horizontal axis
(5) Extend a vertical line to intersect with the diagonal line representing the percentage response rate of the control group (CER)
(6) Extend a horizontal line from the intersection point to the vertical axis and read the required sample size (*n*)

Fig. 12.7 Nomogram for dichotomous variables. If a study found a 20% relative risk reduction and there was a 60% response rate in the control group (vertical line), you would find this effect size statistically significant only if there was a sample size of more than 200 (horizontal line). If the actual study had only 100 patients in each group and found a 20% relative risk reduction, which was not statistically significant, you should wait until a slightly larger study (200 per group) is done. After M. Young, E. A. Bresnitz & B. L. Strom. Sample size nomograms for interpreting negative clinical studies. *Ann. Intern. Med.* 1983; 99: 248–251. (Used with permission.)

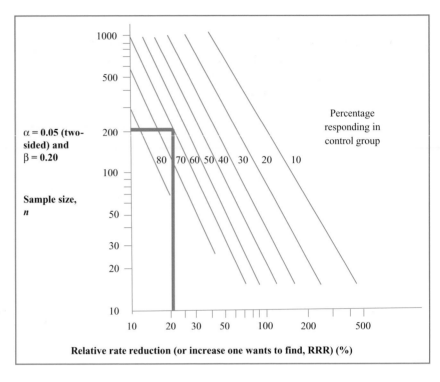

Fig. 12.8 Nomogram for continuous variables. If a study found a difference of 1 unit and the control group had a standard deviation of 2 (vertical line), you would find this effect size statistically significant only if there was a sample size of more than 70 (horizontal line). If the actual study found an effect size of only 0.5, and you thought that was clinically but not statistically significant, you would need to wait for a larger study (about 250 in each group) to be done before accepting that this was a negative study. After M. Young, E. A. Bresnitz & B. L. Strom. Sample size nomograms for interpreting negative clinical studies. *Ann. Intern. Med.* 1983; 99: 248–251. (Used with permission.)

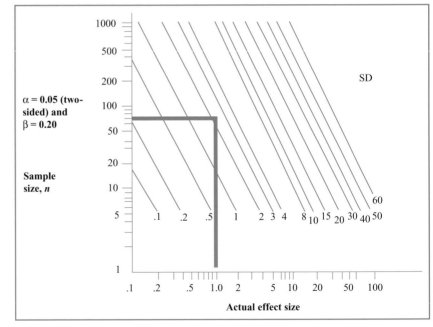

Using a nomogram for continuous variables

Continuous variables – multiple possible values with proportional intervals.
(1) Decide what difference (absolute effect size) is clinically important
(2) Locate this difference on the horizontal axis
(3) Extend a vertical line to the diagonal line representing the standard deviation of the data being measured (can use the SD for either group)
(4) Extend a horizontal line to the vertical axis and read the required sample size

13

Risk assessment

We saw the risk we took in doing good,
But dared not spare to do the best we could.

Robert Frost (1874–1963): The Exposed Nest

Learning objectives

In this chapter you will learn:

- the basic concept and measures of risk
- the meanings, calculations, uses and limitations of
  - absolute risk
  - relative risk
  - odds ratios
  - attributable risk and number needed to harm (NNH)
  - attributable risk percent
- the use of confidence intervals in risk
- how to interpret the concept of "zero risk"

Risk is present in all human activities. What is the risk of getting breast cancer if a woman lives on Long Island and is exposed to organochlorines? What is the risk of getting lung cancer because there is a smoke residue on your co-worker's sweater? What is the risk of getting paralyzed as a result of spinal surgery? How about the risk of getting diarrhea from the antibiotic amoxicillin? Some of these are real and others are at best minimally increased risks of modern life. Risks may be those associated with a disease, with therapy, or with common environmental factors. Physicians must be able to interpret levels of risk for their patients.

Measures of risk

First, a word about **probability**, which has a lot to do with this problem, since risk is a probability. In general, risk is the probability that an event (disease or outcome) will occur in a particular population. The **absolute risk** of an outcome in exposed subjects is defined as the ratio of patients who are exposed and who are affected (who develop the outcome event of interest) to all patients exposed to the risk. For example if we study 1000 people who drink more than two cups of coffee a day and 60 develop pancreatic cancer, the risk of developing pancreatic cancer among people drinking more than two cups of coffee a day is 60/1000 or 6%. This can also be written as a conditional probability, **P\{outcome | risk\} = probability of the outcome if exposed to the risk factor**. The same calculation can be done for people who are not exposed to the risk and who nevertheless get the outcome of interest. Their **absolute risk** is the ratio of those not exposed to the risk factor and who have the outcome to all those not exposed to the risk factor.

Risk calculations can help us in many clinical situations. They can help associate an etiology to an outcome – for example, the connection between smoking and lung cancer. Risk calculations can estimate the probability of developing the outcome because of therapy, as in the example of estrogen use and the increased risk of endometrial cancer. They can demonstrate the effectiveness of an intervention on an outcome such as showing a decreased mortality from measles in children who have been vaccinated against measles. Finally, they can target interventions that are most likely to be of benefit. For example, they can measure the effect of aspirin as opposed to stronger blood thinners (heparin or low-molecular-weight heparin) on mortality from heart attacks.

The data used to estimate risk come from research studies. The **best** estimates of risk come from **randomized clinical trials** or **cohort studies**. These studies can separate groups by the exposure and then measure the risk of the outcome. The exposure also precedes the outcome in these studies. The measure of risk calculated from these studies is the **relative risk**. **Less reliable** estimates of risk come from **case–control studies** or **cross-sectional studies**. These studies start with the assumption that there are more or less equal numbers of subjects with and without the outcome or disease. The estimates of risk from these studies approximate the relative risk calculated from cohort studies using a calculation known as an **odds ratio**.

There are several standardized measures associated with any clinical or **epidemiological** study of risk. Patients are initially identified either by exposure to the risk factor (as in **cohort studies** or **RCTs**) or by their outcome (as in **case–control studies**). The study design determines which way the data are gathered. This in turn determines the type of risk measures that can be obtained from a given study. These are summarized in Fig. 13.1.

Absolute risk

Absolute risk is the probability of the outcome in those exposed or not exposed to the risk factor. It compares those with the outcome and the risk factor (*a*) to all

Fig. 13.1 A pictorial way to look at studies of risk. Note the difference in sampling direction for different types of studies.

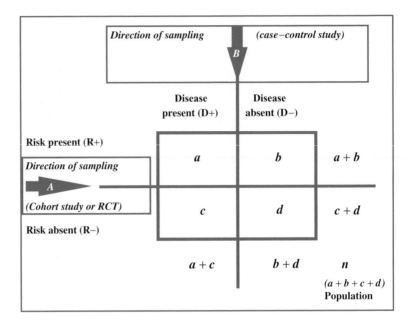

subjects in the population exposed to the risk factor $(a + b)$ or similarly to those in the non-risk exposed group $[c/(c + d)]$. In probabilistic terms, it is the probability of the outcome if exposed to the risk factor, also written as **P{outcome | risk}** = **$P(O+ | R+)$**. Absolute risk only tells you about the risk of one group, either those exposed to the risk factor or those not exposed to the risk factor. It can only be calculated from cohort studies or randomized clinical trials. You must know the relative numbers of the factors in the rows of the 2×2 table in Fig. 13.1 in order to calculate this number.

The absolute risk of the outcome in those not exposed can also be calculated. It is the ratio of the number of patients with the outcome if not exposed to the risk factor and the total number of patients who were not exposed to the risk factor. Probabilistically it is written as **P{outcome | no risk}** = **$P(O+ | R-)$**.

The **absolute risk** is the probability that someone with the risk factor has the outcome. In the 2×2 diagram (Fig. 13.2), patients labeled a are those with the risk factor who have the outcome and those labeled $a + b$ are all patients with the risk factor. The ratio $a/(a + b)$ is the probability that you have the outcome if you were exposed to the risk factor. This is a statement of conditional probability. The same can be done for the row of patients who were not exposed to the risk factor. The absolute risk for them can be written as $c/(c + d)$. These absolute risks are the same as the incidence of disease in the cohort being studied.

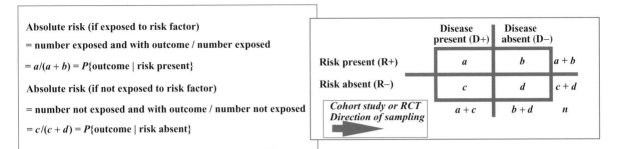

Absolute risk (if exposed to risk factor)

= number exposed and with outcome / number exposed

= $a/(a + b)$ = P{outcome | risk present}

Absolute risk (if not exposed to risk factor)

= number not exposed and with outcome / number not exposed

= $c/(c + d)$ = P{outcome | risk absent}

	Disease present (D+)	Disease absent (D−)	
Risk present (R+)	a	b	$a + b$
Risk absent (R−)	c	d	$c + d$
Cohort study or RCT Direction of sampling	$a + c$	$b + d$	n

Fig. 13.2 Absolute risk.

Relative risk

Relative risk (RR) is the ratio of the two absolute risks. This is the absolute risk of the outcome in subjects exposed to the risk factor divided by the absolute risk of the outcome in subjects not exposed to the risk factor. It tells you whether that risk factor "causes" or "prevents" the index outcome or disease. In other words, it is the probability of the outcome if exposed compared to the probability of the outcome if not exposed. Relative risk can only be calculated from **cohort studies** or **randomized clinical trials**. The larger (or smaller) the relative risk, the stronger the association between the cause (risk) and effect (outcome or disease) variables.

If the RR is greater than 1, the risk factor is associated with an increase in the rate of the outcome. If the RR is less than 1, the risk factor is associated with a reduction in the rate of the outcome. If it is 1, there is no change in risk from the baseline risk level and it is said that the results are not different from baseline. A relative risk (or odds ratio) greater than 4 is usually considered fairly strong. Values below this could have been obtained because of systematic flaws in the study. In studies showing a reduction in risk, look for RR to be less than 0.25 for it to be considered a strong result. A high relative risk does not prove that the risk factor is responsible for outcome: it merely quantifies the strength of association of the two. It is always possible that a third unrecognized factor (**surrogate** or **confounding variable**) is the cause and equally affects both the risk and the outcome.

Relative risk is calculated by taking the ratio of the two absolute risks. This is the ratio of subjects with the outcome and the risk factor (a) to all subjects who possess the risk factor ($a + b$) divided by the ratio of subjects with the outcome and without the risk factor (c) to all subjects without the risk factor ($c + d$) (Fig. 13.3).

Data collected for relative-risk calculations come from **cohort studies**, **nonconcurrent cohort studies**, and **randomized clinical trials**. These studies are the only ones capable of calculating **incidence** (the rate of occurrence of new cases of the outcome). Cohort studies should demonstrate complete follow-up

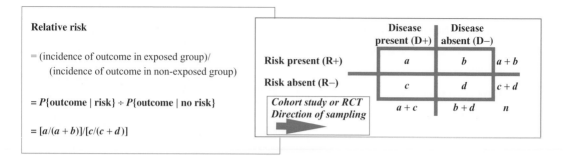

Fig. 13.3 Relative risk.

of all study subjects. If there is too large a drop-out rate, the results may not be valid. The researchers should allow for an adequate length of follow-up in order to ensure that all possible outcome events could have occurred. This is years (or even decades) for cancer while it is usually weeks or days for certain infectious diseases.

Odds ratio

An odds ratio is the calculation used to estimate the relative risk or the association of risk and outcome for **case–control studies**. In case–control studies, subjects are selected based upon the presence or absence of the outcome of interest. Therefore the incidence (the rate of occurrence of new cases of each outcome associated with and without the risk factor) cannot be calculated, and the relative risk cannot be calculated.

Odds are a different way of saying the same thing as probabilities. Odds tell you the number of times an event of interest will happen divided by the number of times it won't happen. As we mentioned in Chapter 9, odds and probability are mathematically related. In these cases, the individual odds of exposure to the risk factor in subjects with the outcome are the ratio of subjects with and without the risk factor among all subjects with that outcome. The same odds can be calculated for those without the outcome. The odds ratio compares the odds of having the risk factor present in the subjects with and without the outcome (disease) under study. This is the odds of having the risk factor if you have the outcome divided by the odds of having the risk factor if you don't have the outcome. It is an estimate of relative risk in case-control studies (Fig. 13.4).

Using the odds ratio to estimate the relative risk

The odds ratio best estimates the relative risk when the disease is very rare. The rationale for this is not intuitively obvious. **Cohort-study** patients are evaluated

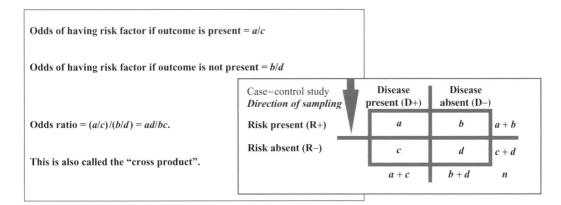

Odds of having risk factor if outcome is present = a/c

Odds of having risk factor if outcome is not present = b/d

Odds ratio = $(a/c)/(b/d) = ad/bc$.

This is also called the "cross product".

Case–control study *Direction of sampling*	Disease present (D+)	Disease absent (D−)	
Risk present (R+)	a	b	$a+b$
Risk absent (R−)	c	d	$c+d$
	$a+c$	$b+d$	n

Fig. 13.4 Odds ratio.

In the cohort study, the **relative risk (RR)** is $[a/(a+b)]/[c/(c+d)]$. If the disease or outcome is very rare, $a <<< b$ and $c <<< d$, making $(a+b) \to$ b and $(c+d) \to d$ and RR $\approx (a/b)/(c/d) = ad/bc$

RR approximates **odds ratio** = $(a/b)/(c/d) = ad/bc$

	Disease present (D+)	Disease absent (D−)	
Risk present (R+)	a	b	$a+b$
Risk absent (R−)	c	d	$c+d$
	$a+c$	$b+d$	n

Fig. 13.5 Odds ratio as estimate of relative risk. From S. B. Hulley & S. R. Cummings. *Designing Clinical Research*. Baltimore, MD, Williams & Wilkins, 1988.

on the basis of **exposure** and outcome is then determined. Therefore, one can calculate the absolute risk, since the incidence is known. The incidence of patients with the risk factor who have the disease and those without the risk factor who have the disease can be known, and relative risk calculated.

Case–control study patients are evaluated on the basis of **outcome** and exposure is then determined. The true ratio of patients with and without the outcome in the general population cannot be known. You can only look at the ratio of the odds of risk in the diseased and non-diseased groups. Hence the odds ratio. In the case–control study, we are looking at the disease as if it were present in a preset ratio (usually half of the population, an equal number of cases and controls). In fact this is not true. In reality, there are many fewer cases (patients with known disease) than controls (people without known disease) in the general population. This fact allows the odds ratio to be close to the relative risk. We can prove this mathematically using two hypothetical studies of the same risk and outcomes (Fig. 13.5).

We assume that the true incidence of disease in the population is represented by the results of the cohort study. In the case–control study, groups with and without outcome are equal. The ratios a/b and c/d approximate the incidences in the general population when the number of cases of the outcome of interest (a and c) is much smaller than the number of cases of no outcome (b and d). Then $a/(a + b)$ becomes a/b and $c/(c + d)$ becomes c/d.

A word of caution is needed here. In order for the above to be absolutely true, the sample must be relatively representative of the population and the outcome must be rare (i.e., rarer than non-disease), and **sampling error** (systematic and random) must be small. When the incidence of disease is high, the odds ratios and relative risk values diverge dramatically. This becomes greater as the value of RR and OR increase above 1 or decrease below 1. The differences are minimal when the RR or OR is equal to 1 regardless of the actual incidence of the outcome.

Attributable risk and the number needed to harm (NNH)

Attributable risk estimates how much of the risk of an outcome in the subjects exposed to the risk factor is attributable to the risk factor. There are two numbers that are called attributable risk. The first is known as the **absolute attributable risk** (AAR) or **absolute risk reduction** (ARR) or **increase** (ARI). This is the difference in absolute risks with and without the risk factors.

The second is the **attributable risk percent**, or **relative attributable risk**. It is calculated by subtracting the absolute risk of subjects not exposed to the risk factor from the absolute risk of subjects exposed to the risk factor and dividing by the absolute risk for those not exposed to the risk factor. Attributable risk can only be calculated from cohort (prospective) studies that provide good estimates of incidence of the outcome of interest. This recognizes that other unidentifiable risk factors account for differences in outcomes between exposed and non-exposed groups.

Attributable risk quantitates the contribution of a risk factor in producing the outcome in those exposed to the risk factor. It is helpful in calculating the **cost–benefit ratio** of eliminating the risk factor from the population. Absolute attributable risk is analogous to absolute risk reduction mentioned in the previous chapters. It is also called the absolute risk increase (ARI) and allows us to calculate the **number needed to harm** (NNH = 1/AAR or 1/ARI). This tells us how many people need to be exposed before harm will befall one additional person, or one additional harmful outcome event will occur (Fig. 13.6).

Putting risk into perspective

A large increase in relative risk may represent a clinically unimportant increase in personal risk. This is especially true if the outcome is relatively rare in the

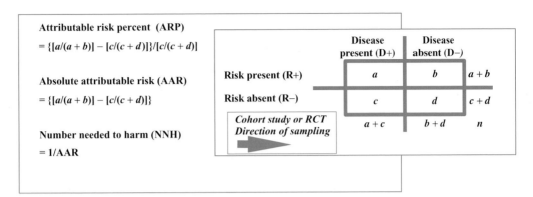

Attributable risk percent (ARP)

$= \{[a/(a + b)] - [c/(c + d)]\}/[c/(c + d)]$

Absolute attributable risk (AAR)

$= \{[a/(a + b)] - [c/(c + d)]\}$

Number needed to harm (NNH)

$= 1/AAR$

	Disease present (D+)	Disease absent (D−)	
Risk present (R+)	a	b	a + b
Risk absent (R−)	c	d	c + d
	a + c	b + d	n

Cohort study or RCT Direction of sampling

Fig. 13.6 Attributable risk and the number needed to harm.

population. For instance, several years ago there was a concern that the influenza vaccine could cause a serious and potentially fatal neurologic syndrome called Guillain–Barré syndrome (GBS). This syndrome consists of progressive weakness of the muscles of the body in an ascending pattern. It is usually reversible, but may require a period of time on a ventilator getting artificial respiration. There were 74 cases of this related to the influenza vaccine in 1993–1994. The odds ratio for that season was 1.5, meaning a 50% increase in the number of cases. Since the base incidence of this disease is approximately two in one million, even a ten-fold increase in risk would have little impact on the general population. This risk needed to be balanced against the number of lives saved by the influenza vaccine. That number is thousands of times greater than the small increased risk of GBS with the vaccine. Although the news of this possible reaction was alarming to many patients, it had no (or little) clinical significance.

Similarly, a small increase in relative risk may represent a clinically important increase in personal risk if the outcome is relatively common in the population. For example, if an outcome has an incidence of 12 in 100, increasing the risk even by 1.5 (the same 50%) will have a significant impact on the general population.

Examination of all possible outcome data is necessary to determine if eliminating the risk is associated with appropriate gains. For example, it is known that conjugated estrogens are associated with an increased risk of endometrial carcinoma. Would the decreased morbidity and mortality due to osteoporosis balance the increase in morbidity and mortality due to endometrial cancer among women using conjugated estrogens? It had previously been thought that the risk of cardiovascular disease was decreased with estrogen use. But recent data has questioned this and the risk may actually be increased. You must be able to interpret these risks for your patient and help her make an informed decision.

Confidence intervals give you an idea of the relative precision of a study result. They represent the "standard error" of the relative risk or odds ratio. They should always be reported whenever relative risk or odds ratios are reported! Small (or as the statisticians say "tight") confidence intervals suggest that the sampling error due to random events is small, leading to a very **precise** result. A large confidence interval (also called "loose") suggests that there is lots of random error leading to a very **imprecise** result. For example if the RR is 2 and the CI is 1.01 to 6, there is an association. However, it may be very strong (6) or very weak (1.01 is almost non-existent). If the confidence interval for a relative risk or odds ratio includes the number 1, there is no statistical association between risk factor and outcome. Statistically this is equivalent to a study result with $P > 0.05$.

The confidence interval allows you to look at the spread of the results. Loose confidence intervals should suggest a need for more research. Usually they represent small samples and the addition of one or two new events could dramatically change the numbers. Very tight intervals that are close to one suggest a high degree of precision in the result, but also a low strength of association which may not be clinically important.

Reporting relative risk and odds ratios

Over the past 10 years most epidemiologic (cohort and case–control) studies have been reporting their results in terms of relative risk and odds ratios. The intelligent consumer of the medical literature will be able to determine whether these were used correctly. Sometimes they are not. A recent example of this was a report in the *New England Journal of Medicine* about the effect of race and gender on physician referral for cardiac catheterization.[1,2]

The original study reported that physicians, when given standardized scenarios, were more likely to refer white men and women and black men than black women for evaluation of coronary artery disease (CAD). The newspapers reported that blacks and women were 40% less likely to be referred for cardiac catheterization than whites and men. The actual study showed that 90.6% of the white men, white women, and black men were referred while 78.8% of the black women were referred. The authors calculated the odds ratios for these numbers and came up with an odds ratio of 0.4. The odds associated with a 90.6% probability are 9.6 to 1 while those associated with a 78.8% probability are 3.7 to 1.

When the data were recalculated for men and women or whites and blacks, the results showed that men were referred more often (90.6%) than women (84.7%) and whites (90.6%) more often than blacks (84.7%). (Strangely, the figures for men vs. women were exactly the same as those for whites vs. blacks.) The odds here were men (9.6), women (5.5), whites (9.6) and blacks (5.5), making the odds ratio for both of these comparisons equal to 0.6.

[1] K. A. Schulman, J. A. Berlin, W. Harless *et al.* The effect of race and sex on physicians' recommendations for cardiac catheterization. *New Engl. J. Med.* 1999; 340: 618–626.
[2] L. M. Schwartz, S. Woloshin & H. G. Welch. Misunderstandings about the effects of race and sex on physicians' referrals for cardiac catheterization. *New Engl. J. Med.* 1999; 341: 279–283.

However, there were two problems with these numbers. First, the outcome was not rare in the diseased group, since all groups were equal in size. This distorts the odds ratio as an approximation of the relative risk. Second, the study was a clinical trial with the risk factor (race and gender) being the independent variable and the outcome (referral) the dependent variable. Therefore, the relative risk and not the odds ratio should have been used. Had this been done, the relative risk for white vs. black and men vs. women was 0.93 with the 95% CI from 0.89 to 0.99. Not only is the risk much smaller than reported in the news, but it approaches lack of statistical significance. The original report using odds ratios led to a distortion in reporting of the study by the media.

What does a zero numerator mean? Is there ever zero risk?

What if you read a study and find no instances of a particular outcome? A zero numerator does not mean that there is no risk. There is an excellent article by Hanley and Lippman-Hand that shows how to handle this eventuality.[3] Their example is used here.

You can still infer an estimate of the potential size of the risk. Suppose a given study shows no adverse events in 14 consecutive patients. What is the largest number of adverse events we can reasonably expect? What we are doing here is calculating the upper limit of the 95% CI for this sample.

You can use the rule of three to determine this risk. The maximum number of events that can be expected to occur when none have been observed is $3/n$. For this study finding no adverse events in a study of 14 patients, the upper limit of the 95% CI is $3/14 = 21.4\%$. You could expect to see as many as one adverse event in every 5 patients and still have come up with no events in the 14 patients in the initial study.

Assume that the study of 14 patients resulted in no adverse outcomes. What if in reality there is an adverse outcome rate of $1:1000$? The probability of no adverse events in one patient is 1 minus the probability of at least one adverse event in one patient. Another way of writing this is P(no adverse event in one patient) $= 1 - P$(at least one adverse event in one patient). This makes the probability of no adverse events $= 1 - 0.001 = 0.999$. Therefore P(no adverse events in n patients) is 0.999^n. For 14 patients this is 0.986, or there is a 98.6% chance that in 14 patients we would find no adverse outcome events.

Now suppose that the actual rate of adverse outcomes is $1:100$. P(no adverse outcomes in one patient) $= 1 - 0.01 = 0.99$. P(no adverse events in 14 patients) $= 0.99^{14}$. This means that there is a 86.9% chance that we would find no adverse

[3] J. A. Hanley & A. Lippman-Hand. If nothing goes wrong, is everything all right? *JAMA* 1983; 249: 1743–1745.

Table 13.1. Actual vs. estimated rates of adverse events if there is a zero numerator

Rate found in study	Exact 95% CI	Rule $3/n$
0/10	26%	30%
0/20	14%	15%
0/30	10%	10%
0/100	0.3%	0.3%

Table 13.2. Approximate maximum event rate for small numerators

Number of events in the numerator	Estimate of maximum number of events
0	3/n
1	4/n
2	5/n
3	7/n
4	9/n

outcome in these 14 patients. We can continue to reduce the actual adverse event rate to $1:10$, and using the same process we get P(no reaction in 14 patients) $=(0.90)^{14}$. Now 22.9% is the chance we would find no adverse outcome events in these 14 patients.

Similarly, for an actual rate of $1:5$ P(no adverse event in 14 patients) $= 0.8^{14}$ or 3.5%, and for an actual rate of $1:6$ you get you will get a potential event rate of 7.7%. Therefore the 95% CI lies between event rates of $1:5$ and $1:6$. The rate estimated by our rule of three for adverse events is $3/n = 1/4.7 = 21.4\%$. When actually calculated the true number is $1/5.5 = 18.2\%$.

Mathematically you must solve the equation $(1-$ maximum risk$)^n = 0.05$ to find the upper limit of 95% CI. Solving the equation for the maximum risk, $1-$ maximum risk $= \sqrt[n]{0.05}$, and maximum risk $= 1-\sqrt[n]{0.05}$. For $n > 30$, $\sqrt[n]{0.05}$ is close to $(n-3)/n$, making the maximum risk $= 1 - [(n-3)/n] = 3/n$. The actual numbers are shown in Table 13.1.

You can use a similar approximation if there are 1, 2, 3, or 4 events in the numerator. Table 13.2 is the estimate of the maximum number of events you might expect if the actual number of events found is from 0 to 4.

For example, studies of head-injured patients to date have shown that none of the 2700 low-risk patients, those with laceration only or bump without loss

Table 13.3. 95% confidence limits on extreme results

If the denominator is	And the % is 0, the true % could be as *high* as	And the % is 100, the true % could be as *low* as
10	26%	74%
20	14%	86%
30	10%	90%
40	7%	93%
50	6%	94%
60	5%	95%
70	4%	96%
80	4%	96%
90	3%	97%
100	3%	97%
150	2%	98%
300	1%	99%

of consciousness, headache, vomiting, or change in neurological status, had any intracranial bleeding or swelling. Therefore, the largest risk of intracranial injury in these low-risk patients would be $3/2700 = 1/900 = 0.11\%$. This is the upper limit of the 95% confidence interval.

To find the upper limit of the 99% CI, use rule of $4.6/n$ – which can be derived in a similar manner. Table 13.3 gives the 95% CIs for extreme results with a variety of sample sizes.

General observations on the nature of risk

Most people don't know how to make reasonable judgments about the nature of risk, even in terms of risks they know they are exposed to. This was articulated in 1662 by the Port Royal monks in their treatise about the nature of risk. If people did have this kind of judgment, no one (or very few people) would be smoking. There are several important biases that come into play when talking about risk. The physician should be aware of this when discussing risks with their patient.

People are more likely to risk a poor outcome if due to voluntary action rather than imposed action. They are likely to smoke because it is (they think) their choice (rather than an addiction). Similarly, they will accept risks that they feel they have control over rather than risks controlled (or decided for them) by others. They are much more likely to be very upset when they find out that their medication causes a very uncommon, but previously known, side effect.

You have only to read the newspapers to know that you will see more stories on page one about catastrophic accidents (plane crashes) than routine accidents (automobile accidents). This is also true of medical situations. Patients are more willing to accept the risk of death from cancer or sudden cardiac death than death due to unforeseen complications of routine surgery. If there is a clear benefit to avoiding a particular risk (don't drink poison), patients are more likely to accept a bad outcome if they engage in that risky behavior. A major exception to this rule is cigarette smoking, because of the social nature of smoking and the addictive nature of nicotine. If the benefit is not really clear or is very small they will be more likely to reject the behavior.

People are democratic about their perception of risk. They are more willing to accept risk that is distributed to all people rather than risk that is biased to some people only. Natural risks are more acceptable than man-made risks. There is a perception that man-made objects ought not to fail, while if there is a natural disaster it is God's will. Risk that is generated by someone in a position of trust (doctor) is less acceptable than that generated by someone not in that position (neighbor). We are more accepting of risks that are likely to affect adults than of those primarily affecting children, risks that are more familiar over those that are more exotic, and random events (struck by lightning) rather than catastrophes (storm without adequate warning).

14

Multivariate analysis

Stocks have reached what looks like a permanently high plateau.

Irving Fisher, Professor of Economics, Yale University, 1929

Learning objectives

In this chapter you will learn:
- the essential features of multivariate analysis
- the different types of multivariate analysis
- the limitations of multivariate analysis

Studies of risk often look at multiple risk factors associated with a disease or other outcome. When analyzing the data, it is hard to determine whether a single statistically significant result is a chance occurrence or a true association. Multivariate analysis is a method of analyzing data which is now used more often to determine the strength of any one of multiple associations uncovered in a study.

What is multivariate analysis?

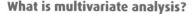

Multivariate analysis answers the question "What is the importance of one risk factor for the risk of a disease, when controlling for all other risk factors that could contribute to that disease?" Ideally, we want to quantitate the added risk for each individual risk factor. For example, in a study of lipid levels and the risk for coronary-artery disease, it was found that after adjusting for advancing age, smoking, elevated systolic blood pressure, and other factors, there was a 19% decrease in coronary heart disease risk for each 8% decrease in total cholesterol level.

In studies of diseases with multiple etiologies the **dependent variable** (disease) is affected by multiple **independent variables** (etiologies). In the example described above coronary heart disease is the dependent variable. Smoking, advancing age, elevated systolic blood pressure, "other factors", and cholesterol levels are the independent variables. The process of multivariate analysis looks at the changes in magnitude of risk associated with each independent variable when all the other contributing independent variables are held fixed.

In studies using multivariate analysis, the dependent variable is most often an outcome variable. Some of the most commonly used outcome variables are incidence of new disease, death, time to death, and disease-free survival. In studies involving small populations or uncommon outcomes, there may not be enough outcome endpoints for analysis. Composite variables are often used to get enough endpoints of interest to enable a valid statistical analysis to be done. The independent variables are the risk factors or treatments that are suspected of influencing the outcome.

How multivariate analysis works: determining risk

Multivariate analysis looks at the changes in magnitude of the risk of an outcome (dependent variable) associated with each suspect risk factor (independent variable) when the other suspect risk factors (independent variables) are held fixed. A schematic example of how this works can be seen in Fig. 14.1.

If more variables are to be adjusted for, further division into even smaller groups must be done. This is shown in Fig. 14.2. You will notice that as more and more variables are added, the number of patients in each "cell" of every 2×2 table gets smaller and smaller. This will result in the confidence intervals of each OR and RR getting larger and larger.

What can multivariate analysis do?

Some studies will look at multiple risk factors to determine which are most important in making a diagnosis or predicting the outcome of a disease. The output of these studies is often the result of a multivariate analysis. Although, this can suggest which variables are most important, those variables should be evaluated in more detail in another study. This is called the **derivation set** and if the statistical significance found initially is still present after the multivariate analysis, it is less likely to be a Type I error. The researchers still need to do a follow-up (**validation set**) study to verify that the association did not occur purely by chance. The analysis can also confirm statistically significant results already found as a result of simple analysis of multiple variables (data dredging). Finally, multivariate analysis can combine different variables and measure the effect of different combinations on the final magnitude of risk factors.

There are four basic types of multivariate analysis depending on the type of outcome variable. **Multiple linear regression** analysis is used when the outcome variable is continuous. **Multiple logistic regression analysis** is used when the

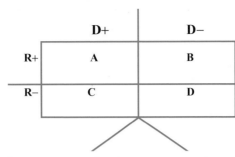

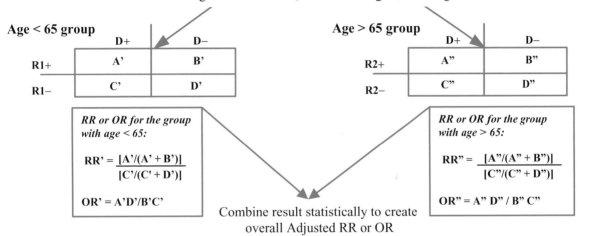

Fig. 14.1 The method of adjusting for a single variable in a multivariate analysis.

outcome variable is a binary event (e.g., alive or dead, disease-free or recurrent disease, etc.). **Discriminate function analysis** is used when the outcome variable is categorical (better, worse, or about the same). **Proportional hazards regression analysis (Cox regression)** is used when the outcome variable is the time to the occurrence of a binary event. An example of this is the time to death or tumor recurrence among treated cancer patients.

Assumptions and limitations

Overfitting occurs when too many independent variables allow the researcher to find a relationship when in fact none exists. This leads to a Type I error. For example, in a cohort of 1000 patients there are 20 deaths due to cancer. If there are 15 multiple baseline characteristics, it is likely that one or two will cause a result which has statistical significance by chance only. As a rule of thumb, there should be at least 10 (and some statisticians say at least 20) outcome events per independent variable of importance for statistical tests to be valid.

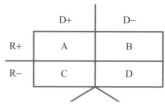

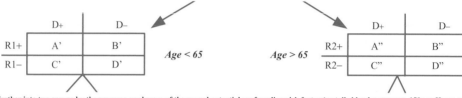

Separate into two groups by the presence or absence of the first potential confounding risk factor (age < 65 or > 65)

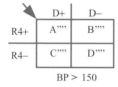

Age < 65   *Age > 65*

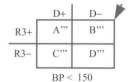

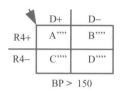

Separate each group further into two groups by the presence or absence of the second potential confounding risk factor (systolic blood pressure > 150mm Hg or <150mm Hg)

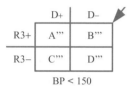

Fig. 14.2 Two confounding variables tested to see if the relationship between risk and outcome would still be true.

Overfitting of variables is characterized by large confidence intervals for each outcome measure.

Underfitting occurs when there are too few outcome events to find a difference that actually exists. This is an example of a Type II error. For example, a study of cigarette smokers followed 200 patients of whom two got lung cancer over 10 years. This may not have been long enough to follow the cohort and the number of cancer cases is too small to find a relationship between smoking and lung cancer. Too few cases of the outcome of interest (lung cancer) may make any statistical relationship with any of the independent variables impossible to find.

Linearity assumes a linear relationship that is not always true. Linearity means that a change in x always produces the same proportional change in y. If this is not true, you cannot use linear regression analysis. In the Cox method of proportional hazards (or risks) the risk of an independent variable is assumed to be constantly proportional over time. This means that when the risks of two treatments are plotted over time, the curves do not cross. If there is a crossover (Fig. 14.3) the early survival advantage of treatment B may not be noted since the initial improvement in survival in that group may cancel out the later reduction in survival.

Interaction between independent variables must be evaluated. For example, smoking and oral contraceptive (OC) use are both risk factors for pulmonary embolism (blood clot in the lungs) in young women. When considering the

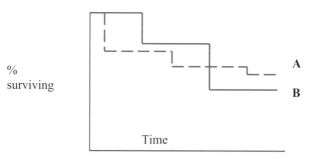

Fig. 14.3 Non-linear curves and the effect of crossing curves.

%
surviving

A

B

Time

risk of either, it turns out that they interact. The risk is greater in smokers using OCs than with either risk factor alone. The adjustment process should include patients with simultaneous presence of both risk factors.

Concomitance refers to a close relationship between variables. Unless there is no relationship between two apparently closely related independent variables being evaluated, only one should be used. If you measure both ventricular ejection fraction and ventricular contractility, correlating them to cardiovascular mortality will yield redundant data. This is an example of **concomitance**. You should use the variable that is most important clinically as the primary predictor of outcome. In our example, ejection fraction is easier to measure clinically and therefore more useful.

Coding of the independent variables can affect the final result. For example, if the age is recorded in one-year or ten-year intervals or as a dichotomous value (< 65 or > 65) the results of a study will be different. There should always be a notation of how the various independent variables are coded for the analysis and why that method of coding was chosen. You should be skeptical when reading studies in which this information is not explicitly given. Post-hoc coding is an example of data dredging.

Outliers are influential observations that occur when one data point or a group of points clearly lie outside the majority of data. These should be explained during the discussion of results and an analysis that includes and excludes these points presented. Outliers can be caused by error in the way the data are measured or by biological variation in the sample. A technique called **stratified analysis** can be used to evaluate outliers.

In evaluation of any study using multivariate analysis, the standard process in critical appraisal should be followed. There should be an explicit hypothesis, the data collection should be done in a non-biased and thorough manner, and the software package used should be specified. Much of the material in this chapter is distilled from an excellent paper on multivariate analysis by J. Concato and others.[1]

[1] J. Concato, A. R. Freinstein & T. S. Halford. The risk of determining risk with multivariate analysis. *Ann. Int. Med.* 1993; 118: 200–210.

15

Randomized clinical trials (RCTs)

One pill makes you larger,
and one pill makes you small.
And the ones your mother gives you,
don't do anything at all.

Grace Slick, The Jefferson Airplane: White Rabbit, from Surrealistic Pillow, 1967

Learning objectives

In this chapter you will learn:
- the unique features of RCTs
- how to undertake critical interpretation of RCTs

The randomized clinical trial (RCT) is the ultimate paradigm of clinical research. Many consider the RCT to be the most important medical development of the twentieth century. These trials have been put on a pedestal and their results used to dictate clinical practice. As with any other experiment, there may be flaws, occasionally fatal ones, in the design, implementation, and interpretation of these trials. The competent reader of the medical literature is able to evaluate the results of a clinical trial in the context of the potential biases introduced into the research experiment.

Introduction

The clinical trial is a relatively recent development in medical research. Prior to the 1950s most research was based upon case series or uncontrolled observations. James Lind, a surgeon in the British Navy, can claim credit for performing the first recorded clinical trial. In 1747, aboard the ship *Salisbury*, he took 12 sailors with scurvy and divided them into six groups of two each. He made sure they were similar in every way except for the intervention, the proposed treatment for scurvy. He found that the two who were given oranges and lemons got better while the other ten did not. The process of the clinical trial was revived with studies of the efficacy of streptomycin for the treatment of tuberculosis done in 1950. The **randomized clinical trial** or **randomized controlled trial** (RCT) has remained the premier source of new knowledge in medicine since then.

Physician decision making and RCTs

There are several ways that physicians make decisions on the best treatment for their patients. **Induction** is the **retrospective** analysis of uncontrolled clinical experience or extension of the expected mechanism of disease as taught in patho-physiology. It is doing that which "seems to work," "worked before," or "ought to work." **Abdication** (or "seduction") is doing something because others tell you it is the right thing to do. These may be teachers, consultants, colleagues, adver-tisements, pharmaceutical representatives, medical textbooks, and others. You accept their analysis of the medical information on faith and this dictates what you actually do for your patient.

Deduction is the **prospective** analysis and application of the results of critical appraisal of formal randomized clinical trials. This method of decision making will successfully withstand formal attempts to demonstrate the worthlessness of a proven therapy. Therapy proven by well-done RCTs is what physicians should be doing for their patients, and it is what you should integrate into your clinical practice for the rest of your professional life.

There are three global issues to identify when evaluating an RCT (Table 15.1). These are (1) the ultimate objective of treatment, (2) the nature of the specific treatment, and (3) the treatment target. The ultimate objective of treatment must be defined up-front. While we want therapy to cure and eliminate all traces of disease, more often than not other outcomes will be sought. Therapy can re-duce mortality (prevent a "treatable" death), prevent recurrence, limit structural or functional deterioration, prevent later complications, relieve the current dis-tress (troubling symptoms of disease), deliver reassurance (confidently know the prognosis), or allow the patient to die with comfort and dignity. These are all very different goals and any study should specify which ones are being sought.

After deciding on the specific outcome you wish to achieve, you must decide which element of sickness (or lack of wellness) your therapy will most affect. These are not always the disease or target disorder, or the pathophysiologic derangement itself. It may be the illness or how that pathophysiologic derangement affects the patient through the production of certain signs and symptoms. Finally, it could also be the predicament or how the illness directly or indirectly affects the patient through disruption of the social, psychological, and economic function of their lives.

Table 15.1. Schema for randomized clinical trials

Ultimate objective	Specific treatment	Target disorder
cure	drug therapy	disease
reduce mortality	surgery	illness
prevent recurrence	other therapies	predicament
limit deterioration	nutrition	
prevention	psychological support	
relieve distress		
deliver reassurance		
allow the patient to die comfortably		

Characteristics of RCTs

The majority of RCTs, and certainly the studies that we are most likely to be evaluating, are **drug studies** or **studies of therapy**. Researchers and drug companies are trying to prove that a new drug is better than drugs that are currently in use for a particular problem. There are some basic rules that apply to your critical evaluation of RCTs. Other specific treatments can be surgical operations, physical or occupational therapy, other procedures or other modalities to modify illness. We will use the example of drug trials in this discussion.

Hypothesis

The study should contain a hypothesis regarding the use of the drug in the general medical population or the specific population tested. There are two basic types of drug (therapy) study hypotheses. The drug can be tested against placebo or against the other regularly used active drug for the same indication. "Does the drug work better than nothing?" looks at how well the drug performs against a placebo (or inert treatment). The placebo effect has been shown to be relatively consistent over many studies and approximates 35%. Unless there is a compelling reason to compare the drug against a placebo, it should always be compared against an active drug that is in current use for the same indication.

The other possibility is to ask "Does the drug work against another drug which has been shown to be effective in the treatment of this disease in the past?" Beware of comparisons of drugs being tested against ones not commonly used in clinical practice or with uncommon or inadequate dosage or routes of administration. These caveats also apply to studies of medical devices, surgical procedures, or other types of therapy. Blinding is difficult in studies of these modalities and should be done by a non-participating outside evaluation team.

When ranking evidence, the well-done RCT with a large sample size is the highest level of evidence. An RCT can reduce the uncertainty surrounding conflicting evidence obtained from lesser quality studies. Over the past 20 years, there were multiple studies that demonstrated decreased mortality if magnesium was given to patients with heart attacks (acute myocardial infarction, AMI). Most of these studies were fairly small and showed no statistically significant improvement in survival. However, when they were combined in a single systematic review (also called a meta-analysis) there was definite statistical and clinical improvement. Since then, a single large randomized trial (called ISIS-4) with thousands of patients showed no beneficial effect of giving magnesium to these patients. It is therefore very unlikely that magnesium therapy would benefit AMI patients.

The unique feature of a clinical trial is the intervention by the investigator in the subject's care for the purposes of the study. These are scientific experiments, using people as subjects! The cause is often the treatment or prevention being studied, and the effect is the outcome of the disease being treated or prevented by early diagnosis. RCTs are the strongest research design capable of proving cause-and-effect relationships. This design alone does not guarantee a quality study and a poorly designed RCT can give false results. Critical evaluation of the study components is necessary before accepting the results of any study. A standardized method of reviewing clinical trails is useful when assessing the quality of a study.

The hypothesis is usually found at the end of the introduction. Each study should contain at least one clearly stated, specific, explicit, and unambiguous hypothesis. A single hypothesis that attempts to prove multiple cause-and-effect relationships cannot be analyzed with a single statistical test and will lead to data dredging. Multiple hypotheses can be analyzed with multivariate analysis and the risks noted in Chapter 14 should be considered when analyzing these studies. The investigation should be a direct test of the hypothesis. Occasionally it is easier and cheaper to test a substitute hypothesis. For example, drug A is studied to determine its effect in reducing cardiovascular mortality, but what is measured is its effect on exercise-stress-test performances, coronary-artery blood flow, or cholesterol level. Those outcomes are not necessarily related to cardiovascular (or all-cause) mortality, the outcome in which most patients are interested.

Inclusion and exclusion criteria

Inclusion and exclusion criteria for subjects should be clearly spelled out so that anyone reading the study can replicate the selection of patients. It ought to be sufficiently broad to allow generalization of the study results from the study sample to a large segment of the population (**external validity**). The source of patients should minimize sampling or referral bias. A full list of exclusions, reasons why people are not allowed to be study subjects, should be given. Commonly accepted exclusions are patients with rapidly fatal diseases that are unrelated to the study, those with absolute or relative contraindications to the therapy, and those unlikely to be followed up (how this was determined must be defined). The reasons for exclusion should have face validity. A full list of the numbers of patients and reasons for their exclusion should be presented. Beware if too many subjects are excluded without sound reasons.

Randomization

The main purpose of randomization is to create study groups that are equivalent in every way except for the intervention. Proper randomization means subjects have an equal chance of inclusion into any of the study groups. By making them as equal as possible the researcher seeks to limit potential **confounding variables** or those associated with both the cause and effect. If these factors are equally distributed in both groups, bias is minimized.

Randomization schemes that have the potential for bias are the date of admission to hospital, location of bed in hospital (Berkerson's bias), and common physical characteristics such as color of eyes, or day of birth. The first table in most research papers is a comparison of baseline variables of the study and control groups. This documents the adequacy of the randomization technique. Statistical tests should be done to show the absence of statistically significant differences between groups. Remember that the more characteristics looked at, the higher the likelihood that one of them will show differences between groups, by chance alone. The characteristics listed in "Table 1" should be the most important ones or those most likely to confound the results of the study.

Blinding

Allocation of patients to the randomization scheme should be **concealed**. This means that the process of randomization is completely blinded. If a researcher knew to which study group the next patient was going to be assigned, it would be possible to withhold that patient or switch their group assignment. This can have profound effects on the study, acting as a form of selection bias. Patients who appeared to be sicker could be assigned to the study group preferred by the researcher, resulting in poorer or better results for that group. Current practice requires that the researcher states whether allocation was concealed. If this is not stated, it should be assumed that it was not done and the effect of that bias assessed.

Blinding prevents confounding variables from affecting the results of a study. If all subjects, treating clinicians, and observers are blinded to the treatment being given during the course of research, any subjective changes are minimized. No

Table 15.2. Effects of acupuncture on short-term outcomes in back pain

Type of study	Number of trials	Improved with acupuncture (%)	Improved with control (%)	Relative benefit (95 % CI)	NNT (95% CI)
Blinded	4	73/127 (57)	61/123 (50)	1.2 (0.9 to 1.5)	13 (5 to no benefit)
Non-blinded	5	78/117 (67)	33/87 (38)	1.8 (1.3 to 2.4)	3.5 (2.4 to 6.5)

matter how pure at heart and honest, researchers may subconsciously tend to find what they want to find. Blinding prevents observer bias, contamination, and cointervention bias in either group. Lack of blinding can lead to finding an effect where none exists, or vice versa.

A recent review of studies of acupuncture for low back pain found that there was a dramatic effect of blinding (yes, it is tricky, but can be done) on the results of the studies. The non-blinded studies found acupuncture to be relatively useful for the short-term treatment of low back pain with a very low NNT. However, when blinded studies were analyzed, no such effect was found and the results (presented in Table 15.2) were not statistically significant. [1]

Description of methods

The intervention must be well described, including dose, frequency, route, precautions, and monitoring. The intervention must be one that is reasonable in terms of current practice. If a non-standard therapy is being compared to the intervention being tested, the results will not be applicable or generalizable. The availability, practicality, cost, invasiveness, and ease of use of the intervention will also determine the generalizability of the study. If the intervention requires special monitoring it may be too expensive and difficult to carry out and therefore, impractical in most ordinary situations.

Instruments and measurements should be evaluated using the techniques discussed in Chapter 7. Search the methods section for potential sources of bias. The appropriate outcome measures should be clearly stated. The way these are measured should be reproducible and free of bias. Blinded observers should record the ideal objectively measured outcomes. Subjective outcomes don't automatically invalidate the study and observer blinding can minimize any bias from subjective outcomes. The measurements should be made in a manner that assures consistency and some objectivity in the way the results are recorded. Beware of composite outcomes, subgroup analysis, and post-hoc cut-off points.

[1] E. Ernst & A. R. White. Acupuncture for back pain: a meta-analysis of randomised controlled trials. *Arch. Intern. Med.* 1998; 158: 2235–2241.

The study should be clear about the method, frequency, and duration of patient follow-up. All patients who began the study should be accounted for at the end of the study. Patients may leave the study for important reasons related to treatment or outcome including those who died as well as those who refused to continue because of complications, ineffectiveness, or compliance issues. While a study attrition rate of > 20% is a rough number that may invalidate or bias the final results even a smaller percentage of patient drop-outs may affect the results of a study if not taken into consideration. The results should be analyzed with an intention-to-treat analysis or using a best case/worst case analysis.

Analysis of results

The preferred method of analysis of all subjects when there has been a significant drop-out or crossover rate is to use an intention-to-treat methodology. In this method, all patient outcomes are counted with the group to which the patient was originally assigned even if the patient dropped out or switched groups. This approximates real life where some patients drop out or are non-compliant for various reasons. Removing patients after randomization for reasons associated with the outcome (e.g., they have advanced stages of the disease not likely to respond as well to therapy) is patently biased and grounds to invalidate the study. Leaving them in the analysis as an intention to treat is honest and won't inflate the results.

A good example of intention-to-treat analysis was in a study of survival after treatment for prostate cancer. The group randomized to surgery (radical prosta-tectomy, or complete removal of the prostate gland) did much better than the group randomized to either radiation therapy or watchful waiting (no treatment). Some patients who were initially randomized to the surgery arm of the trial were switched to the radiation or watchful waiting arm of the trial when, during the surgery, it was discovered that they had advanced and inoperable disease. These patients should have been kept in their original group (surgery) even though their cancerous prostates were not removed. When the study was re-analyzed using an intention-to-treat analysis, the survival in all three groups was identical. Removing those patients biased the original study results since patients with similarly advanced cancer spread were not removed from the other two groups.

In the best case/worst case analysis, the results are re-analyzed considering that all patients who dropped out or crossed over had the best outcome possible or worst outcome possible. This should be done by adding the drop-outs of the intervention group to the successful patients in the intervention group and at the same time subtracting the dropouts of the comparison group from the successful patients in that group. The opposite (subtracting from the intervention group and adding to the comparison group) should then be done. This will give a range of possible values of the final effect size. If this range is very large, we say that the results are **sensitive** to small changes that could result from drop-outs or crossovers. If the range is very small, we call the results **robust**, as they are not likely to change drastically because of drop-outs or crossovers.

Compliance with the intervention should be measured and noted. Lack of compliance may influence outcomes since the reason for non-compliance may be directly related to the intervention. High compliance rates in studies may not be duplicated in clinical practice. Other **clinically important outcomes** that should be measured include adverse effects, cost, invasiveness, and monitoring of an intervention. An independent observer should measure these outcomes. If the outcome is not objectively measured, it may limit the usefulness of the therapy. Remember, no adverse effects among n patients could signify as many as $3/n$ events in actual practice.

Results should be interpreted using the techniques discussed in chapters on statistical significance (Chapters 9–12). Look for both statistical and clinical significance. Look at confidence intervals and assess the precision of the results. Narrow CIs are indicative of precise results while wide CIs are imprecise. Determine for yourself if any positive results could be due to Type I errors. For negative studies determine the relative likelihood of a Type II error.

Discussion and conclusions

The discussion and conclusions should be based upon the study data and limited to settings and subjects with characteristics similar to the study setting and subjects. Good studies will list weakness of the current research and offer directions for future research in the discussion section. The author should compare the current study to other studies done on the same intervention or with the same disease.

In summary, no study is perfect, all studies have flaws, but not all flaws are fatal. After evaluating a study using the standardized format presented in this chapter, you must decide if the merits of a study outweigh the flaws before accepting the conclusions as valid.

Further problems

A study published in *JAMA* in February 1995 reviewed several systematic reviews of clinical trials, and found that if the trials were not blinded or the results were incompletely reported there was a trend to showing better results.[2] This highlights

[2] K. F. Schulz, I. Chalmers, R. J. Hayes & D. G. Altman. Empirical evidence of bias: dimensions of methodological quality associated with estimates of treatment effects in controlled trials. *JAMA* 1995; 273: 408–412.

Fig. 15.1 Effect of blinding and sample size on results in trials of acupuncture for low back pain. From E. Ernst & A. R. White. *Arch. Intern. Med.* 1998; 158: 2235—2241.

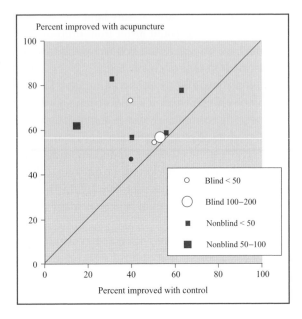

the need for the reader to be careful in evaluating these types of trials. Always look for complete randomization, total double blinding, and reporting of all potentially important outcomes. An example of this phenomenon can be seen in the systematic review of studies of acupuncture for back pain that was described earlier.

L'Abbé plots are a graphic technique for presenting the results of many individual clinical trials.[3] The plot provides a simple visual representation of all the studies of a particular clinical question. It is a way of looking for the presence of bias in the types of studies done on a single question. The plot shows the proportion of patients in each study who improved taking the control therapy against the proportion who improved taking the active treatment. Each study is represented by one point. The size of the circle around that point is proportional to the sample size of the study. In addition to getting an idea of the strength of the difference between the two groups, you can also look for the effects of blinding, sample size, or any other factor on the study results.

Fig. 15.1 shows the results of studies of the effectiveness of acupuncture on short-term improvements in back pain. The studies are divided by blinded vs. non-blinded and by size of sample. You can clearly see that the results of the blinded trials were less spectacular than the unblinded ones. The studies closest to the diagonal show the least effect of therapy.

---

[3] K. A. L'Abbé, A. S. Detsky & K. O'Rourke. Meta analysis in clinical research. *Ann. Intern. Med.* 1987; 107: 224–233.

The n-of-1 trial

An n-of-1 trial is done like any other experiment, but with only one patient as a subject. It is a useful technique to determine optimal therapy in a single patient when there appears to be no significant advantage of one therapy over another based on reported clinical trials. In order to justify the trial, the effectiveness of therapy must really be in doubt, the treatment should be continued long-term if it is effective, and the patient must be highly motivated to allow you to do an experiment on them. It is helpful if there is a rapid onset of action of the treatment in question and rapid cessation when treatment is discontinued. There should be easily measurable and clinically relevant outcome measures and sensible criteria for stopping the trial.

The patient should give informed consent before beginning the trial. You must have a willing pharmacist and pharmacy that can dispense identical, unlabeled active and placebo medications. Endpoints must be measurable with as much objectivity as possible. The patient should be asked if they knew which of the two treatments they were taking. A statistician should be available to help evaluate the results.[4]

A user's guide to the randomized clinical trial of therapy or prevention

The following is a standardized set of methodological criteria for the critical assessment of a randomized clinical trial article looking for the best therapy which can be used in your practice. It is based (with permission) upon the Users' Guides to the Medical Literature published by *JAMA*.[5] The University of Alberta (www.med.ualberta.ca.ebm) has online worksheets for evaluating articles of therapy that use this guide.

(1) **Was the study valid?**
    (a) Was the assignment of patients to treatments really randomized?
        (i) Was similarity between groups documented?
        (ii) Was prognostic stratification used in allocation?
        (iii) Was there allocation concealment?
        (iv) Were both groups of patients similar at the start of the study?
    (b) Were all patients who entered the study accounted for at its conclusion?
        (i) Was there complete follow-up of all patients?
        (ii) Were drop-outs, withdrawals, non-compliers, and those who crossed over handled appropriately in the analysis?

[4] For more information on the n-of-1 RCT, consult D. L. Sackett, R. B. Haynes, G. H. Guyatt & P. Tugwell. *Clinical Epidemiology: a Basic Science for Clinical Medicine.* 2nd edn. Boston, MA: Little Brown, 1991, pp. 225–238.
[5] G. Guyatt & D. Rennie (eds.). *Users' Guides to the Medical Literature: a Manual for Evidence-Based Practice.* Chicago: AMA, 2002. See also Bibliography.

    (c) Were the patients, their clinicians and the study personnel (recorders or measurers of outcomes) blind to the assigned treatment?

    (d) Were the baseline factors the same in both groups at the start of the trial?

    (e) Aside from the intervention being tested, were the two groups of patients treated in an identical manner?

        (i) Was there any contamination?

        (ii) Were there any cointerventions?

        (iii) Was the compliance the same in both groups?

(2) **What are the results?**

    (a) How large was the effect size and were both statistical and clinical significance considered? How large is the treatment effect?

        (i) If statistically significant, was the difference clinically important?

        (ii) If not statistically significant, was the study big enough to show a clinically important difference if it should occur?

        (iii) Was appropriate adjustment made for confounding variables?

    (b) How precise are the results? What is the size of the 95% confidence intervals?

(3) **Will the results help me care for my patient?**

    (a) Were the study patients recognizably similar to my own?

        (i) Are reproducibly defined exclusion criteria stated?

        (ii) Was the setting primary or tertiary care?

    (b) Were all clinically relevant outcomes reported or at least considered?

        (i) Was mortality as well as morbidity reported?

        (ii) Were deaths from all causes reported?

        (iii) Were quality-of-life assessments conducted?

        (iv) Was outcome assessment blind?

    (c) Is the therapeutic maneuver feasible in my practice?

        (i) Is it available, affordable, and sensible?

        (ii) Was the maneuver administered blind?

        (iii) Was compliance measured?

    (d) Are the benefits worth the costs?

        (i) Can I identify all the benefits and costs, including non-economic ones?

        (ii) Were potential harms considered?

Ethical issues

Finally, there are always ethical issues that must be considered in the evaluation of any study. Informed consent must be obtained from all subjects. This is a problem in some resuscitation studies, where other forms of consent such as substituted or implied consent may be used. Look for Institutional Review Board

(IRB) approval of all studies. If it is not present, it may be an unethical study. It is the responsibility of the journal only to publish ethical studies. Most journals will not publish studies without IRB approval. Decisions about whether or not to use the results of unethical studies are very difficult and beyond the scope of this book. As always, in the end, you must make your own ethical judgment about the research.

All the major medical journals now require authors to list potential conflicts of interest with their submissions. These are important to let the reader know that there may be a greater potential for bias in these studies. However, there is always potential for bias based upon other issues. These include the author's need to "publish or perish," desire to gain fame, and belief in the correctness of a particular hypothesis. A recent study on the use of bone-marrow transplantation in the treatment of stage 3 breast cancers showed a positive effect of this therapy. However, some time after publication, it was discovered that the author had fabricated some of his results, making the therapy look better than it actually was.

The question of placebo (Latin for "I will please") controls is one ethical issue which is constantly being discussed. Since there are therapies for almost all diseases, is it ever ethical to have a placebo control group? This is still a contentious area with strong opinions on both sides. One test for the suitability of placebo use is "clinical equipoise." If the clinician is unsure about the suitability of a therapy and there is no other therapy that works reasonably well to treat the condition, placebo therapy can be used. Both the researcher and the patient must be similarly inclined to choose either the experimental or a standard therapy. If this is not true, placebo ought not to be used.

16

Scientific integrity and the responsible conduct of research

John E. Kaplan, Ph.D.

Professor of Cardiovascular Sciences, Albany Medical College, New York, USA

> Physical science will not console me for the ignorance of morality in the time of affliction.
> But, the science of ethics will always console me for the ignorance of the physical sciences.
>
> Blaise Pascal (1623–1662)

Learning objectives

In this chapter you will learn:
- what is meant by "responsible conduct of research"
- how to be a responsible consumer of research
- how to define research misconduct and how it is dealt with
- how conflicts of interest may compromise research, and how they are managed
- why and how human participants in research studies are protected
- what constitutes responsible reporting of research findings
- how peer review works

The responsible conduct of research

The practice of evidence-based medicine requires high-quality evidence. A primary source of such evidence is from scientifically based clinical research. To be able to use this evidence you must be able to believe what you read. For this reason it is absolutely necessary that the research be trustworthy. Research must be proposed, conducted, reported, and reviewed responsibly and with integrity. Research and indeed the entire scientific enterprise are based upon trust. In order for that trust to exist the consumer of the biomedical literature must be able to assume that the researcher has acted responsibly and conducted the research honestly and objectively.

The process of science and proper conduct of evidence-based medicine are equally dependent on the consumption and application of research findings being conducted responsibly and with integrity. This requires readers to be knowledgeable and open-minded in reading the literature. They must know the factual base and understand the techniques of experimental design, research, and statistical analysis. It is as important that the reader consumes and applies research without bias as it is that the research is conducted and reported without bias. Responsible use of the literature requires that the reader be conscientious in obtaining a broad and representative, if not complete, view of that segment. Building one's knowledge-base on reading a selected part of that literature (e.g., abstracts) risks incorporating incomplete or wrong information and may lead to bias. Worse would be to act on pre-existing bias and selectively seek out or use only those studies in the literature that you agree with or that support your point of view, and to ignore those parts that disagree. It is, of course, essential that when one uses or refers to the work of others their contribution be appropriately referenced and credited.

The conduct and ethics of biomedical researchers began to receive increased attention after World War 2. This occurred in part as a response to the atrocities of Nazi medicine and in part because of the increasing rate of technological advances in medicine. This interest intensified in the USA in response to the publicity surrounding improper research practices, particularly the Tuskeegee syphilis studies, studies of the effects of LSD on unsuspecting subjects, and studies of radiation exposure. While these issues triggered important reforms the focus was largely restricted to protection of human experimental subjects.

The conduct of scientists again became an area of intense interest in the 1980s after a series of high-profile cases of scientific misconduct attracted the attention both of the public, through the media, and of the US Congress, which conducted a series of investigations and hearings. These included the misconduct cases regarding Robert Gallo, a prominent AIDS researcher, and Nobel Laureate David Baltimore. Even cases that were not found to be misconduct increased public and political interest in the behavior of researchers. This interest resulted in the development of federally prescribed definitions of scientific misconduct. There are now requirements that federally funded institutions adopt policies for responding to allegations of research fraud and protect the whistle-blowers. This was followed by the current requirement that certain researchers be given ethics training with funding from federal research training grants.

This initial regulation was scandal-driven and was focused on preventing wrong or improper behavior. As these policies were implemented it became apparent that this approach was not encouraging right or proper behavior. This new focus on fostering proper conduct by researchers lead to the emergence of the field now generally referred to as **responsible conduct of research**. This development is not the invention of the concept of scientific integrity, but it has significantly increased the attention bestowed on adherence to existing rules, regulations, guidelines, and commonly accepted professional codes or norms for the proper conduct of research. It has been noted that much of what constitutes responsible conduct of research would be achieved if we all adhered to the basic code of conduct we learned in kindergarten: "play fair, share, and tidy up."

Scientists behaving responsibly and with integrity constitute the first line of defense in assuring the truth and accuracy of biomedical research. It is important to recognize that the accuracy of scientific research does not depend upon the integrity of any single scientist or study. The process of science depends on findings being reproduced and reinforced by other scientists, a mechanism that protects against a single finding or study being uncritically accepted as fact. The process of peer review is another mechanism that further protects the integrity of the scientific record.

Research misconduct

Research or scientific misconduct represents events in which error is introduced into the body of scientific knowledge knowingly, through deception and misrepresentation. Research misconduct does not mean honest error or differences in opinion. Errors occurring as the result of negligence in the way the experiment is conducted are also not generally considered research misconduct. But they do fall outside the scope of responsible conduct of science guidelines.

In many respects research misconduct is a very tangible concept. This contrasts to other areas within the broad scope of responsible conduct of research. Both the agencies sponsoring research and the institutions conducting research develop policies to deal with research misconduct. This requires that a specific definition of research misconduct be developed. This effort has been fraught with difficulty and controversy and has resulted in a proliferation of similar but not identical definitions from various government agencies that sponsor research. Nearly all definitions agree that three concepts underlie scientific misconduct. These include **fabrication**, **falsification** and **plagiarism**. In a nutshell, definitions agree that scientists should not lie, cheat, or steal.

It is likely that the vast majority of scientists (and people in general) know that it is wrong to lie, cheat, or steal. This probably includes those who engage in such behavior. There are clearly numerous motivations that lead people to engage in such practices. These may include, but are not limited to, acting on personal or political biases, having personal financial incentives, personal and professional ambition, and fear of failure. In our system of research, the need for financial support and desire for academic advancement as measures of financial and professional success are dependent upon the productivity of a research program. Until there are some fundamental changes in the way research is funded, these questionable incentives are likely to remain in place.

The definition from the **National Institutes of Health**, the agency sponsoring most US-government-funded biomedical research, also includes a statement prohibiting "other serious deviations from accepted research practices." This statement is difficult to define specifically but reflects the belief that there are other behaviors besides fabrication, falsification, and plagiarism that constitute research misconduct.

A government-wide definition has been developed and is pending approval. According to this policy "research misconduct is defined as fabrication, falsification, or plagiarism in proposing, performing, or reviewing research, or in reporting research results." These three types of misconduct are defined as follows:

Fabrication is making up data or results and recording or reporting them.

Falsification is manipulating research materials, equipment, or processes, or changing or omitting data or results such that the research is not accurately represented in the research record.

Plagiarism is the appropriation of another person's ideas, processes, results, or words without giving appropriate credit.

Many people believe that a substantial amount of research misconduct goes unreported because of concerns that there will be consequences to the whistle-blower. All institutions in the USA that engage in federally supported research must now have in place formal policies to prevent retaliation against whistle-blowers. Unfortunately it is unlikely that you will be able to recognize scientific misconduct simply by reading a research study unless the misconduct is plagiarism of work you did or are familiar with. Usually such misconduct, if found at all, is discovered locally or in the review process.

Conflict of interest

Conflicts of interest may provide the motivation for researchers to act outside of the boundaries of responsible conduct of research. Webster's dictionary defines conflict of interest as "A conflict between the private interests and professional responsibilities of a person in a position of trust." A useful definition in the context of biomedical research and patient care was stated by D. F. Thompson who stated that "a conflict of interest is a set of conditions in which professional judgement concerning a primary interest (such as patient welfare or the validity of research) tends to be unduly influenced by secondary interest (such as financial gain)."[1] These relationships are diagrammed in Fig. 16.1. It is very important to recognize that conflicts of interest *per se* are common among people with complex professional careers. Simply having conflict of interest is not necessarily wrong and is often unavoidable. What is wrong is when one is inappropriately making

[1] D. F. Thompson. Understanding financial conflicts of interest. *N. Engl. J. Med.* 1993; 329: 573–576.

Fig. 16.1 Conflict of interest
schematic.

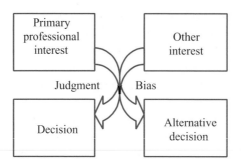

decisions founded on these conflicts or when one accepts a new responsibility (part-ownership of a clinical lab) to which one would defer over a previous professional interest (patient care). Decisions that are made based upon the bias produced by these other interests are especially insidious when they result in the compromise of patient care or in research misconduct.

Many of the rules regarding conflict of interest focus on financial gain, not because it is worse but because it is more objective and regulable. There is substantial reason for concern that financially based conflicts of interest have affected research outcomes. Recent studies of calcium channel blockers,[2] non-steroidal anti-inflammatory drugs,[3] and health effects of secondhand smoke[4] each found that physicians with financial ties to manufacturers were significantly less likely to criticize safety or efficacy. A study of clinical-trial publications[5] determined a significant association between positive results and pharmaceutical-company funding. Analysis of the cost-effectiveness of six oncology drugs[6] found that pharmaceutical company sponsorship of economic analyses led to a reduced likelihood of reporting unfavorable results.

Most academic institutions attempt to "manage" potential researcher conflict of interest. This is justified as an attempt to limit the influence of those conflicts and protect the integrity of research outcomes and patient-care decisions. Surprisingly some academicians have argued against such management on the grounds that it impugns the integrity of honest physicians and scientists. Some institutions have decided that limiting the opportunity for outside interests prevents recruitment and retention of the best faculty.

Nearly all academic institutions engaging in research currently have policies to manage and/or limit conflicts of interest. Most of these focus exclusively on

[2] H. T. Stelfox, G. Chua, K. O'Rourke & A. S. Detsky. Conflict of interest in the debate over calcium-channel antagonists. *N. Engl. J. Med.* 1998; 338: 101–106.
[3] P. A. Rochon, J. H. Gurwitz, R. W. Simms, P. R. Fortin, D. T. Felson, K. L. Minaker & T. C. Chalmers. A study of manufacturer-supported trials of nonsteroidal anti-inflammatory drugs in the treatment of arthritis. *Arch. Intern. Med.* 1994; 154: 157–163.
[4] R. M. Werner & T. A. Pearson. What's so passive about smoking? Secondhand smoke as a cause of atherosclerotic disease. *JAMA* 1998; 279: 157–158.
[5] R. A. Davidson. Source of funding and outcome of clinical trials. *J. Gen. Intern. Med.* 1986; 1: 155–158.
[6] M. Friedberg, B. Saffran, T. J. Stinson, W. Nelson & C. L. Bennett. Evaluation of conflict of interest in economic analyses of new drugs used in oncology. *JAMA* 1999; 282: 1453–1457.

financial conflicts and are designed primarily to protect the institutions financially. Increased awareness of the consequences of conflict of interest will hopefully result in the development of policies that offer protection to research subjects and preserve the integrity of the research record.

There are several ways that institutions choose to manage conflict of interest. The most common has been requiring disclosure of conflicts of interest with the rationale that individuals are less likely to act on conflicts if they are known. Other methods include limitations on the value of outside interests. Examples include limiting the equity a researcher could have in a company they work with or limiting the amount of consultation fees they can collect. Recently some professional organizations have suggested that the only effective management for potential conflicts of interest is their complete elimination.

Some of the most difficult conflicts occur when physicians conduct clinical studies where they enroll their own patients as research subjects. This can place the performance of the research and patient care in direct conflict. Another common area of conflict is in studies funded by pharmaceutical companies. Often they desire a veto in all decisions affecting the conduct and publication of the results.

Research with human participants

In order to obtain definitive information on the pathophysiologic sequelae of human disease, as well as to assess risk factors, diagnostic modalities, and therapeutic interventions, it is necessary to use people as research subjects. After several instances of questionable practices in studies using human subjects, the US Congress passed the **National Research Act** in 1974. One outcome of this legislation was the publication of the Belmont Report that laid the foundation of ethical principles which govern the conduct of human studies and provide protection for human participants. These principles are respect for personal autonomy, beneficence, and justice.

The principle of **respect for persons** manifests itself in the practice of **informed consent**. Informed consent requires that individuals be made fully aware of the risks and benefits of the experimental protocol and that they be fully able to evaluate this information. Consent must be fully informed and entirely free of coercion.

The principle of **beneficence** manifests itself in the **assessment of risk and benefit**. The aim of research involving human subjects is to produce benefits to either the research subject, society at large, or both. At the same time, the magnitude of the risks must be considered. The nature of experimental procedures generally dictates that everything about them is not known and so risks, including some that are unforeseen, may occur. Research on human subjects should only take place when the potential benefits outweigh the potential risks. Another way of looking at this is the **doctrine of clinical equipoise**. At the onset, the research aims (treatment and control) are equally likely to result in the best outcome. At the very least, the comparison group must be receiving a treatment consistent with the current standard of care.

The principle of **justice** manifests itself in the selection of research subjects. This principle dictates that the benefits and indeed the risks of research be distributed fairly within the population. There should be no favoritism shown when enrolling patients into a study.

The responsibilities for assuring that these principles are applied rest with **Institutional Review Boards** (IRBs). IRBs must include members of varying background, both scientific and non-scientific, who are knowledgeable of the institution's commitments and regulations, applicable law and ethics, and standards of professional conduct and practice. The IRB must approve both the initiation and continuation of each study involving human participants. The IRB seeks to insure that risk is minimized and reasonable in relation to the anticipated benefit or value of the knowledge gained.

The IRB evaluates whether selection of research subjects is equitable, and ensures that consent is informed and documented, that provisions are included to monitor patient safety, and that privacy and confidentiality are protected.

One of the most difficult roles for the physician is the potential conflict between patient care responsibilities and the objectivity required of a researcher. Part of the duty of the IRB ought to be an evaluation of the methodology of the research study. While many researchers disagree with this role, it assures that subjects (patients) are not subjected to useless or incompetently done research.

Peer review and the responsible reporting of research

Peer review and the responsible reporting of research are two important and related subjects that impact directly on the integrity of the biomedical research record. Peer review is the mechanism used to judge the quality of research and is applied in several contexts. This review mechanism is founded on the premise that a proposal or manuscript is best judged by individuals with experience and expertise in the field.

The two primary contexts are the evaluation of research proposals and manuscript reviews for journals. This mechanism is used by the National Institutes of Health and nearly every other nonprofit sponsor of biomedical research (e.g., American Heart Association, American Cancer Society) to evaluate research proposals. Nearly all journals also use this mechanism. In general you should be able to assume that journal articles are peer-reviewed. It is important to be aware of those that are not. You should have a lower level of confidence in research reported in journals that are not peer-reviewed. In general society-sponsored and "high-profile" journals are peer-reviewed. If you have doubts check the "information for authors" section, which should describe the review process.

To be a responsible peer reviewer one must be knowledgeable, impartial, and objective. It is not as easy as it might seem to meet all of these criteria. The more knowledgeable a reviewer is in the field of a proposal or manuscript the more likely they are to be a collaborator, competitor, or friend of the investigators. These factors, as well as potential conflicts of interest, may compromise their objectivity. Prior to publication or funding, proposals and manuscripts are considered privileged confidential communications that should not be shared. It is the responsibility of the reviewer to honor this confidentiality. It is similarly the responsibility of the reviewer not to appropriate any information gained from peer review into his or her own work.

As consumers and, perhaps, contributors to the biomedical literature we need research to be reported responsibly. Responsible reporting of research includes making each study a complete and meaningful contribution as opposed to breaking it up to achieve as many publications as possible. Also important is the making of responsible conclusions and issuing appropriate caveats on the limitations of the work. It is necessary to offer full and complete credit to all those who have contributed to the research, including references to earlier works. It is necessary always to provide all information that would be essential to others who would repeat or extend the work.

17

Applicability and strength of evidence

Find out the cause of this effect,
Or rather say, the cause of this defect,
For this effect defective comes by cause.

William Shakespeare (1564–1616): Hamlet

Learning objectives

In this chapter you will learn:
• the different levels of evidence
• the principles of applying the results of a study to a patient
The final step in the EBM process is the application of the evidence found to a patient. In order to do this, the reader of the medical literature must understand that all evidence is not created equal and that some forms of evidence are stronger than others. Once a cause-and-effect relationship is discovered, can you always apply it to your patient? What if your patient is of a different gender, socioeconomic, ethnic, or racial group than the study patients? This chapter will summarize these levels of evidence and help to put the applicability of the evidence into perspective. It will also help you decide how to apply lower levels of evidence to everyday clinical practice.

Applicability of results

Application of the results of a study is often difficult and frustrating for the clinician. You must consider the generalizability or particularizability of the results to your patient. Is a study of the risk of heart attack in men applicable to a woman in your practice? This means inducing the strength of a presumed cause-and-effect relationship in that patient based upon uncertain evidence. This is the essence of the art of medicine and is a blend of the available evidence, your clinical experience, the clinical situation, and the patient's preferences (Fig. 17.1).

Table 17.1. Criteria for application of results (in decreasing order of importance)

Strength of research design
Strength of result
Consistency of studies
Specificity (confounders)
Temporality (time–related)
Dose–response relationship
Biological plausibility
Coherence (consistency in time)
Analogous studies
Common sense

Source: After Sir Austin Bradford Hill. *A Short Textbook of Medical Statistics.* Oxford: Oxford University Press, 1977, pp. 309–323.

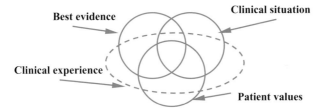

Fig. 17.1 The application of evidence to a particular clinical situation.

You must consider the strength of the evidence for a particular intervention or risk factor. The stronger the study, the more likely it is that those results will be borne out in practice. A well-done RCT with a large sample size is the strongest evidence for the efficacy of a practice in a defined population. However, these are very expensive and difficult to perform, and we often must make vital clinical decisions based upon less stringent evidence.

Sir Austin Bradford Hill, the father of modern biostatistics and epidemiology, developed a useful set of rules to determine the strength of causation based upon the results of a clinical study. These are summarized in Table 17.1.

Levels of evidence

Strength of the research design

The strongest design for evaluation of a clinical question is a systematic review (SR) of multiple randomized clinical trials. The studies in these reviews must be homogeneous and done with carefully controlled methodology. The process of data analysis is complex. This is the basis of the Cochrane Collaboration, a loose network of physicians who systematically review various topics and publish the results of their reviews. We will discuss these further in Chapter 31.

The randomized clinical trial with human subjects is the strongest single research design capable of proving causation. It is least likely to have methodological confounders and is the only study design that can show that altering the cause alters the effect. Confounding variables (recognized and unrecognized) can and should be evenly distributed between control and experimental groups (randomization), minimizing the likelihood of bias due to these differences. Ideally the study should be double-blinded. In studies with strong results, those results should be accompanied by narrow confidence intervals. Clearly, the strongest evidence is the RCT in the exact population that fits your patient. However, such a study is rarely available and we must use what evidence we can find, combined with our previous knowledge, to determine how the evidence produced by the study should be used.

The next best level of evidence comes from observational studies. The results of such studies may only represent association and can never prove that an intervention can change the effect. The strongest observational-study research design supporting causation is a cohort study. This can be done with either a prospective or a non-concurrent design. Cohort studies can show that cause precedes effect but not that altering the cause alters the effect. Bias due to unrecognized confounding variables between the two groups might be present and should be sought.

A case–control study is a weaker research design that can still support causation. Cause cannot be shown to precede effect and altering the cause cannot alter the effect. It is subject to many methodological problems that may bias the outcome. However, for uncommon and rare diseases or outcomes this may be the strongest evidence possible and can provide high-quality evidence if the study is done correctly.

Finally, case reports and descriptive studies (case series and cross-sectional studies) cannot prove cause and effect. They are only useful to suggest an association between two variables and point the way towards further directions of research. For very rare conditions, they can be the only and therefore the best source of evidence. This is true when they are the first studies to call attention to a particular disorder or phenomenon or when they are of the "all-or-none" type.

Hierarchies of research studies

There are several published hierarchies of classification for research studies. A system graded in levels I through V is one hierarchy that is the basis of the current grading scheme for clinical studies. This system grades studies by their overall quality and design. Level I studies are very large RCTs or systematic reviews. Level II studies are smaller RCTs (less than 50 subjects) or those with lower quality, or large high-quality cohort studies. Level III are smaller cohort or case–control studies. Level IV evidence comes from case reports and low-level case–control and cohort studies. Finally, Level V is expert opinion or consensus based upon experience, physiology, or biological principles. EBM resources must be evaluated on their own merits and should be peer-reviewed.

Another classification scheme uses levels A through D to designate the strength of the evidence. Grade A is the strongest evidence and D the weakest. These levels of evidence are cataloged for articles of therapy or prevention, etiology or harm, prognosis, diagnosis, decision and economic analyses. This scheme was developed at the Centre for Evidence-Based Medicine at Oxford University and is shown in Appendix 1. For studies of therapy or prevention, the following is a brief description of this classification.

Grade A is the strongest study design and consists of sub-levels 1a to 1c. 1a is systematic reviews with homogeneity, free of worrisome variations (hetero-geneity) in the direction and degree of the results between individual studies. Heterogeneity, whether statistically significant or not, does not necessarily disqualify a study and should be addressed on an individual basis. 1b is an individual randomized clinical trial with narrow confidence intervals. Trials or studies with wide confidence intervals should be viewed with care and would not qualify as A1b levels of evidence. Finally, the inclusion of the all-or-none case series as 1c evidence is somewhat controversial. They may be helpful for studying new, uniformly fatal, or very rare disorders, but should be viewed with care.

Grade B is the next level of strength of design and includes 2a, systematic reviews of homogeneous cohort studies; 2b, strong individual cohort studies or (weak) RCTs with < 80% follow-up; and 2c, "outcomes" research. Also included are 3a, systematic reviews of homogeneous case–control studies, and 3b, individual case–control studies.

Grade C has the weakest study designs and includes level 4, case series and lower-quality cohort and case–control studies. These studies fail clearly to define comparison groups or to measure exposures and outcomes in the same (preferably blinded) objective way in both groups, or to identify or appropriately control known confounding variables, or carry out a sufficiently long and complete follow-up of patients.

Finally, grade D is evidence not based upon any studies and is therefore the lowest level of evidence. Also called level 5, it consists of expert opinion without explicit critical appraisal. It is based solely upon personal experience, applied physiology, or the results of bench research.

These strength-of-evidence recommendations apply to "average" patients. The individual practitioner should modify them in light of a patient's uniqueness (risk factors, responsiveness, etc.) and preferences about the care they receive. A level that fails to provide a conclusive answer can be preceded by a minus sign −. This may occur because of wide confidence intervals that result in a lack of statistical significance but which fail to exclude a clinically important benefit or harm, or as a result of a systematic review with serious (and statistically significant) heterogeneity. Evidence with these problems is inconclusive and can only generate Grade C recommendations.

Strength of results

The actual strength of association or causation is the next important issue to consider. This refers to the clinical and statistical significance of the results. It is reflected in the magnitude of the effect size or the difference found between the two groups studied. The larger the effect size and lower the P value, the more likely that the results did not occur by chance alone and there is a real difference between the groups. Other common measures of association are odds ratios and relative risk: the larger they are, the stronger the association. A relative risk or odds ratio over 4 (or over 2 with very narrow confidence intervals) should be considered strong. Confidence intervals (CI) quantify the precision of the result. These give the potential range of this strength of association and should be routinely given in the study.

Even if the effect size, odds ratio, or relative risk is statistically significant, you must decide if this result is clinically important. Lower levels of RR or OR may be important in situations where the baseline risk level is fairly high. If the CI for these measures is overly wide, the results are less precise and therefore less meaningful. Finding no effect size or one that was not statistically significant may have occurred because of lack of power. The skew of the CI may give a subjective sense of the power of a negative study. Other measures of strength of association include the number needed to treat (NNT), obtained from randomized clinical trials, and the number needed to screen (NNS) and number needed to harm (NNH), obtained from cohort or case–control studies.

John Snow performed what is acknowledged as the first modern recorded epidemiologic study in 1854. Known as the Broad Street Pump study, he proved that the cause of a cholera outbreak in London was the pump on Broad Street. This was supplied by water from one company while a pump supplied by water from a rival company fed houses that had a much lower rate of infection. The relative risk (a term not used by John Snow) of death was 14, suggesting a very strong association between consumption of water from the tainted pump and death due to cholera. Similar high strengths of association have been found in the connection between smoking and lung cancer. Here the relative risk in heavy smokers is about 20. With results this high, competing hypotheses are unlikely and the course for the clinician should be obvious.

Consistency of evidence

The next feature to consider is the consistency of the results. There should be similar results from other studies of the same problem. It is critical that different researchers in different settings and at different times should have done research on this topic. If the effect size is similar in these studies, the evidence is stronger. Less consistency exists in those studies that use different research designs, clinical settings, or study populations.

A single study that shows results that are discordant from many other studies suggests the presence of bias in that study. However, sometimes a single large study will show a discordant result compared with multiple small studies. This may be due to lack of power (if the small studies were all negative) or differing methodology from study to study. Carefully evaluate the methodology of all the studies and use those studies with the best and least-biased methodology. In general, large studies result in more believable results. If a study is small, a change in the outcome status of one or two patients could change the study conclusion from positive to negative. For the association between smoking and lung cancer, prior to the 1965 Surgeon General's report, there were 29 retrospective and 7 prospective studies, all of which showed an association.

Specificity

The next characteristic to consider is the specificity of the results. Often the putative risk factor is confused with a confounding factor. In some circumstances another unrecognized factor called a surrogate marker may produce both cause and effect.

This can be a problematic feature of generalization as there are usually multiple sources of causation in chronic illness and multiple effects from one type of cause. For example, before the advent of milk pasteurization, there were many and diverse diseases associated with the consumption of milk. A few of these were tuberculosis, undulant fever, typhoid, and diphtheria. To attribute the cause of all these diseases to the milk ignores the fact that what they have in common is that they are all caused by bacteria. The milk is simply the vehicle and once the presence of bacteria and their role in human diseases was determined, it could be seen that ridding milk of all bacteria was the solution to preventing milkborne transmission of these diseases. The next step was inspecting the cows for those same diseases and eradicating them from the herd.

We can relate this to cancer of the lung in smokers. Overall the death rate in smokers is higher than in non-smokers. However, for most causes of death, the increase in death rate is about double (100%). For cancer of the lung, the increase in the death rate in smokers is almost 2000%, an increase of 20 times. This is more specific than the increased death rate for other diseases. In those other diseases, smoking is less of a significant factor, since there are multiple other factors that contribute to the death rate for those diseases. However, it is still a factor!

Temporal relationship

The next characteristic that should be considered is the temporal relationship between the purported cause and effect. There should be an appropriate temporal sequence of events found by the study. This should follow a predictable path from risk-factor exposure to the outcome. That pattern should be reproducible from study to study. It is also possible that the effect may produce the cause. For example, some smokers quit smoking just prior to getting sick with lung cancer. While they may attribute their illness to quitting, the illness was present long before they finally decided to quit. Is quitting smoking the "cause" and lung cancer the "effect," or neither? In this case, the cancer may be the cause and the cessation of smoking the effect. This may be difficult to determine in many cases, especially with slowly progressive and chronic diseases.

Dose–response

The dose–response gradient can help define cause and effect if there are varying concentrations of the cause and varying degrees of association with the effect. Usually, the association becomes stronger with increasing amounts of exposure. However, some cause-and-effect relationships show the opposite relationship, with increasing strength of association when exposure decreases. The relationship of vitamin intake with birth defects is an example of this. As the consumption of folic acid increased in a population, the incidence of neural tube birth defects decreased. The direction and magnitude of the effect should also show a consistent dose–response gradient. This can be demonstrated in randomized clinical trials and cohort studies but not in case–control or descriptive studies.

In general, we would expect that an increased dose or duration of the cause would produce an increased risk or severity of the effect. The more cigarettes smoked the higher the risk of lung cancer. The risk of lung cancer decreases among smokers who stop smoking as the time from giving up smoking increases. Some phenomena produce a J-shaped curve relating exposure to effect or outcome. In these cases the risk is higher at both higher and lower rates of exposure while it is lowest in the middle. A recent study of the effect of obesity on mortality showed a higher mortality among patients with the highest and lowest body mass index with the lowest mortality among people with the mid-range levels of body mass index.

Biological plausibility

When trying to decide on applicability, biological plausibility or consistency should be considered. The results of the study should be consistent with what we know about the biology of the body, cells, tissues, organs, etc., and with data from various branches of biological sciences. There should be some basic science (*in-vitro* or animal) studies to support the conclusions, and previously known biologic mechanisms should be able to explain the results. Is there a reason in biology that men and women smokers will have different rates of lung cancer? For some medical issues gender, ethnic group, or cultural background has a huge influence while for others the influence is very little. To determine which areas fall into each category requires more studies of gender and other differences for various medical interventions.

Coherence (or consistency) of the evidence over time

There should be coherence of the evidence over varying types of studies. The results of a cohort study should be similar to those of case–control or cross-sectional studies done on the same cause-and-effect relationship. Studies that show consistency with previously known epidemiological data are said to evidence epidemiological consistency. Results should agree with previously discovered relationships between the presumed cause and effect in studies done on other populations around the world. An association of high cholesterol with increased deaths due to myocardial infarction (heart attack) was noted in several epidemiological studies in Scandinavian countries. A prospective study in the USA found similar results. However, a potential confounding factor is the increase in cigarette smoking and related diseases in men after World War 1 and women following World War 2.

Analogy

Reasoning by analogy is one of the weakest criteria allowing generalization. Knowing that a certain vitamin deficiency predisposes women to deliver babies with certain birth defects will marginally strengthen the evidence that another vitamin or nutritional factor has a similar effect. The proposed cause-and-effect relationship is supported by findings from studies using the same methods but different independent or dependent variables. For example, multiple studies using the same methodology have demonstrated that aspirin is an effective agent for the secondary prevention of myocardial infarction (MI). From this one could infer that a potent anticoagulant like warfarin ought to have the same effect. However, it may increase mortality because of side effects and other factors. How about suggesting that warfarin use decreases the risk of stroke in patients who have had transient ischemic attacks (reversible strokes or TIAs), or MI in patients with unstable angina (worsening of a coronary pain syndrome)? Again, although it is suggested by the initial study, the proposed new intervention (warfarin) may not prove beneficial when studied alone for another indication.

Common sense

Finally, the association should make sense. Competing explanations associating risk and outcome should be ruled out. For instance, very sick patients are likely to do poorly even if given a very good drug. Conversely, if most patients with a disease do well without any therapy, it may be very difficult to prove that one drug is better than another (Pollyanna effect). In this case, an inordinately large number of patients would be necessary to prove a beneficial effect. The "overselling" of potent drugs may result in clinical researchers neglecting simpler, more common, cheaper, and better forms of therapy. Similarly, patients thinking that a new "wonder drug" will cure them may delay seeking care at a time when a potentially serious problem is easily treated and complications averted.

Finally, it is up to the individual physician to determine how a particular piece of evidence should be used in a particular patient. As I said earlier, this is the art of medicine. There are many that decry the slavish use of EBM in patient-care decisions. There are also those who demand that we use only the highest evidence. There is a middle ground. We must learn to use the best evidence in the most appropriate situations. There is a real need for more high-quality evidence for our practice. However, we must treat our patients now, with the highest-quality evidence available. I believe that we are in a period of rapid transition towards this goal and will continue in this mode until "all is known." This is longer from now than I care to predict.

18

An overview of decision making in medicine

Nothing is more difficult, and therefore more precious, than to be able to decide.

Napoleon I (1769–1821)

Learning objectives

In this chapter you will learn:

- how to describe the decision-making strategies commonly used in medicine
- the process of formulating a differential diagnosis
- how to define pretest probability of disease
- the common heuristics (modes of thought) which can aid or detract from good decision making
- the problem associated with premature closure of the differential diagnosis and some tactics to avoid that problem

This part of the book (Chapters 18 to 30) teaches the process involved in making a diagnosis, thereby determining the best course of treatment or management for your patient. First you will learn the principles of how to use diagnostic tests efficiently and effectively. Then we will present some mathematical techniques that can help the clinician make the most appropriate medical decisions for both individuals and populations of patients.

Medical decision making

Medical decision making is more complex now than ever before. The way you use clinical information will affect the accuracy of your diagnosis and ultimately the outcome for your patient. Incorrect or improper use of data will lead you (the physician) away from the correct diagnosis. It will also result in excess pain, suffering, and expense for your patient as well as increased cost and decreased efficiency of the health-care system.

Clinical diagnosis requires early hypothesis generation called the differential diagnosis. This is a list of plausible diseases from which the patient may be suffering, based upon the information gathered in the history and physical examination. Gathering more clinical data, usually obtained by performing (or ordering) diagnostic tests, refines this list.

However, using diagnostic tests without paying attention to their reliability (precision and reproducibility) and validity (measuring what is intended) can lead to poor decision making and ineffective care of the patient. We can measure the ability of each element of the history, physical examination, and laboratory and other diagnostic testing accurately to distinguish patients who have a given disease from those without that disease. The quantitative measure of this is expressed mathematically as the likelihood ratios of a positive or negative test. This tells us how much more likely a disease is if the test is positive or how much less likely if it is negative.

These diagnostic-test characteristics are relatively stable characteristics of a diagnostic test and must be considered in the overall process of diagnosis and management of a disease. The most commonly measured diagnostic-test characteristics are the sensitivity (ability of a test to find disease when present) and specificity (ability of a test to find a patient without disease among non-diseased people). Positive (test's ability to predict disease when it is positive) and negative predictive values (test's ability to predict lack of disease when it is negative) depend on the disease prevalence (percentage of people in a population with the disease), which is also called the pretest probability. The likelihood ratios can be used to adjust and revise the original diagnostic impression to come to a statistical likelihood of the final diagnosis, the post-test probability (likelihood of disease after doing the test). This can be calculated using a simple equation or nomogram.

The characteristics of tests can be used to find the treatment threshold (pretest probability above which we would treat without testing) and testing threshold (pretest probability below which we would neither treat nor test) for a particular disease and diagnostic test. Finally, the receiver operating characteristic (ROC) curves (graphs which summarize sensitivity and specificity over a series of cutoff values) are used to determine the overall value of a test, the best cutoff point for a test, and the best test when comparing two diagnostic tests.

More advanced mathematical constructs for making medical decisions involve the use of decision trees, which illustrate diagnostic and treatment pathways using branch points to help choose between treatment options. Ideally they will show the most effective care process. This is heavily influenced by patient values, which can be quantified for this process. Finally, the cost-effectiveness of a given treatment can be determined and it will help choose between treatment options when making decisions for a population.

Variation in medical practice and the justification for the use of practice guidelines

More than ever in the current health-care debate, physician decisions are being challenged. One major reason is that not all of these decisions are correct or even consistent. A recent study of managed care organization (MCO) physicians showed that only half of the physicians studied treated their diabetic and heart-attack patients with proven lifesaving drugs or tests. A recent estimate of medical errors suggested that up to 98 000 deaths per year in the USA were due to preventable medical errors. This leads to the perception that many physician decisions are arbitrary and highly variable.

Several studies done in the 1970s showed a marked geographic variation in the rate of common surgeries. In Maine, hysterectomy rates varied from less than 20% in one county to greater than 70% in another. This was true despite similar demographic patterns and physician manpower in the two counties. Studies looking at prostate surgery, heart bypass, and thyroid surgery show variation in rates of up to 300% in different counties in New England. Among Medicare patients, rates for many procedures in 13 large metropolitan areas varied by greater than 300%. Rates for knee replacement varied by 700% and for carotid endarterectomies by greater than 2000%.

How well do physicians agree among themselves about treatment or diagnosis? Cardiologists given angiograms (x-rays with contrast showing coronary artery anatomy) could not reliably agree upon whether there was a blockage. Sixty percent disagreed on whether the blockage was at a proximal or distal location. There was a 40% disagreement on whether the blockage was greater or less than 50%. In another study, the same cardiologists disagreed with themselves from 8% to 37% of the time when re-reading the same angiograms. Given a hypothetical patient and asked to give a second opinion about the need for surgery, half of the surgeons asked gave the opinion that no surgery was indicated. When asked about the same patient two years later, 40% had changed their mind.

Physicians routinely treat high intraocular pressure because if intraocular pressure is high it could lead to glaucoma and blindness. How high must the intraocular pressure be in order to justify treatment? In 1961 the ophthalmologic textbooks said 24 mm Hg. In 1976 it was noted to be 30 mm Hg without any explanation or justification for this change based upon clinical trials.

Physician experts asked to give their estimate of the effect on mortality of screening for colon cancer varied from 5% to 95%. Heart surgeons asked to estimate the 10-year failure rates of implanted heart valves varied from 3% to 95%. These data suggest that physician decision making is not standardized. Evidence-based decision making in medicine, the conscientious application of the best possible evidence to each clinical encounter, can help us regain the confidence of the public and the integrity of the profession.

More standardized ways in which to practice can help reduce second-guessing of physician decisions. This commonly occurs with utilization review of physician decisions by MCOs or government payors. This can lead to rejection of coverage for "excess" hospital days or refusal of payment for recommended surgery or other (usually expensive) therapy. It also occurs in medical malpractice cases where an expert reviews care through a retrospective review of medical records. Second-guessing, as well as the marked variation in physician practices, can be reduced through the use of practice guidelines for the diagnosis and treatment of common disorders. When used to improve diagnosis, we refer to these guidelines as diagnostic clinical prediction rules.

A primary cause of physician variability lies in the complexity of clinical problems. Clinical decision making is both multifaceted and practiced on highly individualized patients. We can't know the outcomes of our decisions beforehand, but must act anyway. Clinical research is imperfect. In most situations, medical practices work (or seem to work) and are effective (or not harmful). In many situations, when something goes wrong, no one is at fault. Physicians are well-meaning and confront not only biological but also sociological and political variability. These include patient expectations, changing reimbursement policies, competition, malpractice threat, peer pressure, and incomplete information.

There are some barriers to the process of using best evidence in medical decision making. The quality of evidence is often only fair or poor. Some physicians believe that if there is no evidence from well-done randomized control trials, a practice should not be used. The lack of evidence is not equal to evidence of lack of effect. Most physicians gladly accept much weaker evidence, yet don't have the clinical expertise to put that evidence into perspective for that clinical encounter. They also may not be able to discern well-done RCTs or even observational studies from those that are heavily biased. This points up the need for clinical expertise as part of the EBM process.

Some of the reasons for the high degree of uncertainty in our decision making are noted in Table 18.1. We want some certainty before we are willing to use an intervention, yet tend to do what we learned in medical school or follow the actions of the average practitioner. The rationalization is that if everyone is doing the treatment it must be appropriate. Some physician treatment decisions are based on the commonness or severity of the disease. If a disease is common, or the outcome severe, we are more willing to use whatever treatment is available. There are even times when physicians feel the need simply to do something, and the proposed treatment is all we have. There is also a certain amount of novelty or technical fascination with some diagnostic or treatment modalities that result in wholesale increases in usage.

One way we can do better is by having better clinical research and improved quality of evidence for clinical decisions. We must also increase our ability to use

Table 18.1. Causes of variability in physician performance

(1) **Complexity of clinical problem**	multiple factors influence actions
(2) **Uncertainty of outcomes** **of decisions**	variability of outcomes in studies
(3) **Need to act**	feeling on our part that we have to "do something"
(4) **Large placebo effect**	spontaneous cures (sometimes doing nothing but educating is the best thing)
(5) **Patient expectations**	expectation from patients and society that what we do will work
(6) **Political expectations**	do what is cheapest and best
(7) **Malpractice threat**	don't make any mistakes
(8) **Peer pressure**	do things the same way that other physicians are doing them
(9) **Technological imperative**	we have a new technology so let's use it

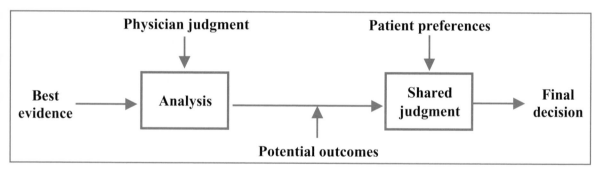

Fig. 18.1 Anatomy of a decision.

the available evidence through improving individual and collective reasoning and actions. Fig. 18.1 shows the anatomy of a clinical decision, a simplified look at decision making in general and the factors that influence the process. Reduction of error in the decision-making process requires better training of physicians in all three parts of EBM: evaluating the evidence, understanding the clinical situation, and having good patient communications. Another way to reduce error is by "automating" the decision process. If there is good evidence for a certain practice, it ought to be done all the time in that (best) way. Practice guidelines are one way of automating part of the decision-making process for physicians.

In 1910 Abraham Flexner asked physicians and medical schools to stop teaching empiricism and rely on solid scientific information. In those days, empiric "facts" were usually based on single-case testimonials or poorly documented case presentations. He proposed teaching and applying the pathophysiological approach to diagnosis and treatment. The medical establishment endorsed this, and the modern medical school was born. Currently we are in the throes of a new paradigm shift. In some ways this involves a return to empiricism. We want to see the evidence (empirical data) and ought to act only on evidence that is of high quality.

The clinical examination (history and physical)

In most cases in medicine, a patient does not walk into your office and present with a pre-made diagnosis. They arrive with a series of signs and symptoms that you must interpret for them (to make a diagnosis). When you have correctly done this, you can determine the best course of action (decide on the best treatment). The process by which this occurs begins with the clinical examination. Traditionally this consists of several components collectively called the history and physical or H&P (Table 18.2).

The chief complaint is the stated reason that the patient comes to medical attention in the first place. It is often the disorder of their normal functioning that alarms the patient and tells the physician in which systems to look for the pathology.

The history of the present illness is a chronological description of the chief complaint. The physician seeks to determine the onset of the symptoms, their quality, frequency, duration, associated symptoms, and exacerbating and alleviating factors. For a chief complaint of chest pain, the acronym PQRST stands for Position, Quality, Radiation, Severity, and Timing. A brief review of symptoms of dysfunction in systems that could be associated with the potential disease is included in this part of the H&P. It is important to include all the pertinent positives and negatives in reporting the history of the present illness.

The past medical history, family history, social and occupational history, and the medication and allergy history are all designed to get a picture of the patient's medical and social background. This puts the illness into the context of the patient's life. The accuracy and adequacy of this part of the history is extremely important. It appears to some that this is the most important part of the practice of "holistic" medicine, the process of looking at the whole patient and his or her environment. It must be an integral part of any medical history.

The review of systems gives the physician an overview of any additional medical conditions that the patient has. These may or may not be related to the chief

Table 18.2. Components of the H&P (with a clinical example)

Chief complaint	Why the patient sought medical care (e.g., coughing up blood, hemoptysis)
History of present illness	Description of symptoms: what, when, where, how much, etc. (e.g., coughing up spots of bright red blood four or five times a day for three days associated with some shortness of breath, fever, poor appetite, occasional chest pain, and fatigue)
Past medical history	Previous illness and operations, medications and allergies, including herbal, vitamin, and supplement use (e.g., seizure disorder, on phenytoin daily, no operations or allergies)
Family and social histories	Hereditary illness, habits and activities, diet, etc. (e.g., iv drug abuser, homeless, poor diet, adopted and does not know about his or her family medical history)
Review of systems	Review of all possible symptoms of all bodily systems. (e.g., recent weight loss and night sweats for the past three weeks, occasional indigestion)
Physical examination	(e.g., somewhat emaciated male in minimal respiratory distress, cervical lymphadenopathy, dullness to percussion at right upper lobe area and few rales in this area, multiple skin lesions consistent with needle marks and associated sclerosis of veins, remainder of examination normal)

complaint. It helps to give the physician other hypotheses to look into as being the cause of the patient's problem. It also gives the physician more insight into the patient's overall well-being, attitudes towards illness, and comfort level with various symptoms.

Finally, the physical examination is an attempt to elicit objective signs of disease in the patient. The physical exam usually helps to confirm or deny the physician's suspicions based upon the history.

An old adage states that in 80% of patients the final diagnosis comes solely from the history. In another 15% it comes from the physical examination, and only in the remaining 5% from additional diagnostic testing. This may appear to overstate the value of the history and physical, but not by much.

Clinical observation is a powerful tool for deciding what diseases are possible in a given patient, and most of the time the results of the H&P determine which additional data to seek. The clinician must know how to obtain the required data in a reliable and accurate way by using diagnostic tests appropriately to achieve the best outcome for the patient. For the health-care system, this must also be done at a reasonable cost not only in dollars, but also in patient lives, time, and anxiety if an incorrect diagnosis is made.

Hypothesis generation in the clinical encounter

While performing the H&P the clinician develops a set of hypotheses about what diseases could be causing the patient's problem. This list is called the differential diagnosis and some diseases on this list are more likely than others to be present in that patient. When finished with the H&P, the clinician estimates the probability of each of these diseases in this patient and rank-orders this list. The probability of a patient having a particular disease on that list is referred to as the prior probability (a-priori or pretest probability) of disease. It may be equivalent to the prevalence of that disease in the population of patients with the same or a similar result on the medical history and physical examination.

The numbers for pretest probability come from your knowledge of medicine and from studies of disease prevalence in the medical literature. Let's use the example of a 50-year-old alcoholic with no history of liver disease who presents to an emergency department in North America with digested blood in the stool (melena or black tarry stools). This symptom is likely caused by varices of the esophagus (dilated veins in the esophagus), by gastritis (inflammation of the stomach), or by an ulcer of the stomach. The prevalence in this population (pretest probability) for varices is 5%, for ulcer 55%, and for gastritis 40%. In this case the probabilities add up to 100% since there are virtually no other diagnostic possibilities. A rare person fitting this description will turn out to have gastric cancer, which occurs in much less than 1% of patients like this and can be left off the list for the time being. If none of the other diseases turn out to be correct, then you need to look for this rare disease. In this case a single diagnostic test, upper gastrointestinal endoscopy, is the test of choice for all four diagnostic possibilities and would address the issue outright.

There are other situations where the presenting history and physical are much more "vague" and non-specific. In these cases, it is very likely that the total pretest probability can add up to more than 100%. This occurs because of the desire on the part of the physician not to miss an important disease. Therefore each disease must be considered by itself when determining the probability of its occurrence. In our desire not to miss an important disease, probabilities that may be much greater than the true prevalence of the disease in the population will be assigned to each diagnosis on the list. Also, we must assume that any patient may have more than one cause of their symptoms. A patient with chest pain can have coronary artery disease and anxiety or panic disorder simultaneously. In general, anxiety or panic disorder is much more likely in a 20-year-old and coronary artery disease more likely in a 50-year-old. Here the pretest probabilities reflect

	Common presentation	Rare presentation
Common disease	90%	9%
Rare disease	0.9%	0.09%

Fig. 18.2 2×2 table view of pretest probabilities.

the likelihood of considering the disease in a single patient rather than the true prevalence.

Constructing the differential diagnosis

The differential diagnosis begins with diseases that are very likely and for which the patient has many of the classical symptoms and signs. These are also known as the leading hypotheses or working diagnoses. Next, diseases that are possible are included on the list if they are serious (potentially life- or limb-threatening) or easily treated. These are active alternatives to the leading hypothesis and must be ruled out of the list. This means we must be relatively certain from the H&P that they are not present. If not, we must do a diagnostic test that can reliably rule them out.

Next are diseases that are very unlikely and not serious, or are more difficult (and potentially dangerous) to treat, and which need not be immediately excluded, but ought to be kept in mind for future consideration if the initial working diagnosis turns out to be wrong. Initially these are excluded hypotheses, diseases that are possible based on the chief complaint but have already been ruled out by the history and physical.

When considering a diagnosis, it is helpful to have a framework for considering likelihood of each disease on your list. This depends upon the relative frequency with which a disease occurs. One schema for classifying this is shown in Fig. 18.2, which describes the overall probability of diseases using a 2×2 table. This only helps to get an overview and does not help you determine the pretest probability of each disease you are considering for the differential diagnosis on your patient. In this schema, each disease is considered as if the total probability of disease adds up to 100%. You must tailor the probabilities in your differential diagnosis to the patient in front of you at that moment. You should be less likely to consider a particular disease that is a common presentation of a rare disease, when the patient is more likely to present with a rare presentation of a common disease.

The first step in generating a differential diagnosis is systematically to make a list of all the possible causes of your patient's symptoms. This skill is learned through extensive study of diseases and clinical experience and practice. When

Table 18.3. Mnemonic to remember classification of disease for a differential diagnosis

V	Vascular
I	Inflammatory / Infectious
N	Neoplastic / Neurologic and psychiatric
D	Degenerative / Dietary
I	Intoxication / Idiopathic / Iatrogenic
C	Congenital
A	Allergic / Autoimmune
T	Trauma
E	Endocrine & metabolic

you first start doing this, it is useful to make the list as exhaustive as possible to avoid missing some disease. Think of all possible diseases by category or pathophysiologic process causing the disease. There are several helpful mnemonics that can get you started. One is VINDICATE (Table 18.3).

Initially list all possible diseases for a chief complaint by category. After you have created the list, assign a pretest (a-priori) probability for each item on the differential. The values of pretest probability are relative and can be assigned according to the scale shown in Table 18.4.

You must consider the ramifications of missing the diagnosis. If the disease is immediately life- or limb-threatening, it should be ruled out, virtually regardless of the probability you assign. We will use this schema for selecting pretest probabilities for the rest of the book.

For example, if you were in the emergency department and a 21-year-old man came in complaining of chest pain, you would first perform a complete history and physical examination. Following this you might suspect that anxiety or a pectoralis muscle strain are the cause of his pain. These would have very high pretest probabilities (50–90%). You also consider slightly less likely and more serious causes which are easily treatable such as pericarditis (inflammation of the pericardium), spontaneous pneumothorax (collapse of the lung due to a weakness of the lung tissue and leak of air into the pleural space), pneumonia (infection of the lung tissue), or esophageal spasm secondary to reflux of stomach acid into the esophagus. These would have variably lower pretest probabilities (1–50%). Next, there are hypotheses that are very much less likely such as myocardial infarction (heart attack), dissecting thoracic aortic aneurysm (tear of the inside wall of the aorta), and pulmonary embolism (blood clot in the lungs). The

Table 18.4. Useful schema for assigning pretest (a-priori) probabilities

Pretest probability		Action	Interpretation
	<1%	Off the list – for now	**Rare disease** (rare presentation)
	1%	Can't exclude, but very unlikely (effectively **ruled out**)	**Rare disease** (common presentation)
Low	10%	Should be **ruled out**	**Common disease** (rare presentation)
	25%	Possible	
Moderate	50%	50–50 (toss-up)	
	75%	Probable	
High	90%	Very likely	**Common disease** (common presentation)
	99%	Almost certain – **ruled in**	
	99.9%	**Pathognomonic** – there is no other disease which will present like this. This is a unique presentation of this disease, and therefore the patient can only have this disease.	

pretest probabilities of these are less than 1%. And then, you must think of and consider some disorders such as lung cancer that are so rare and not immediately life- or limb-threatening that they are pretty much ruled out.

If you had a 39-year-old man with the same complaint (chest pain) and the pain was similar, but not typical of angina pectoris (squeezing, pressure-like pain in the chest characteristic of coronary artery disease) you could look up the pretest probability of coronary artery disease. You would find this in an article by Patterson, which would tell you that the probability he had this disease was about 22%.[1] This means that about 1/5 of all 39-year-old men with this presentation will have

---

[1] R. E. Patterson & S. F. Horowitz. Importance of epidemiology and biostatistics in deciding clinical strategies for using diagnostic tests: a simplified approach using examples from coronary artery disease. *J. Am. Coll. Cardiol.* 1989; 13: 1653–1665.

significant coronary artery disease. That would change your list and put myocardial infarction higher up on the list.

Making the differential diagnosis means considering diseases from three perspectives: likelihood of the disease (probability), severity of the disease (prognosis), and ease of treatment of the disease (pragmatism). The differential diagnosis is a complex interplay of these factors and the patient's signs and symptoms.

Narrowing the differential

Let's look at a more common, everyday example. You are examining a seven-year-old child who is sick with a sore throat. You suspect that this child might have strep throat, a common illness in children (high pretest probability of disease). This is your working diagnosis. Your differential diagnosis also includes another common disease, viral pharyngitis (inflammation of the pharynx caused by a virus). Also included are uncommon diseases like epiglottitis (severe and life-threatening inflammation of the epiglottis) and mononucleosis (another viral illness), and extremely rare diseases such as diphtheria and gonorrhea. The more serious (and in this example very uncommon) ones must be actively ruled out. In this case, that can almost certainly be done with an accurate history (lack of sexual abuse and oral–genital contact for gonorrhea) and physical examination (child is immunized and there is a lack of the typical "pseudomembrane" in the hypopharynx for diphtheria).

If you find none of the characteristic signs and symptoms of epiglottitis, mononucleosis, gonorrhea, or diphtheria your differential diagnosis narrows down to strep throat and viral pharyngitis. You apply a published decision rule to differentiate strep throat from viral pharyngitis. If it is positive, you treat for strep throat with antibiotics; if negative, you treat symptomatically for viral pharyngitis. If the rule comes up inconclusive you must consider doing a diagnostic test. Therefore, to make a final diagnosis, you decide to do a throat culture.

In this case, you believe that doing this test will make a difference. You must also decide what kind of culture to take, since the type of culture that will demonstrate strep is different from one that will grow gonorrhea. Since you know that gonorrhea is extremely rare in children, especially when there is no evidence of sexual abuse in the history, you decide against culturing the child for gonorrhea bacteria and do a strep throat culture.

You have just made several decisions about this child's illness. First, you set up a differential diagnosis (in descending order) and assigned a pretest probability to each disease on that list (Table 18.5). None of the diseases on the list had a pretest probability of 100%, so you decided to do some tests to determine which diagnosis was most likely. Additional tests must be done in order to rule in or out any disease not excluded in the original differential and important for us to

Table 18.5. Differential diagnosis of sample patient

Disease	Pretest probability of disease	
Streptococcal infection	50%	Likely, common, and treatable
Viruses	50%	Likely, common, and self-limiting
Mononucleosis	1%	Unlikely, uncommon, and self-limiting
Epiglottitis	<1%	Unlikely and uncommon
Gonorrhea	<<1%	Rare
Diphtheria	<<<1%	Very rare

Table 18.6. Relative costs of tests

Disease	Test	Cost
Streptococcal infection	Rapid strep antigen or throat culture	$
Viruses	Viral culture	$$$
Epiglottitis	Neck x-ray	$$
Mononucleosis	Epstein–Barr antigen test	$$
Diphtheria	Culture or diphtheria serology	$$$$
Gonorrhea	Gonorrhea culture	$$

diagnose. The tests vary in their cost – in dollars, ease of performance, patient discomfort, potential complications, and many other factors. For our example of a sore throat, these are listed in Table 18.6.

You must determine which of all these tests is worthy of doing in order to make the diagnosis most efficiently. This is determined by the cost (both money and other factors) of the test, the ability of the test to identify the clinical disease with accuracy, and whether identifying the test will make a difference for the patient. If the diagnosis were in question, a rapid strep antigen would be the test of choice to rule in or out strep throat. We usually don't do viral cultures since the treatment is the same whether the patient is known to have a virus or not.

For our 39-year-old man with chest pain, the differential diagnosis would initially include all the diseases (anxiety, musculoskeletal, aneurysm, pneumothorax, etc.) we listed. For anxiety and musculoskeletal causes, the pretest probability is pretty high, as these are common in this age group. In fact, the most likely cause of chest pain in a 39-year-old is going to be pain of musculoskeletal origin. For the other diseases on the list, their pretest probabilities would be approximately similar to that of coronary artery disease. However, because of the potential severity of heart disease and most of the other diseases on your differential, you will need to do some diagnostic testing to rule out that possibility. For some of them (pneumothorax, dissecting aortic aneurysm, and pneumonia) a single diagnostic test (chest x-ray) can rule them out if the test is normal. For others (coronary artery disease or pulmonary embolism) a more complex algorithmic scheme is necessary.

Strategies for making a medical diagnosis

There are several diagnostic strategies that clinicians employ when using patient data to make a diagnosis. These are presented here as unique methods even though most clinicians use a combination of them to make a diagnosis.

Pattern recognition is the spontaneous (instantaneous) recognition of a previously learned pattern. It is usually the starting point for creating a differential diagnosis and determines the diagnoses that will be at the top of the list. This method is employed by the seasoned clinician for most patients. Most of the time, an experienced clinician will be able to "sense" when the pattern is not characteristic of the disease (e.g., rare presentation of common disease or common presentation of a rare disease). A really experienced and "good" doctor knows when to look beyond the apparent pattern and when to search for clues that the patient is presenting with a rare or unusual disease. Premature closure of the differential diagnosis is a pitfall of pattern recognition that is more common to neophytes and will be discussed at the end of this chapter.

Multiple branching strategy is an algorithmic approach using a preset path with multiple branching nodes to lead to a correct final conclusion. Examples of this are diagnostic clinical guidelines or decision rules. They are tools to assist the clinician in remembering the steps to making a proper diagnosis. If they are simple, they are easily memorized and can be very useful. More complex diagnostic decision tools can be of greater help when used with a computer.

Strategy of exhaustion is also called diagnosis by possibility and involves "the painstaking and invariant search for (but paying no immediate attention to the importance of) all medical facts about the patient."[2] This is followed by carefully sifting through the data for a diagnosis. Although it will usually (much more often than not) come up with the correct diagnosis, the process is time consuming and not cost-effective. A good example of this can be found in the Case Records of the Massachusetts General Hospital feature found in each issue of the *New England Journal of Medicine*. This strategy is most helpful in diagnosing very uncommon diseases.

---

[2] D. L. Sackett, R. B. Haynes, G. H. Guyatt & P. Tugwell. *Clinical Epidemiology: a Basic Science for Clinical Medicine*. 2nd edn. Boston: Little Brown, 1991.

The hypothetico-deductive strategy is also called diagnosis by probability. This is the way diagnoses have typically been made in clinical medicine. It involves the formulation of a short list of potential diagnoses or actions from the earliest clues about the patient (differential diagnosis) followed by the performance of those clinical maneuvers and diagnostic tests that will increase or decrease the probability of each item on the list. This process may reduce or increase the length of the list. This is the best strategy to learn to use and will also lead to a correct diagnosis in most cases. Initial hypothesis generation is based on "triggering" or the use of pattern recognition to suggest certain diagnoses. Further refinement results in a shortlist of diagnoses and further testing or initiation of treatment will lead to the final diagnosis. A good example of this can be found in the Clinical Decision Making feature found frequently (but irregularly) in the *New England Journal of Medicine*.

Heuristics: how we think

Heuristics are cognitive shortcuts used in prioritizing diagnoses. They help you deal with the magnitude and complexity of clinical data. They are not always helpful but you should recognize the way you use them in order to solve problems effectively and prevent clinical mistakes. There are three important heuristics that are used in medical diagnosis. They are representativeness, availability, and competing hypotheses heuristics.

    Representativeness heuristic. The probability that a diagnosis is thought of is based upon how closely its essential features resemble the essential features of a typical (textbook) description of the disease. This is the process of pattern recognition and works fine if you have seen many atypical as well as typical cases of common diseases. It can lead to erroneous diagnosis if you initially think of rare diseases based upon the patient presentation. Because the child's sore throat is described as very severe, you immediately think of gonorrhea which you remember as being particularly painful. The pain of the sore throat represents gonorrhea in your diagnostic thinking. You ignore or minimize the more common causes of sore throat, thinking of a rare disease more often than a common one. Remember: unusual or rare presentations of common diseases (strep throat) occur more often than common presentations of rare diseases (pharyngeal gonorrhea).

    Availability heuristic. The probability of a diagnosis is judged by the ease with which the diagnoses is remembered. The diagnoses of patients you most recently cared for are the ones most easily remembered and brought to the forefront of your consciousness. This can be thought of as a form of recall bias. If you recently took care of a patient with a sore throat who had gonorrhea,

Fig. 18.3 Hypothetico-deductive strategy using anchoring and adjustment.

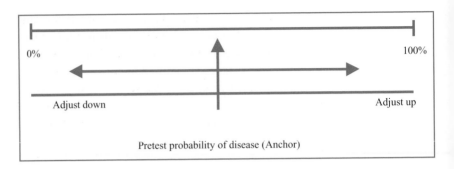

you will be more likely to look for that cause of sore throat in the next patient (or series of patients) even though this is a very rare cause of sore throat. The availability heuristic is much more problematic and likely to occur if the missed diagnosis was of a rare and serious disease.

Anchoring and adjustment. The special characteristics of a patient are used to estimate the probability of a given diagnosis. Additional information is used to adjust the probability of disease up or down. This is the way we think about most diagnoses. Your patient presents with a sore throat. You think of common causes of sore throat and come up with diagnoses of either a viral pharyngitis or strep throat (anchor). After getting more history and doing a physical examination you decide that the characteristics of the sore throat are more like a viral pharyngitis than strep throat (adjustment), and other diagnoses are extremely unlikely. This adjustment is based on more diagnostic information from the H&P and diagnostic tests. The process is shown in Fig. 18.3. This is also called the **competing hypotheses heuristic**. New information is compared against all diagnoses being considered to change the probability estimates for each diagnosis on the list. The differential diagnosis list is then reordered and new hypotheses generated, which are again tested when more new information (diagnostic tests) is gathered. This is contrasted to searching for all signs and symptoms known to be associated with a given diagnosis and then moving on to the next possible diagnosis, the strategy of exhaustion.

The problem of premature closure of the differential diagnosis

One of the most common problems novices have with diagnosis is that they are unable to recognize atypical patterns. This common error in diagnostic thinking occurs when the novice jumps to the conclusion that a pattern exists when it doesn't. There is a tendency to attribute illness to a common and often less serious problem rather than search for a less likely, but potentially more serious illness. This is called premature closure of the differential diagnosis. It represents removal from consideration of many diseases from the differential diagnosis list because the clinician jumped to an early conclusion on the nature of the patient's illness.

Sadly this phenomena is not limited to neophytes. Even experienced clinicians can make this mistake, thinking that a patient has a common illness when in fact it is a more serious but less common one. No one expects the clinician to always immediately come up with the correct diagnosis of a rare presentation of a rare disease. However, the key to good diagnosis is recognizing when a patient's presentation or response to therapy is not following the pattern that was expected.

This can be avoided by following two simple rules. The first is always to include a healthy list of possibilities in the differential diagnosis for any patient. Don't be seduced with an apparently obvious diagnosis. When you find yourself diagnosing the patient within the first minutes of the history (a common occurrence), step back and look for other clues that could dismiss that diagnosis and add others to the list. Then ask yourself whether you can exclude those other diseases simply through the history and physical examination. Since most common diseases do occur commonly, in many cases the common disease you first thought of will turn out to be correct. However, you will be more likely to miss important clues of the presence of another (and less common disease) if you focus only on that diagnosis.

The second step is to avoid modifying the final list until you have collected all the relevant information. When you have completed the history, make a detailed and objective list of all the diseases for consideration and determine their relative probabilities. The formal application of such a list will be invaluable for the novice (student and intern) and will be done in a less and less formal way by the expert. Again, looking for clues of the presence of other diseases will help avoid this error.

19

Sources of error in the clinical encounter

Here is my secret, it is very simple: it is only with the heart that one can see rightly; what is essential is invisible to the eye.

Antoine de Saint-Exupéry (1900–1944): The Little Prince

Learning objectives

In this chapter you will learn:
- the measures of precision in clinical decision making
- how to identify potential causes of "clinical disagreement" and inaccuracy in the clinical examination
- strategies for preventing error in the clinical encounter

The clinical encounter between doctor and patient is the start of the process of medical decision making. This is where the physician has the opportunity to gather the most accurate information about the nature of the illness and the meaning of that illness to the patient. If this is not done well and there are errors made in processing this information, the resulting decisions may be wrong and not in the patient's best interests. This can lead to over-, under- and misuse of therapies and increased error in medical practice.

Measuring clinical consistency

Precision is synonymous with consistency and is the extent to which multiple examinations of the same patient or specimen agree with one another. Each part of the clinical examination should be accurately reproducible by a second examiner. Accuracy is the closeness of a given clinical observation to the true clinical state. The synthesis of all the clinical findings should represent the actual clinical or pathophysiological derangement possessed by the patient.

If two people measure the same parameter several times, for instance the temperature of a sick child, we can determine the consistency of this measurement. The kappa statistic is a statistical measurement of the precision of a clinical finding and measures inter-observer consistency between measurements. Different observers can obtain different results when they measure the temperature of a child using a thermometer because they use slightly different techniques (time thermometer left in the patient) or different ways to read the mercury level. Kappa can also measure intra-observer consistency, the ability of the same observer to reproduce a measure.

We often assume that all diagnostic tests are precise. Many studies have demonstrated that most non-automated tests have some some degree of subjectivity in their interpretation. This has been seen in commonly used x-ray tests such as CT scan, mammography, and angiography. It is also present in tests commonly considered to be the gold standard such as the interpretation of tissue samples from biopsies or surgery. The kappa statistic is described in detail in Chapter 7 and should be calculated and reported in any study of the usefulness of a diagnostic test.

There are many potential sources of error and clinical disagreement in the process of the clinical examination. If the examiner is not aware of these, they will lead to incorrect and inaccurate data. A broad classification of these sources of error includes the examiner, the examinee and the environment.

The examiner

Tendencies to record inference rather than evidence

The examiner should record actual findings (both subjective ones told you by the patient and objective ones detected by your own senses) and not make assumptions about the meaning of these findings. In examining a patient's abdomen if you feel a mass in the right upper quadrant and record that you felt the gall bladder, you may be incorrect, and in fact the mass could be a liver cancer.

Ensnarement by diagnostic classification schemes

Jumping to conclusions about the nature of the diagnosis based on an incorrect coding scheme. If you hear wheezes in the lungs and assume that the patient has asthma or emphysema when in fact they have congestive heart failure (all of which can cause wheezing) you will make a serious error. The diagnosis of heart failure can be made from other features of the history and clues in the physical exam.

Entrapment by prior expectation

Jumping to conclusions about the diagnosis based upon a first impression of the chief complaint without considering other diagnoses. Also called premature closure of the differential diagnosis, and discussed in Chapter 18. If you examine a patient who presents with a sore throat, fever, aches, nasal congestion, and cough and think it is a cold (upper respiratory infection), you may miss hearing the wheezes in the chest. This occurs because you didn't expect them to be present, and in fact the patient has acute bronchitis. The symptoms (wheezing and coughing) can be easily and effectively treated, but the therapy will be ineffective if the diagnosis is incorrect.

Bias

You bring an internal set of biases based upon your upbringing, schooling, training, and experiences to each clinical encounter. These biases can easily lead to erroneous diagnoses. If you assume without further investigation that a disabled man with alcohol on his breath is simply a drunk who needs a place to stay, you can easily miss a significant head injury. Denying pain medication to someone whom you think may be a drug abuser based upon his or her attitude or appearance will result in unnecessary suffering for the patient.

Biologic variations in the senses

Hearing, sight, smell, and touch will vary between examiners and will change with age of the examiner. As your hearing decreases, it will become harder for you to hear heart murmurs or gallop sounds.

Not asking

If you don't ask, you won't find out! Many clinicians don't ask newly diagnosed cancer patients about the presence of depression. At least one-third of cancer patients are depressed and treating this may make it easier to treat the cancer. It will also make the patient feel more in control and less likely to look for other methods of therapy (alternative or complementary medicine to the exclusion of proven chemotherapy). Many physicians don't ask a sexual history, about alcohol use, or domestic violence. They may be afraid of opening a Pandora's box. Most patients are reluctant to give important information spontaneously about these issues, and need to be asked in a non-threatening way. When asked in an honest and respectful manner, almost all are very pleased that you asked and will give you accurate and detailed information. This is part of the art of medicine.

Simple ignorance

You have to know what you are doing in order to be able to do it well. Poor history and physical examination skills will lead to incorrect diagnoses. If you don't know the significance of straight leg raising in the back examination, you won't do it or will do it incorrectly. This can lead to a missed opportunity to make a correct diagnosis of herniated lumbar disc on your patient.

Level of risk

You must be aware of your level of risk taking. This will directly affect the amount of risk you project on your patient. If you don't like taking risks yourself, you may try to minimize risk for your patient. If you don't mind taking risks, you may not try to minimize risk for your patient. Physicians can be classified by their risk-taking behavior into **risk minimizers** or **test minimizers**. Risk-taking physicians are less likely to admit patients with chest pain to the hospital than physicians who are risk averse.

Risk minimizers or risk-averse physicians tend to order more tests (or therapy) than might be necessary in order to minimize missing the diagnosis. They are more likely to order tests or recommend treatments when the risk of missing a diagnosis or the potential benefit from the therapy is small. Test minimizers may order fewer tests (or therapy) than might be necessary and thereby increase the risk of missing a diagnosis in the patient. This can make you less likely to recommend certain tests or treatments, thinking your patient would not want to take the risk associated with the test or therapy, but will be willing to take the risk associated with an error of omission in the process of diagnosis or treatment. You project that you would be willing to take the risk of missing this diagnosis for yourself (since you consider it very unlikely) and would not want any additional tests performed. To minimize the bias associated with risk-taking behavior, ask yourself what you would do if this patient were your close family member or loved one who presented with these signs and symptoms. Then do that to your patient. Scrupulous honesty and open communications with your patient are a must here.

Know when you are having a bad day

Everyone has off days. If things aren't working right for you because of extraneous issues (fight with your spouse, kids, or partners, problems paying your bills, etc.) don't take it out on your patients. It is better to reschedule or ask for more help on those days. If this is not possible, you must learn to overcome your own feelings and not let them get in the way of good and empathic communications with your patients.

The examinee

Biologic variation in the system being examined

This is the main source of random error in medicine. People are complex biological organisms and all physiological responses vary from person to person or from time to time in the same person. Some patients with chronic bronchitis will have audible wheezes and rhonchi. Others won't have wheezes but will only have a cough on forced expiration. Some people with heart attacks have typical crushing substantial chest pain while others have a fainting spell, weakness, or shortness of breath as their only symptom.

Effects of illness and medication

Ignoring the effect of medication or illness on the physiologic response of the patient may result in an inaccurate examination. Patients who take beta-blocker drugs for hypertension will have a slowing of the pulse. The drug may prevent the expected speeding up of the pulse if the patient is in shock from bleeding or hypoxic from heart failure.

Memory and rumination

A form of recall bias. Patients will remember the history differently at different times. This explains the commonly observed phenomenon that the attending seems to obtain the most "accurate" history. The intern (or student) obtains the first history. When the attending gets the history later (and after several others have obtained the same information by asking the same questions), the patient will have had time to reconsider their answers to the questions and may give a different (and usually more accurate) history. They have recalled things they either did not remember or thought were not important during the first questioning. A way to reduce this is by summarizing the history obtained several times during your initial encounter.

Filling in

Sometimes patients will "invent" parts of the history because they cannot recall what actually happened. This commonly occurs with dementia patients and alcoholics during withdrawal or other patients with organic brain syndromes. In most of these cases, orientation to time and place is also lost. However, sometimes otherwise oriented patients will be unable to recall an event because they were briefly "impaired" and actually don't recall what happened. This is common in the elderly who fall as a result of a syncopal episode (brief loss of consciousness or fainting spell). They may fill in a plausible explanation for their fall such as "I must have tripped." Try to get an explicit description of the entire event step by step before simply attributing their fall to tripping over something.

Toss-ups

A question can be answered correctly in many different ways. The way a question is worded may result in the patient giving apparently contradictory answers.

Descriptors of pain and discomfort are notoriously vague in their presentation and will change from telling to telling by the patient. Asking "do you have pain" could be answered "no" by the patient who describes their pain as "pressure" and doesn't equate that with pain. The examiner will not find out that this person has "chest pain" without asking more specific questions using other common descriptors of "chest pain" such as aching, burning, pressure, or discomfort.

Patient ignorance

The patient may not be able to give accurate and correct answers due to lack of understanding of the examiner's questions. The average patient understands at the level of a tenth-grade student (meaning half are below that level). They may not understand the meaning of a word as simple as congestion, and answer no, when they have a cough and stuffed nose. Avoid using "complex" medical or non-medical terminology.

Patient speaks different language

Situations in which the patient and physician cannot understand each other often lead to misinterpretation of the communications. Federal law requires US hospitals to have translators available for any patient that cannot speak or understand spoken English. This includes deaf patients. In situations where a translator is not immediately available, a translation service sponsored by AT&T is available by phone. Patients who do not speak English are more likely to be admitted from the emergency department and to have additional (and often unnecessary) diagnostic testing done.

Patient embarrassment

Patients will not usually volunteer sensitive information and they may be very anxious to discuss these same topics when asked directly. This includes questions about sexual problems, domestic violence, and alcohol or drug abuse. Even though teenagers are engaged in sexual activity, they may not know how to ask about protection from pregnancy or sexually transmitted diseases. Ask yourself if you as a "scared person" (teenager, older person, etc.) would volunteer certain information without being asked. It is better to assume that most patients will not and ask directly in an empathetic and non-judgmental manner.

Denial

Some patients will minimize certain complaints because they are afraid of finding out they have a bad disease. They may say that their pain is really not so bad and that the tests or treatments you are proposing are not necessary. Your job is to find out what their fear is due to, educate them about the nature of the illness, and help them make an informed decision.

Patient assessment of risk and level of risk taking

Some patients will reject your interpretation or explanation of the nature of their complaint because of their own risk-taking behavior. They may be more willing to take a risk than you think is reasonable. You must follow the precept of patient autonomy here. Your job is to educate them about the nature of their illness and the level of risk they are assuming by their behavior and then help them make an informed decision.

Lying

Finally there are occasions when a patient will simply lie to you. Questions about alcohol or drug abuse, child abuse, and sexual activity are common areas where this occurs. You may detect inconsistencies in the history or pick up secondary clues that give you an idea that this may be happening. The best way to handle this is to get corroborating evidence from the family, current and previous physicians, and medical records. Sometimes you must simply "believe them and treat them anyway."

The environment

Disruptive environments for the examination

Excess noise or interruptions, including background noise or children in the examination room, make it hard to be accurate in your examination. This may be unavoidable in some circumstances. Consider the emergency department (ED) with its chaotic environment and constant noise from disruptive patients or a large clinic space where noise carries from room to room. If it is impossible to remove the noise, make sure you compensate for it in some other way. It may take you longer to gather your information in these circumstances but you will be rewarded with increased accuracy.

Disruptive interactions between the examiner and the examined

Patients who are in severe pain, uncooperative, delirious, or agitated and crying children are in this category. You simply must try your best to do a competent examination over the interruptions. Occasionally in the ED we have to sedate patients in order to examine them properly. Providing pain relief for patients with severe pain early in the encounter will usually help you to obtain a better history and more accurate examination.

Reluctant co-workers

Nurses, residents, other allied health workers, and other physicians may disagree with your evaluation. If you believe that your evaluation is correct and evidence-based, their opinions should not stand in the way. This could be very problematic with managed care organizations. You should be confident in your skills and that on the average you are ordering tests appropriately. If a patient comes to the ED with the worst headache of their life, the correct medical action is to rule out a subarachnoid hemorrhage (bleed in the brain). This is done with a CT scan and, if that is negative, a spinal tap. The fact that this occurs at 0200 in the morning should not make a difference in your decision to order the CT scan. This is true even if the radiologist asks you to wait until the morning to do the procedure or if the nurses tell you that the spinal tap is unnecessary (since it takes more nursing time). Know when to stand your ground. Know when your staff are having a bad day.

Incomplete function or use of diagnostic tools

Diagnostic instruments and tools should be functioning properly and the examiner should be an expert in their use.

Strategies for preventing or minimizing error in the clinical examination

The following suggestions will help you avoid making errors in the examination. The examination is a tool for making an accurate final diagnosis. In order to do this, you must obtain accurate information. This must be done in a meticulous and systematic way.

(1) **Match the diagnostic environment to the diagnostic task**. Make sure the environment is "user friendly" to you and the patient. Wherever possible, get rid of noisy distractions. Obviously there are some situations in which this would be difficult, for example the ED.

(2) **Repeat key elements of your examination**. Review and summarize the history with patients to make sure the data are correct. Make sure your physical examination findings are accurate by repeating them and observing how they change with time and treatment.

(3) **Corroborate important elements of the patient history with documents and witnesses**. Make sure that you have all the information. Personally

Table 19.1. Problem-oriented medical record: the SOAP format

S	**Subjective** information from the patient – the history.
O	**Objective** information gathered in the patient examination and from diagnostic tests.
A	**Assessment** of the patient's problem. This is where inference should be noted. Make a determination of the nature of the patien's problem and your interpretation of that problem, the diagnosis. Initially this will be a provisional diagnosis, differential diagnosis, or just a summary statement of the problem.
P	**Plan** of treatment or further diagnostic testing.

question witnesses. Don't rely only on secondhand information about the history. If the patient does not speak English well or is deaf, get a translator. Don't make clinical decisions based on an incomplete history due to your inability to understand the patient accurately.

(4) **Confirm key clinical findings with appropriate tests**. Determine what tests are most useful in order to refine the diagnosis. You will learn about medical decision making from the next several chapters.

(5) **Ask "blinded" colleagues to examine your patient**. Corroborate your findings and make sure they are accurate. This will occur more often during medical school and residency. However, even experienced physicians will occasionally ask colleagues to check part of their clinical examination when things don't quite "add up." Obtaining reasonable and timely consultation with a specialist is one way of doing this. Remember that you are learning how to be the best doctor possible and sometimes that means getting a "better" doctor (consultant) to help you.

(6) **Report evidence as well as inference, making a clear distinction between the two**. Initially, record the facts only. When this is done, clearly note your interpretations. Use the problem-oriented medical record (POMR) and the SOAP format in making your notes (Table 19.1).

(7) **Use appropriate technical tools**. Make sure your tools (stethoscope, otoscope, ophthalmoscope, etc.) are working properly and that you know how to use them well.

(8) **"Blind" your assessment of raw diagnostic test data**. Look at the results of diagnostic tests objectively, applying the principles you will learn in medical decision making. Don't be overly optimistic or pessimistic about the value of a single lab test and apply rigorous methods of decision making in determining the meaning of the diagnostic test result.

(9) **Apply social sciences, as well as biologic sciences of medicine**. Remember that your patient is functioning within a social context. Emotional, cultural,

and spiritual components of health are important in getting an accurate picture of the patient. These can easily affect the interpretation of the information you gather.

(10) **Write legibly**. Others will read your notes and prescriptions. If you cannot write legibly, mistakes will occur. If this is a serious problem for you, consider dictating your charts or using a computer or typewriter for your medical charting.

20

The use of diagnostic tests

Science is always simple and always profound. It is only the half-truths that are dangerous.
George Bernard Shaw (1856–1950): The Doctor's Dilemma, 1911

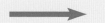 **Learning objectives**

In this chapter you will learn:
- the uses and abuses of diagnostic tests
- the hierarchical nature of features that determine the usefulness of a diagnostic test

The Institute of Medicine has determined that error in medicine is due to over-, under-, and misuse of medical resources. These include diagnostic tests. In order to understand the best way to use diagnostic tests, it is helpful to have a hierarchical format within which to view them.

The use of medical tests in making a diagnosis

Before deciding on ordering a diagnostic test, you should have a good reason for doing the test. There are four general reasons for ordering a diagnostic test.

(1) To establish a diagnosis in a patient with signs and symptoms. Examples are a throat culture in a patient with a sore throat to look for the presence of strep throat, or a mammogram in a woman with a palpable breast mass to look for a cancer.

(2) To screen for disease among asymptomatic patients. Examples are a PKU (phenylketonuria) test in a healthy newborn to look for the presence of this (rare) genetic disorder, a mammogram in a woman without signs or symptoms of a breast mass, or a PSA (prostate specific antigen) test in a healthy asymptomatic man to look for a (common) prostate cancer. Screening tests will not benefit the majority of people who get them and who don't have the disease. In general there are five criteria that must be met for a screening test – burden of suffering, early detectability, test validity, acceptability, and improved

outcome – and unless all these are met the test should not be recommended. We will discuss these in Chapter 26.

(3) To provide prognostic information on patients with established disease. Examples are a CD-4 count or viral load in a patient with HIV infection to look for susceptibility to opportunistic infection, or a CA-27.29 or 15.3 in a woman with breast cancer to look for a recurrence of the cancer.

(4) To monitor ongoing therapy, maximize effectiveness, and minimize side effects. Examples are the prothrombin time in patients on warfarin therapy to monitor level of anticoagulation and prevent either too high or too low levels, and gentamycin level in patients on this antibiotic to reduce the likelihood of toxic levels causing renal failure.

Important features to determine the usefulness of a diagnostic test

There are several ways of looking at the usefulness of diagnostic tests. This hierarchical evaluation uses six possible endpoints to determine a test's utility. The more criteria in the schema that are fulfilled, the more useful the test. Tests that fulfill fewer criteria have only limited usefulness. These criteria are based on an article by Pearl.[1]

(1) **Technical aspects**. What are the technical performance characteristics of the test? How easy and cheap is it to perform? How reliable are the results?

(a) **Reliable and precise** – results should be reproducible, giving the same result when the test is repeated on the same individual under the same conditions. This is usually a function of the instrumentation or operator reliability (e.g., of the person reading an x-ray) of the test. In the past, precision was assumed to be present for all diagnostic tests. Many studies have demonstrated that with most non-automated tests there is some degree of subjectivity in test interpretation. This has been seen in x-ray tests such as CT scan, mammography, and angiography. It is also present is tests commonly considered to be the "gold standard" such as the interpretation of tissue samples from biopsies or surgery.

(b) **Accurate** – the test should produce the correct result (the actual value of the variable it is seeking to measure) all the time. The determination of accuracy depends upon the ability of the result of the test found by the instrument to be the same as the result determined using a standardized specimen and instrument.

(c) **Operator dependence** – test results may depend on the skill of the person performing the test. A person with more experience, better training or more talent will get more precise and accurate results on the test.

---

[1] W. S. Pearl. Hierarchy of outcomes approach to test assessment. *Ann. Emerg. Med.* 1999; 33: 77–84.

(d) **Feasibility and acceptability** – how easy is it to do the test? Is there a large and expensive machine that must be bought? Is the test invasive or uncomfortable to perform? For example, many patients cannot tolerate being in an MRI machine because they have claustrophobia. For them this would be an unacceptable test. If a test is very expensive and not covered by health insurance, the patient may not be able to pay for it, making it a useless test for them.

(e) **Interference and cross-reactivity** – are there any substances (bodily components, medications, foods, etc.) that will interfere with the results? These may create false-positive test results (a positive test in a person with a normal value of the variable being tested). They may also prevent the test from picking up true positives (making them false negatives). For example, eating poppy-seed bagels will give a false-positive urine test for narcotics.

(f) **Inter- and intra-observer reliability** – previously discussed in the section on the kappa statistic (Chapter 7), this is related to operator dependence.

(2) **Diagnostic accuracy**. How well does the test help in making the diagnosis of the disease? This includes the concepts of validity, likelihood ratios, sensitivity, specificity, predictive values, and area under the ROC curve. These concepts will be discussed in later chapters.

(a) **Validity** – the test should discriminate between individuals with and without the disorder in question. How does the test result compare to that obtained using the "gold standard?" **Criterion-based validity** describes how well the measurement agrees with other approaches for measuring the same characteristic. This is what we measure in studies of diagnostic tests.

(b) **The "gold standard"** – this is also known as the **reference standard**. The result of a gold-standard test defines the presence or absence of the disease (i.e., all patients with the disease have a positive test and all patients without the disease have a negative test). All tests must be compared to a gold standard for the disease. There are very few true gold standards in medicine and some are better (scientifically purer) than others. Some typical gold standards are:

(i) Surgical or pathological specimens. These are traditionally considered to be the ultimate gold standard. But their interpretations can vary with different pathologists.

(ii) Blood culture for bacteremia. Theoretically, all bacteria that are present in the blood should grow on a suitable culture medium. Sometimes for technical reasons the culture does not grow bacteria even though they were present in the blood. This can occur because the technician doesn't plate the culture properly, it is stored at an incorrect temperature for a while, or there just happened to be no bacteria in the particular 10-cc vial of blood that was sampled.

(iii) Jones criteria for rheumatic fever. This is a set of fairly objective criteria for making this diagnosis. But one or another component of the criteria (e.g., temperature) may be measured incorrectly in some patients, while another criterion (arthritis) may be interpreted incorrectly by the observer.

(iv) DSM IV criteria for major depression. These criteria are somewhat objective yet depend on the clinician's interpretation of the patient's description of their symptoms.

(v) X-rays. But they are open to variation in the reading even by experienced radiologists.

(vi) Long-term follow up. The ultimate fall-back or de-facto gold standard. If we are ultimately interested in finding out how well the test works to separate diseased from healthy, we can follow all patients with the test for a specified period of time and see who has what outcome. This works as long as the time period is long enough to see all the possible disease outcomes.

(3) **Diagnostic thinking**. Does the result of the test cause a change in diagnosis after testing is complete? This includes concepts of incremental gain and confidence in the diagnosis. If we are almost certain that a patient has a disease based upon one test result or the history and physical exam, we don't need a second test to confirm that result. It only considers how the test performs in making the diagnosis in a given clinical setting and therefore is closely related to diagnostic accuracy.

(4) **Therapeutic effectiveness**. Is there a change in management as a result of the outcome of the test? The outcome can be initiation or cessation of therapy, reassurance, or avoidance of further testing. This must also consider if the test is cost-effective in the management of the particular disease. For example, the venogram is the gold-standard test in the diagnosis of deep venous thrombosis (blood clots in the legs). It is an expensive and invasive test and can cause some side effects, although they are rarely lethal. Is this test worth it if an ultrasound is almost as accurate? Part of the art of medicine is determining which patients with one negative ultrasound can safely wait for a second and confirmatory ultrasound three days later and which ones need to have an immediate venogram.

(5) **Patient outcomes**. Does the result of the test mean that the patient will feel or be better? This considers biophysiological parameters, symptom severity, functional outcome, patient utility, expected values, morbidity avoided, mortality change, and cost-effectiveness of outcomes. We will discuss some of these issues in the chapter on decision trees and patient values (Chapter 28).

(6) **Societal outcomes**. Is the test effective for the society as a whole? Even a cheap test if done to excess may result in prohibitive costs to society. This includes the additional cost of evaluation or treatment of patients with false-positive test results and the psychosocial cost of these results on the patient and community. It also includes the risk of missing the correct diagnosis with patients who are falsely negative and may suffer negative outcomes as a result of the diagnosis being missed. You may need also to consider a cost analysis for evaluating the test. However, the perspective of the analysis can be the patient, the payor, or society as a whole. Patient or societal outcomes ultimately determine the usefulness of a test as a screening test.

21

Utility and characteristics of diagnostic tests: likelihood ratios, sensitivity and specificity

It seems to me that science has a much greater likelihood of being true in the main than any philosophy hitherto advanced.

Bertrand Russell (1872–1970): The Philosophy of Logical Atomism, 1924

Learning objectives

In this chapter you will learn:

- the characteristics and definitions of normal and abnormal diagnostic test results
- how to define, calculate, and interpret likelihood ratios
- the process by which diagnostic decisions are modified in medicine and the use of likelihood ratios to choose the most appropriate test for a given purpose
- how to define, calculate, and use sensitivity and specificity
- how sensitivity and specificity relate to positive and negative likelihood ratios
- the process by which sensitivity and specificity can be used to make diagnostic decisions in medicine and how to choose the most appropriate test for a given purpose

In this chapter we will be talking about the utility (or the usefulness) of a diagnostic test. This is a mathematical expression of the ability of a test to find persons with disease or exclude persons without disease. In general, a test's utility will depend on two factors. These are the likelihood ratios and the prevalence of disease in the target population. Additional test characteristics that will be introduced are the sensitivity and specificity. These factors will tell you how useful the test will be in the clinical setting. Using a test without knowing these characteristics will result in problems. These include missing correct diagnoses, over-ordering tests, increasing health care costs, reducing trust in physicians (who over- or under-order tests), and increasing discomfort and side effects for your patient. Once you understand these properties of diagnostic tests, you will be able to determine when to best order them.

Why order a diagnostic test?

The indications for ordering a diagnostic test can be distilled into two simple rules. They are:

(1) When the characteristics of that test give it validity in the clinical setting. Will a positive (or negative) test be a true positive (or negative)? Will the result help in correctly identifying a diseased patient from one without disease?

(2) When the test result will change the probability of the disease leading to a change of clinical strategy. What will a positive or negative test result tell me about this patient that I don't already know and that I need to know? Will the test results change my treatment plan for this patient?

If the test you are contemplating ordering does not fall into one of these categories, it should not be done!

What do diagnostic tests do?

Diagnostic tests are a way of obtaining information that provides a basis for revising disease probabilities. When a patient presents with a clinical problem you first create your differential diagnosis. You attempt to reduce the number of diseases on this list by ordering diagnostic tests. Ideally, each test will either rule in or rule out one or more of the diseases on the differential diagnosis list. Diseases which are common, have serious sequelae (e.g., death or disability), or can be easily treated are usually the ones which must initially be ruled in or out.

We rule in disease when a positive test for that disease increases the probability of disease making it so likely that we would treat the patient for that disease. This should also make all the other diseases on the differential diagnosis list so unlikely that we would no longer consider them. We rule out disease when the test reduces the probability of that disease making it so unlikely that we would no longer look for that disease.

After setting up a list of possible diseases we can assign a **pretest probability** to each disease on the differential. This is the estimated **likelihood** of disease in a patient before any testing is done. As we discussed earlier, it is based on the history and physical examination as well as on the prevalence of the disease in the population. It is also called the **prior** or **a-priori probability** of disease in that patient.

After doing a diagnostic test, we are able to calculate the **post-test probability** of disease. This is the estimated likelihood of the disease in a patient after testing is done. This is also called the **posterior** or **a-posteriori probability** of disease. We can do this whether the test result is positive or negative. A positive test tends to rule in the disease while a negative test tends to rule out the disease. We normally

Post-test probability	∝	Pretest probability	×	Test factor
What we know after doing the test	=	What we knew before doing the test	×	How much the test results change the likelihood of what we knew before

Fig. 21.1 Bayes' theorem.

think of a test as being something done by a lab or radiologist. However, the test can be an item of history, part of the physical examination, a laboratory test, a diagnostic x-ray, or any other diagnostic maneuver (such as pulmonary function testing or EKG).

Mathematically, the pretest probability of the disease is modified by the application of a diagnostic test to yield a post-test probability of the disease. This revision of the (pretest) disease probabilities is done using a number called the likelihood ratio (LR). Likelihood ratios are stable characteristics of a diagnostic test and give the "strength" of that test. The likelihood ratio can be used to revise disease probabilities using a form of Bayes' theorem (Fig. 21.1). We will return to Bayes' theorem in Chapter 22. Before looking at likelihood ratios, it is useful to look at the definitions of normality in diagnostic tests.

Types of test result

Dichotomous test results can have only two possible values. Typical results are yes or no, positive or negative, alive or dead, better or not. A common dichotomous test is x-ray results which are read as either normal (showing no abnormality) or abnormal. There is also the middle ground or grey zone in these tests as sometimes they will be unreadable (poor quality) or indeterminate (not clearly normal or abnormal). There are of course many subtle gradations that can appear on an x-ray and lead to various specific readings, but they may not pertain to the disease for which the patient is being evaluated.

Continuous test results can have more than two possible values. The serum sodium level or the level of other blood components is an example of a continuous test. A patient can have any of a theoretically infinite number of values for the test result. In life serum sodium can take any value from about 100 to 170, although at the extremes the person is near death. In practice, we often take continuous tests and select a set of values for the variable that will be considered normal (135–145 mEq/dL), turning this continuous test into a dichotomous test (normal or abnormal). Values of the serum sodium below 135 mEq/dL or above 145 mEq/dL are abnormal. Clearly the farther from the normal range, the more serious the problem.

Fig. 21.2 Gaussian results of a diagnostic test.

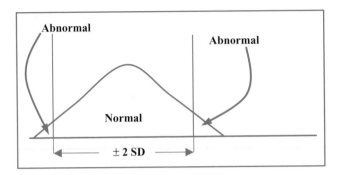

Definitions of a "normal" test result

There have been many mathematical ways to describe the results of a diagnostic test as normal or abnormal. In the method of **percentiles**, cutoffs are chosen at preset percentiles of the diagnostic test results. These preset percentiles are chosen as the upper and lower limits of normal. All values above (or below) the relevant percentile are abnormal. This method assumes that all diseases have the same prevalence. A special case of this method is the **Gaussian** method. In this method, normal is 95% (± 2 SD) of the values observed of all tests done (Fig. 21.2). Results are therefore only specific to the population being studied.

In reality, there are two normal distributions of test results. One is for patients who are afflicted with the disease being sought and the other is for those free of disease. There is usually an overlap of the distributions of test values for the sick and not-sick populations. Some "normal" (non-sick or disease-free) patients will have "abnormal" test results while some "abnormal" (sick or diseased) ones will have "normal" results. The goal of the diagnostic test is to differentiate between the two groups. Setting any single value of the test as the cutoff between normal and abnormal will usually misclassify some patients. The ideal test, the gold standard, will have none of this overlap between diseased and non-diseased populations and will therefore be able to differentiate between them perfectly all the time.

For almost all tests that are not a gold standard there are four possible outcomes. True positives (TP) are those patients with disease who have a positive or abnormal test result. True negatives (TN) are those without the disease who have a negative or normal test. False negatives (FN) are those with disease who have a negative or normal test. False positives (FP) are those without disease who have a positive or abnormal test. We can look at this graphically in Fig. 21.3.

Ideally, when a study of a diagnostic test is done, patients with and without the disease are all given both the diagnostic test and the gold-standard test. The results will show that some patients with a positive gold-standard test (they all actually have the disease) will have a positive diagnostic test and some won't. The ones with a positive test are the true positives and those with a negative one

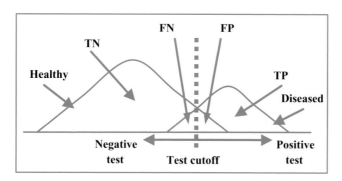

Fig. 21.3 The "real-life" results of a diagnostic test.

are false negatives. A similar situation exists among patients who have a negative gold-standard test (they are all actually disease-free). Some of them will have a negative diagnostic test result (and are called true negatives) and some will have a positive test (and are called false positives).

Strength of a diagnostic test

The results of a clinical study of a diagnostic test can determine the "strength" of the test. We are looking for a mathematical function that describes the ability of the test to change the pretest probability and better distinguish patients with and without the disease. The ideal diagnostic test (the gold standard) will always discriminate "diseased" from "non-diseased" individuals in a population. This test is 100% accurate. The diagnostic test we are comparing to the gold standard is a test that is easier, cheaper, or safer than the gold standard, and we want to know its accuracy. That tells us how often it is correct (either true positive or true negative) and incorrect (either false positive or false negative).

From the results of this type of study, we can create a "2 × 2 table" that divides a real or hypothetical population into four groups depending on their disease status (D+ or D−) and test results (T+ or T−). Patients are either diseased (D+) or free of disease (D−) as determined by the gold standard test. The diagnostic test is applied to the sample, and patients have either a positive (T+) or negative (T−) diagnostic test. We can then create a 2 × 2 table to evaluate the mathematical characteristics of this diagnostic test. This 2 × 2 table (Fig. 21.4) is the conceptual basis for almost all calculations made in the next several chapters.

We can calculate the likelihood (or probability) of having a positive test if a person has or does not have the disease. Similarly we can calculate the likelihood of having a negative test if a person has or does not have the disease. Comparing these likelihoods can give a ratio that shows the strength of the test. Likelihoods are calculated for each of the four possible outcomes. They can be compared in two ratios and are analogous to the relative risk in studies of risk (harm). These

Fig. 21.4 Results of a study of a diagnostic test.

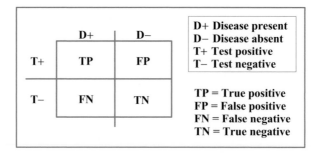

Fig. 21.5 Positive likelihood ratio (LR+) calculations.

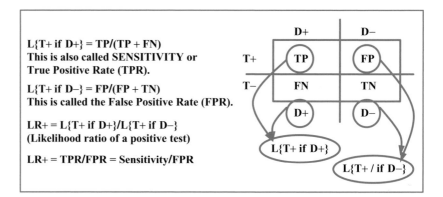

are called the **positive** and **negative likelihood ratios**. In studies of diagnostic tests, we are looking at the probability that a person with the disease will have a positive test. Compare that to the probability that a person without the disease has a positive test and you can calculate the likelihood ratio of a positive test (LR+ in Fig. 21.5).

The likelihood that a patient with the disease has a positive test is also known as the sensitivity or the true positive rate (TPR). It tells you how good (or sensitive) the test is for finding those persons with disease when only looking at those with disease. This tells us how often the result is a true positive (person with disease and a positive test) compared to a false negative (person with disease and a negative test). **Sensitivity can only be calculated from among people who have the disease**. It is the fraction (or percentage) of people with the disease who test positive. Probabilistically it is expressed as $P[T+|D+]$, the probability of a positive test if the person has disease.

If the result of a very sensitive test is negative, it tells us that the patient doesn't have the disease (the test is Negative in Health, NIH) and the disease has been excluded (ruled out). This is because there are very few false negatives and therefore virtually all negative tests must occur in non-diseased people. The clinician has reduced the number of diagnostic possibilities and it would be unlikely that the patient has the disease in question. When two or more tests are available, the most sensitive should be done to minimize the number of false negatives, or

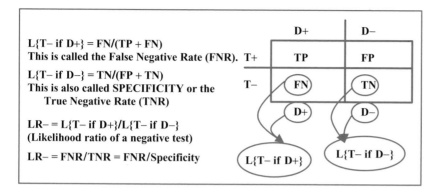

L{T− if D+} = FN/(TP + FN)
This is called the False Negative Rate (FNR).

L{T− if D−} = TN/(FP + TN)
This is also called SPECIFICITY or the
True Negative Rate (TNR)

LR− = L{T− if D+}/L{T− if D−}
(Likelihood ratio of a negative test)

LR− = FNR/TNR = FNR/Specificity

Fig. 21.6 Negative likelihood ratio (LR−) calculations.

missed cases. This is especially true for serious diseases that are easily treated. An example of a very sensitive test is the TSH (thyroid simulating hormone) test for hypothyroidism. A normal TSH test makes it extremely unlikely that the patient has hypothyroidism. Hypothyroidism is ruled out. A sensitive test rules out disease – and the mnemonic is SnOut (**Sen**sitive = ruled **out**).

Similarly, the likelihood that a patient without disease has a positive test is also known as the false positive rate (FPR). It is equal to one minus the specificity. It tells us how often the result is a false positive (person without disease and a positive test) compared to a true negative (person without disease and a negative test). FPR = FP/(FP + TN). This is the proportion of non-diseased people with a positive test.

The LR+ (positive likelihood ratio) tells us by how much a positive test increases the "likelihood" of disease in a person who is having the test done. We start with the likelihood of disease, do the test, and as a result of a positive test that likelihood increases. The LR+ tells us how much of an increase in this likelihood we can expect.

We can do the same thing for a negative test. In this case we are looking at the likelihoods of having a negative test in people with and without the disease. The LR− (likelihood ratio of a negative tests) tells us by how much a negative test decreases the "likelihood" of disease in persons who are having the test done. Fig. 21.6 describes these calculations.

The likelihood that a patient without the disease has a negative test is also known as the specificity or the true negative rate (TNR). It tells you how specific the test is for finding those persons without disease when only looking at those without disease. This tells us how often the result is a true negative (person without disease and a negative test) compared to a false positive (person without disease and a positive test). **Specificity can only be calculated from among people who don't have the disease**. It is the fraction (or percentage) of people without the disease who test negative. Probabilistically it is expressed as $P[T - \mid D -]$, the probability of a negative test if the person does not have disease.

If the result of a very specific test is positive, it tells us that the patient has the disease (the test is Positive in Disease, PID) and the disease has been verified

Table 21.1. Strength of test by likelihood ratio

Qualitative strength	LR+	LR−
Excellent	10	0.1
Very good	6	0.2
Fair	2	0.5
Useless	1	1

(ruled in). This is because there are very few false positives and therefore any positive tests must occur in diseased people. The clinician has reduced the number of diagnostic possibilities and it would be unlikely that the patient doesn't have the disease in question. When two or more tests are available, the most specific should be done to minimize the number of false positives, or mislabeled cases. This is especially true for diseases that are not easily treated or for which the treatment is potentially dangerous. An example of a very specific test is the ultrasound for deep venous thrombosis (blood clot) of the leg. If the ultrasound is positive, it is extremely unlikely that there is no clot in the vein. A deep vein thrombosis is ruled in. A specific test rules in disease – and the mnemonic is SpIn (**Sp**ecificity = ruled **in**).

Similarly, the likelihood that a patient with disease has a negative test is also known as the false negative rate (FNR). It is equal to one minus the sensitivity. It tells us how often the result is a false negative (person with disease and a negative test) compared to a true positive (person with disease and a positive test). FNR = FN/(FN + TP). This is the proportion of diseased people with a negative test.

The LR− tells us by how much a negative test decreases the "likelihood" of disease in a person who is having the test done. We start with the likelihood of disease, do the test and as a result of a negative test, that likelihood decreases. The LR− tells us how much of a decrease in this likelihood we can expect.

Likelihood ratios are called stable characteristics of a test. This means that they do not change with the prevalence of the disease. Their values are determined by clinical studies against a gold standard. Therefore, published reports of likelihood ratios are only as good as the gold standard against which they are based and the quality of the study that determined their value.

The likelihood ratios are the strength of the diagnostic test. The larger the value of LR+, the more a positive test will increase the probability of disease in a patient to whom the test is given. In general, you would like the likelihood ratio of a positive test to be very high (ideally over 10) to maximally increase the probability of disease after doing the test and getting a positive result. Similarly, you want the likelihood ratio of a negative test to be very low (ideally less than 0.1) to maximally decrease the probability of disease after doing the test and getting a negative result A qualitative list of LRs has been devised to show the "strength" of a test based upon LR values. These are listed in Table 21.1.

Table 21.2. Mnemonics for sensitivity and specificity

(1)   SeNsitive tests are **N**egative in health (**NIH**)
       SPecific tests are **P**ositive in disease (**PID**)
(2)   Sensitivity: **SnOut** – sensitive tests rule out disease
       Specificity: **SpIn** – specific tests rule in disease
(3)   SeNsitivity includes False **N**egatives
       SPecificity includes False **P**ositives

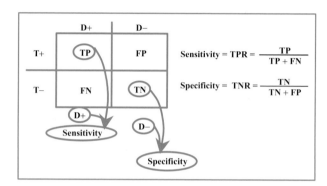

Fig. 21.7 Sensitivity and specificity calculations.

Using sensitivity and specificity

The sensitivity and specificity are the mathematical components of the likelihood ratios. They are the diagnostic-test characteristics that are most often measured and reported in studies of diagnostic tests in the medical literature. Like the likelihood ratios they are also intrinsic characteristics of a diagnostic test. From the study results, we can use our 2×2 table (Fig. 21.7) that divided a real or hypothetical population into four groups depending on their disease status (D+ or D−) and test results (T+ or T−) as a starting point to evaluate these characteristics of the diagnostic test.

There are two other important definitions of stable characteristics of diagnostic tests. The **false negative rate** (FNR) is the same as the likelihood of a negative test if the person has disease. This is the proportion of diseased people with a negative test. The **false positive rate** (FPR) is the same as the likelihood of a positive test if the person does not have disease. This is the proportion of non-diseased people with a positive test. Three mnemonics can help you remember the difference between sensitivity and specificity. These are listed in Table 21.2.

We have previously noted the mathematical relationship between sensitivity and specificity and the likelihood ratios. You can calculate the likelihood ratios from sensitivity and specificity. The formulas are as follows:

Fig. 21.8 The effect of changing the cutoff point for a diagnostic test.

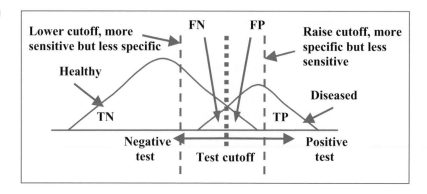

$$LR+ = \text{sensitivity}/(1 - \text{specificity})$$

$$LR- = (1 - \text{sensitivity})/\text{specificity}$$

There is also a dynamic relationship between sensitivity and specificity. As the sensitivity of a test increases, the cutoff point moves to the left in Fig. 21.8. The number of true positives increases compared to the number of false negatives. At the same time, the number of false positives will increase compared to the number of false negatives. This will result in a decrease in the specificity. Notice what happens to the sensitivity and specificity in Fig. 21.8 when the test cutoff moves to the right. Now the sensitivity decreases as the specificity increases. We will see this dynamic relationship better when we discuss receiver operating characteristic (ROC) curves in Chapter 23.

Sample problem

Diarrhea in children is usually caused by viral infection. However in some cases, bacterial infection causes the diarrhea and these cases should be treated with antibiotics. A study was done in which 156 young children with diarrhea had stool samples taken. All of them were tested for the presence of polymorphonuclear leukocytes (white blood cells) in the stool. A positive test was defined as one in which there were >5 white blood cells per high power field. All the children had a stool culture done and that was the gold standard. There were 27 children who had positive cultures and 23 of these had smears that were positive for fecal leukocytes. Of the 129 who had a negative stool culture, 16 had smears that were positive for fecal leukocytes. What are the likelihood ratios of the stool leukocyte test?

First make your 2×2 table (Fig. 21.9). Prevalence $= 27/156 = 0.17$.

$$L\{T+ \mid D+\} = \textbf{sensitivity} \text{ or } \textbf{TPR} = TP/(TP + FN) = 23/(23 + 4) = 0.85$$

$$L\{T+ \mid D-\} = \textbf{FPR} = FP/(TN + FP) = 16/(113 + 16) = 0.12$$

	D+	D−	Totals
T+	23 (TP)	16 (FP)	39
T−	4 (FN)	113 (TN)	117
Totals	27	129	156 (N)

Fig. 21.9 2×2 table using data from the study of the use of fecal leukocytes in the diagnosis of bacterial diarrhea in children. The prevalence of disease is 27/156 = 0.17. From: T. G. DeWitt *et al.* Clinical predictors of acute bacterial diarrhea in young children. *Pediatrics* 1985; 76: 551–556.

From these we can calculate the likelihood ratio of a positive test:

LR+ = L{T+ | D+ }/L{T+ | D− } = 0.85/0.12 = 7.08

Doing the same for a negative test leads to the following results:

L{T− | D+ } = **FNR** = FN/(TP + FN) = 4/(23 + 4) = 0.15

L{T− | D− } = **specificity** or **TNR** = TN/(TN + FP) = 113/(113 + 16) = 0.88

LR− = L{T− | D+ }/L{T− | D− } = 0.15/0.88 = 0.17

These likelihood ratios are pretty good and this is a fairly good test since the LR+ = 7.08 and the LR− = 0.17 are very close to a strong test (LR+ > 10 and LR− < 0.1). This is a test that will increase the likelihood of disease by a lot if the test is positive and decrease the likelihood of disease by a lot if the test is negative. We will talk about applying these numbers in a real clinical situation in a later chapter.

There were some potential biases in the performance of the study. It was done on 156 children who presented to an emergency department with severe diarrhea and were entered into the study. This meant that someone (the resident or attending physician on duty at the time) thought that the child had infectious (bacterial) diarrhea. They were screened before both the test and gold standard were run on them. Therefore the study is subject to filter or selection bias. This simply means that the population in the study may not be representative of the population of all children with diarrhea (the ones you are seeing in your pediatric or family-practice office). The next chapter will deal with this problem and how to generalize the results of this study to your patients.

22

Bayes' theorem, predictive values, post-test probabilities, and interval likelihood ratios

As far as the laws of mathematics refer to reality, they are not certain; and as far as they are certain, they do not refer to reality.

Albert Einstein (1879–1955)

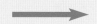

Learning objectives

In this chapter you will learn:
- how to define predictive values of positive and negative test results and how they differ from sensitivity and specificity
- the difference between odds and probability and how to use each correctly
- Bayes' theorem and use likelihood ratios to modify the probability of a disease
- how to define, calculate, and use interval likelihood ratios for a diagnostic test
- how to calculate and use positive and negative predictive values
- how to use predictive values to choose the appropriate test for a given diagnostic dilemma
- how to apply basic test characteristics to solve a clinical diagnostic problem
- the use of interval likelihood ratios in clinical decision making

In this chapter we will be talking about the application of likelihood ratios, sensitivity, and specificity to a patient.

Introduction

Likelihood ratios, sensitivity, and specificity of a test are derived from studies of patients with and without disease. They are essential characteristics of the test that are related to the disease. They give us the probabilities of a positive or negative test if the patient does or does not have disease. This is not the information a clinician needs to know to apply the test to a patient.

What the clinician needs to know is: if a patient has a positive test, what is the likelihood that patient has the disease? The clinician is interested in how the test result relates to the patient. For a given patient, how will the probability of disease change given a positive or negative test result? Applying likelihood ratios or sensitivity and specificity to a selected pretest probability of disease will give you the post-test probability of disease. There are two methods for doing this calculation. The first uses Bayes' theorem while the second calculates the predictive values of a positive and negative test directly from sensitivity, specificity, and prevalence.

Predictive values

Positive predictive value (PPV) is the proportion of patients with the disease among all those who have a positive test. If the test comes back positive, what is the probability that this patient really has the disease? Probabilistically it is expressed as $P[D+|T+]$, the probability of disease if a positive test occurs. It is also called the post-test or posterior probability of a positive test. A related concept is the false alarm rate (FAR), which is equal to $1 - $ PPV. That is the proportion of people with a positive test who don't have disease (and will be falsely alarmed by a positive test result).

Negative predictive value (NPV) is the proportion of patients without the disease among all those who have a negative test. If the test comes back negative, what is the probability that this patient really does not have the disease? Probabilistically it is expressed as $P[D-|T-]$, the probability of not having disease if a negative test occurs. It is also called the post-test or posterior probability of a negative test. A related concept is the false reassurance rate (FRR), which is equal to $1-$ NPV. That is the proportion of people with a negative test who have disease (and will be falsely reassured if the test result is negative).

Bayes' theorem

Thomas Bayes was an English clergyman with broad talents. His famous theorem was presented posthumously in 1763. In eighteenth-century English, it said: "The probability of an event is the ratio between the value at which an expectation depending on the happening of the event ought to be computed and the value of the thing expected upon its happening." Now, aren't you glad you know that! In simple language, the theorem was a way of updating a previously held belief (odds of an event happening) when confronted with new information (evidence). In statistics, this new information is that gained in the research process. In clinical medicine this new information is the likelihood ratio. Bayes' theorem is a way of using likelihood ratios (LRs) to revise disease probabilities.

Bayes' theorem was put into mathematical form by Laplace (remember his other law?). Its use in statistics was supplanted at the start of the twentieth century

Black and white blocks in a jar	Odds	Probability
■ ■ ■ ■ ■ ■ ■ ■ ■ □	9/1 = 9	9/10 = 0.9
■ ■ ■ □	3/1 = 3	3/4 = 0.75
■ ■ □ □	2/2 = 1	2/4 = 0.5
■ □ □ □	1/3 = 0.33	1/4 = 0.25
■ □ □ □ □ □ □ □ □ □	1/9 = 0.11	1/10 = 0.1

Fig. 22.1 Relationship between odds and probability. As the odds and probabilities get smaller, they also approximate each other. As they get larger, they become more and more different.

by Sir Ronnie Fisher's ideas of statistical significance (remember he decided on $P < 0.05$ for statistical significance?). It was kept in the dark until revived in the 1980s. (Are we lucky, or what?) We won't get into the actual formula in its usual and original form here because it only involves another very long and useless formula. A derivation and the full mathematical formula for Bayes' theorem are given in Appendix 5, if you are interested. In it's simplest form it states:

Post-test odds = pretest odds × LR

Odds and probabilities

In order to use Bayes' theorem and likelihood ratios, you must first convert the probability of disease to the odds of disease. (Sorry, you probably suspected that there had to be a hitch here.) Odds describe the chance that something will happen against the chance it won't happen. Probability describes the chance that something will happen against the chance that it will or won't happen. The odds of an outcome are the number of people affected divided by the number of people not affected. In contrast, the probability of an outcome is the number of people affected divided by the number of people at risk (affected plus not affected). Probability is what we are estimating when we select a pretest probability of disease for our patient. We next have to convert this to odds.

Let's use a simple example to show the relationship between odds and probability. If we have 5 white blocks and 5 black blocks in a jar, we can calculate the probability or odds of picking a black block at random (without looking, of course). The odds of the outcome of interest (picking a black block) is 5/5 = 1. There are equal odds of picking a white and black block. For every one black block, you will likely pick one white block (on average). The probability of the outcome of interest (picking a black block) is 5/10 = 0.5. Half of all your picks will be a black block. Fig. 22.1 shows this relationship.

> **To convert odds to probability:**
> Probability = Odds/(1 + Odds)
>
> **To convert probability to odds:**
>
> Odds = Probability/(1 – Probability)

Fig. 22.2 Converting odds to probability (and back).

In our society, odds are usually associated with gambling. In horse racing or other games of chance, the odds are usually given backwards by convention. For example, the odds against Dr. Disaster winning the fifth race at Saratoga are 7 : 1. This means that this horse is likely to lose 7 times for every eight races he enters. In usual medical terminology, these numbers are reversed. We put the outcome we want on top and the one we don't on the bottom. Therefore, the odds of him winning would be 1 : 7, or 1/7 or 0.14. He will win one time in eight. (I actually bet on him and he won!)

The probability of him winning is different. Here we answer the question of how many times will Dr. Disaster have to race in order to win once? He will have to race eight times in order to have one win. The probability of him winning any one race is 1 in 8 or 1/8 or 0.125. Since the odds and probabilities are small numbers, they are very similar. If he were a better horse and the odds of him winning were 1 : 1, or one win for every loss, the odds could be expressed as 1/1 or 1.0. Here the probability would be that he would win one race in every two he starts. The probability of winning is 1/2 or 0.5.

The language for odds and probabilities differs. Odds are expressed as one number to another: for example, odds of 1 : 2 are expressed as "one to two" and equal the fraction 0.5. This is the same as saying the odds are 0.5 to 1. Probability is expressed as a fraction. The same 1 : 2 odds would be expressed as "one in three" = 0.33. These two expressions and numbers are the same way of saying that for every three attempts, there will be one "successful" outcome.

There are mathematical formulas for converting odds to probability and vice versa. They are listed in Fig. 22.2.

Using likelihood ratios to revise pretest probabilities of disease

LRs can be used to revise disease pretest probabilities when test results are dichotomous, using Bayes' theorem. This says post-test odds of disease equals pretest odds of disease times the likelihood ratio. We get the pretest probability of disease from our differential list and our estimate of the likelihood of disease in our patient. Pretest probability is converted to pretest odds and multiplied by the likelihood ratio. This results in the post-test odds, which are converted back to a probability, the post-test probability.

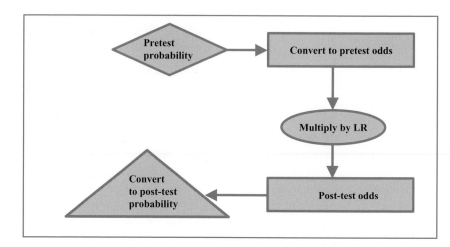

The end result of using Bayes' theorem when a positive test occurs is the post-test probability of disease. This is also called the positive predictive value (PPV). For a negative test, Bayes' theorem calculates the probability that the person still has disease even if a negative test occurs. This is called the false reassurance rate (FRR). From this you can calculate the negative predictive value (NPV), which is the probability that a person with a negative test does not have the disease. Mathematically it is 1 minus the FRR. The process is represented graphically in Fig. 22.3.

We will demonstrate this with an example. A study was done to evaluate the use of the urine dipstick in testing for urinary tract infections (UTI) in children seen in a pediatric emergency department.[1] A positive leukocyte esterase and nitrite test on a urine dipstick was to be diagnostic of a UTI. The urine culture done on all the children was the gold standard. The positive test on both indicators (leukocyte esterase and nitrite) had a positive likelihood ratio (LR+) of 20 but a negative likelihood ratio (LR−) of 0.61. In the study population, the probability of a urinary tract infection in the children being evaluated in that setting was 0.09 (9%).

Suppose you are in a practice and estimate that a particular child whom you are seeing for fever has a pretest probability of 10% of having a UTI. This is equivalent to a low pretest probability of disease. If you want to find out what the post-test probabilities of a urinary tract infection are after using the dipstick test, use Bayes' theorem and do the following steps:

(1) **Convert probability to odds**. Pretest probability $= 0.1$, therefore, Pretest odds $= 0.1/(1 − 0.1) = 0.11$. (Remember, for low values you could use the same number and get results that are close enough.)

[1] From K. N. Shaw, D. Hexter, K. L. McGowan & J. S. Schwartz. Clinical evaluation of a rapid screening test for urinary tract infections in children. *J. Pediatr.* 1991; 118: 733–736.

(2) **Apply Bayes' theorem**. Multiply pretest odds by the likelihood ratio for a positive test (LR+). In this case, LR+ = 20, a very high LR+, so the test is very powerful if positive. Post-test odds = pretest odds × LR+ = 0.11 × 20 = 2.2.

(3) **Convert odds back to probability**. Post-test probability = odds/(odds +1) = 2.2/3.2 = 0.69. (Here we have to do the formal calculation back to probability to get a reasonable result.)

(4) **Interpret the result**. Post-test probability (positive predictive value, PPV) of disease is 69%. In other words, a positive urine dipstick has increased the probability of a urinary tract infection from 0.1 to 0.69. This is a big jump! Most tests have much less ability to jump the patient's pretest probability.

Using the same example for a negative test:

(1) Pretest probability and odds of disease are unchanged. Pretest odds = 0.11.

(2) LR− = 0.61, and post-test odds = 0.11 × 0.61 = 0.067.

(3) Post-test probability = 0.067/1.067 = 0.063.

In other words, a negative urine dipstick has reduced the probability of urinary tract infection from 0.1 to 0.06. This is the false reassurance rate (FRR), and tells us how many children (6 out of 100) we will falsely tell not to worry. We are falsely telling them that they don't have a urinary tract infection when in fact they do. We can also calculate the negative predictive value, which is 1 − FRR, or 1 − 0.06. The NPV is, therefore, 0.94, or 94% of children with a negative test are free of disease.

When we get a negative test result, we have to make a clinical decision. Should we do the urine culture (gold standard) for all children who have a negative dipstick test in order to pick up the 6% who actually have an infection, or should we just reassure them and repeat the test if the symptoms persist? This must be accurately communicated to the patient (in this case the parents) and plans made for all contingencies. Choosing to do the urine culture on all children with a negative test will result in a huge number of unnecessary cultures. They are expensive and will result in a large expenditure of effort and money for the health-care system. Whether or not to do them depends on the consequences of not diagnosing this condition at the time the child presents with their initial symptoms. At the present time, it is not known if these undetected children progress to kidney damage. But the available evidence suggests that there is no significant delayed damage and that (at least) most of these infections will spontaneously clear or show up with persistent symptoms and be treated at a later time.

The nomogram

A nomogram to calculate post-test probability using likelihood ratios was developed in 1975 by Fagan (Fig. 22.4). Begin by marking the LR and pretest probability on the nomogram. Connect these two points, and continue the line until you

Fig. 22.4 Nomogram for Bayes' theorem. From T. J. Fagan. [letter.] *N. Engl. J. Med.* 1975; 293: 257. Used with permission.

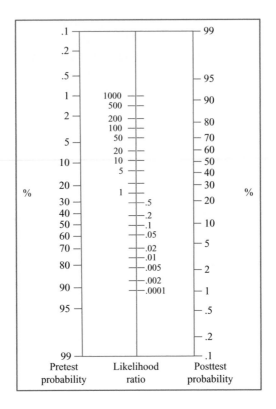

reach the post-test probability. This obviates the need to calculate pretest odds and post-test probability.

Let's return to our example of a child with signs and symptoms of a urinary tract infection. The plot of the post-test probability for this clinical situation is shown in Fig. 22.5.

Calculating post-test probabilities using positive and negative predictive values

The other way of calculating post-test probabilities uses sensitivity and specificity directly to calculate the predictive values. Positive and negative predictive values of the test are related to the sensitivity and specificity, but are also dependent on the prevalence of disease, or the pretest probability. The prevalence is the pretest or prior probability of disease in your patient or the population of interest. The history and physical exam give you an estimate of the pretest probability. Simply knowing the sensitivity and specificity of a test without knowing the prevalence

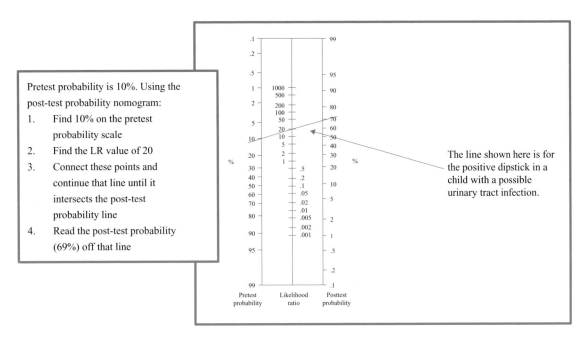

Pretest probability is 10%. Using the post-test probability nomogram:
1. Find 10% on the pretest probability scale
2. Find the LR value of 20
3. Connect these points and continue that line until it intersects the post-test probability line
4. Read the post-test probability (69%) off that line

The line shown here is for the positive dipstick in a child with a possible urinary tract infection.

Fig. 22.5 Using the Bayes' theorem nomogram in the example of UTI in children.

of the disease in the population you are interested in will not allow you to differentiate between disease and non-disease in your patient. Now go back to Table 18.4 in Chapter 18 and look at the table of pretest probabilities again. This ought to help it make more sense.

Clinicians can use pretest probability (for disease and non-disease respectively) along with the test sensitivity and specificity to calculate the post-test probability that the patient has the disease (post-test probability = predictive value). This is shown graphically in Fig. 22.6.

Calculating predictive values

(1) Pick a likely pretest probability (P) of disease using the rules we discussed in Chapter 18. Moderate errors in the selection of this number will not significantly affect the results or alter the interpretation of the result.
(2) Set up a cohort of 1000 (N) patients (or a similarly convenient number to make the math as easy as possible) and divide them into diseased (D+ $= P \times N$) and non-diseased (D− $= (1 − P) \times N$) groups based on the estimated pretest probability (prevalence, P). Use the 2×2 table.
(3) Multiply to get the contents of the boxes TP and TN:

Sensitivity $\times$ D+ $=$ TP

Specificity $\times$ D− $=$ TN

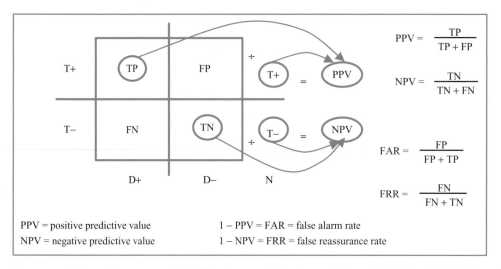

$$PPV = \frac{TP}{TP + FP}$$

$$NPV = \frac{TN}{TN + FN}$$

$$FAR = \frac{FP}{FP + TP}$$

$$FRR = \frac{FN}{FN + TN}$$

PPV = positive predictive value   1 − PPV = FAR = false alarm rate
NPV = negative predictive value   1 − NPV = FRR = false reassurance rate

Fig. 22.6 Predictive values calculations.

(4) Fill in the remaining boxes, FN and FP. FN = (D+) − TP and FP = (D−) − TN.
(5) Calculate predictive values using the formulas

$$PPV = TP/(TP + FP)$$
$$NPV = TN/(TN + FN).$$

Let's go back to the 156 young children with diarrhea whom we met at the end of Chapter 21.[2] Recall that we calculated the sensitivity and specificity of the stool sample test for polymorphonuclear leukocytes (> 5 cells/high power field) and got 85% and 88% respectively. We have already decided that this study population does not represent all children with diarrhea who present to a general pediatrician's office. In this setting, we (the pediatrician) estimate the prevalence of bacterial diarrhea is closer to 0.02 than 0.17 (as it was in the study: 27/156). How does the lower prevalence change the predictive values of the test? What is the likelihood of disease in a child with a positive or negative test?

(1) First, use 1000 patients (N) to set up the 2×2 table using the new (estimated) clinical prevalence of bacterial diarrhea of 0.02 or 20 out of 1000 (Fig. 22.7).
(2) Next, multiply the number with disease by the sensitivity and without disease by the specificity to get the values of TP and TN. Round off decimals (Fig. 22.8).
(3) Fill in the FP and FN boxes and add the lines across (Fig. 22.9).
(4) Calculate PPV, NPV, FAR, and FRR:

$$PPV = TP/T+ = 17/135 = 0.13$$
$$NPV = TN/T- = 862/865 = 0.996$$
$$FAR = FP/T+ = 1 - PPV = 0.87$$
$$FRR = FN/T- = 1 - NPV = 0.004$$

[2] T. G. Dewitt *et al. Pediatrics* 1985; 76: 551–556.

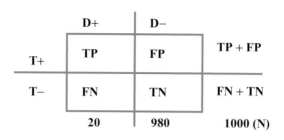

Fig. 22.7 Set up the 2×2 table using a population of 1000 patients (N) and an estimated clinical prevalence (P) of bacterial diarrhea of 0.02.

	D+	D−	
T+	TP	FP	TP + FP
T−	FN	TN	FN + TN
	20	980	1000 (N)

Fig. 22.8 Multiply the number with disease (D+ = P × N) by the sensitivity and the number without disease (D− = (1 − P) × N) by the specificity to get the values of TP and TN.

	D+	D−	
T+	20 × 0.85 = 17	FP	
T−	FN	980 × 0.88 = 862	
	20	980	1000 (N)

Fig. 22.9 Subtract TP from D+ and TN from D− to get the values of FP and FN, and add the lines across.

	D+	D−	
T+	17	118	135
T−	3	862	865
	20 (P)	980 (N − P)	1000 (N)

(5) Interpret the results and decide how you are going to use them.

Compared to the original population (with a prevalence of 17.3%), we can see that the PPV drops significantly when the prevalence decreases. This is a general rule of the relationship between PPV and prevalence.

PPV of 13% means that most positives are not true positives: they are children who don't have bacterial diarrhea. For every seven children you treat with antibiotics (thinking they had bacterial diarrhea), only one really needed it. The others got no benefit from treatment. You have to decide whether it is better to treat six children without bacterial diarrhea in order to treat the one with the disorder, to treat no one, or to order another test to further eliminate the false positives. Bacterial diarrhea will get better quicker with antibiotics. The downsides of antibiotic use include rare side effects (allergic reactions) and problems that are removed from the individual (increased bacterial resistance with high rate of antibiotic usage), so you decide this is a reasonable trade-off. If, on the other hand, you decide that antibiotic resistance is a real problem (and I believe it is) and treatment will not change the course of the illness in a dramatic manner (alleviate much suffering), you would choose not to treat. In that case, you would decide not to do the test (stool WBCs) since even with a positive result you wouldn't treat with antibiotics.

NPV of 99.6% means that if the test is negative, you will miss only 4 in 1000 (FRR) children with true bacterially caused infectious diarrhea, so you can safely avoid treating them. This is especially true since the result of non-treatment is simply prolonging the diarrhea by a day. It would be different if the results of non-treatment were serious (prolonged disease with significant complications or mortality). In that case missing even 4 out of 1000 could be too many to miss and you should do the gold standard test (stool culture) on all the children.

Predictive values are the numbers that we (clinicians) need in order to determine the likelihood of disease in a patient with a positive (or negative) test result and a given pretest probability. We use these numbers to modify the differential diagnosis and change the pretest probabilities that we assigned to the patient.

Finally, we can do the same problem with likelihood ratios. The calculations are as follows:

$$LR+ = \text{sensitivity}/(1 - \text{specificity}) = 0.85/0.12 = 7.08$$

$$LR- = (1 - \text{sensitivity})/\text{specificity} = 0.15/0.88 = 0.17$$

Using a pretest probability of 2%, the probability and odds are the same: 0.02. Applying Bayes' theorem, post-test odds $= LR+ \times 0.02 = 7.08 \times 0.02 = 0.14$, and post-test probability $= 0.124$. Compare this to the PPV of 0.13.

Similarly for a negative test: post-test odds $= LR- \times 0.02 = 0.17 \times 0.12 = 0.0034$. Compare this to the FRR of 0.004.

You now have two ways of calculating the post test probability of disease given the operating characteristics of the tests.

Finally, we must add a word about accuracy. This term has been used more in the past to designate the strength of a diagnostic test. Simply, it is the true positives and true negatives divided by the total population (to whom the test was applied). However, this can be a grossly misleading number. If there are many more without the disease, a very specific test (few false positives) will be very accurate even with poor sensitivity. It says nothing about the sensitivity and should not be used as the measure of a test's performance.

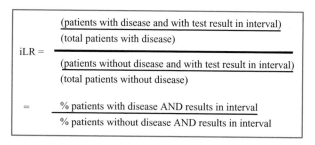

$$iLR = \cfrac{\dfrac{\text{(patients with disease and with test result in interval)}}{\text{(total patients with disease)}}}{\dfrac{\text{(patients without disease and with test result in interval)}}{\text{(total patients without disease)}}}$$

$$= \frac{\text{\% patients with disease AND results in interval}}{\text{\% patients without disease AND results in interval}}$$

Fig. 22.10 Interval likelihood ratio (iLR).

Interval likelihood ratios (iLR)

Likelihood ratios allow us to calculate post-test probabilities when continuous rather than just dichotomous test results are used. Single cutoff points of tests with continuous variable results set potential "traps" for the unwary clinician. Often in studies where the outcome variable of interest is a continuous variable, a single dichotomous cutoff point is selected as the best single-point cutoff between normal and abnormal patients. Valuable data are disregarded if the results of such a test are considered only "positive" or "negative." We can obviate this problem using interval likelihood ratios.

The "interval" LR (iLR) is the probability of a test result in the interval under consideration among diseased subjects, divided by the probability of a test result within the same interval among non-diseased subjects. Simply put, the interval likelihood ratio is the percentage of patients with disease who have test results in the interval divided by the percentage of patients without disease with test results in the interval (Fig. 22.10). If the iLR associated with an interval is less than 1 the probability of disease decreases, and if greater than 1 the probability of disease increases.

When data are gathered for results of a continuous variable, predetermined cutoff points should be set. Then the number of people with and without disease in each interval can be determined. Many authorities believe that these results are more accurate and represent the true state of things better than a single cutoff point. The following illustration with the white cell count in appendicitis will illustrate this issue.

A 16-year-old girl comes to the emergency department complaining of right-lower-quadrant abdominal pain for 14 hours and a decreased appetite. Her physical examination reveals right-lower-quadrant tenderness and spasm and the clinician thinks that she might have appendicitis. You obtain a white blood count and get a level of 10 200 cells/μL ("normal" range is 4500–11000 cells/μL). Although this test result is "normal," it is just below the cutoff for an elevated WBC count. You know that a mildly decreased WBC count has a different implication than a highly elevated WBC count of 17000 cells/μL. Interval likelihood ratios can help attack this question quantitatively.

Table 22.1. Distribution of white-blood-cell count in patients with and without appendicitis

WBC/μL	With appendicitis (% of 59)	Without appendicitis (% of 145)	iLR+ (95% CI)
4000–7000	1 (2%)	30 (21%)	0.1 (0–0.39)
7000–9000	9 (15%)	42 (29%)	0.52 (0–1.57)
9000–11 000	4 (7%)	35 (24%)	0.29 (0–0.62)
11 000–13 000	22 (37%)	19 (13%)	2.8 (1.2–4.4)
13 000–15 000	6 (10%)	9 (6%)	1.7 (0–3.6)
15 000–17 000	8 (14%)	7 (5%)	2.8 (0–6.0)
17 000–19 000	4 (7%)	3 (2%)	3.5 (0–10)
19 000–22 000	5 (8%)	0 (0%)	Infinite (NA)
Total	59 (100%)	145 (100%)	

Example: For WBC from 4000 to 7000, iLR $= (1/59)/(30/145) = 2\%/21\% = 0.1$
From S. Dueholm *et al*. Laboratory aid in the diagnosis of acute appendicitis. A blinded prospective trial concerning diagnostic value of leukocyte count, neutrophil differential count, and C-reactive protein. *Dis. Colon Rectum* 1989; 32: 855–859.

Table 22.1 represents the distribution of WBC count results among 59 patients with confirmed appendicitis and 145 patients without appendicitis. For each interval, the probabilities for results within the interval were used to calculate an iLR.

Note that in this study the interval likelihood ratio is lower for the third interval (9k–11k) than for the second interval (7k–9k), and similarly for the intervals 11k–13k and 13k–15k. The 95% CIs overlap in each case and include the point estimate of the other group's iLR. Therefore the iLR differences found for these intervals are not statistically different. This is the result of the small sample size in this study, and probably a Type II error. This value of LR+ would more likely be in line (positive dose–response relationship) if there were more patients.

Ideally, 95% CI should always be given for each LR. This allows the reader to determine the statistical significance of the results. In initial studies, researchers often "data dredge" by using several different cutoff points to see which gives the best iLR and which are statistically significant. These results must be verified in a second and new validation study.

Given this girl's symptoms and physical findings, we estimate that her pretest (before obtaining results of WBC count) probability of appendicitis is about 0.50. (We're not sure and it is a toss-up.) What is the probability of appendicitis if our

	D+	D−
WBC > 9K T+	49	73
WBC < 9K T−	10	72
Totals	59	145

Fig. 22.11 2×2 table for the use of a white-blood-cell count of greater than 9000 as a cutoff for diagnosing appendicitis. Data from S. Dueholm *et al. Dis. Colon Rectum* 1989; 32: 855–859.

patient had a WBC count of 10200? We will demonstrate how to determine this using Bayes' theorem.

Start with the pretest probability of 50% and calculate the odds. These are $0.5/(1 − 0.5)$. Pretest odds (appendicitis) $= 0.5/0.5 = 1$ and iLR $= 0.29$. Therefore post-test odds (appendicitis) $= 1 × 0.29 = 0.29$, and post-test probability (appendicitis) $= 0.29/1.29 = 0.22$. This is less than before, but not low enough to rule out the diagnosis. We must therefore decide either to do another test or to observe the patient.

What happens if her white-cell count is 7500 (iLR $= 0.52$)? The pretest odds are unchanged and the post-test odds (appendicitis) $= 1 × 0.52 = 0.52$. Post test probability (appendicitis) $= 0.52/1.52 = 0.33$, leading to the same problem as with a white-cell count of 10200.

What if her white-cell count is 17500 (iLR $= 3.5$)? Again, the pretest odds are unchanged and the post-test odds (appendicitis) $= 1 × 3.5 = 3.5$. Post-test probability (appendicitis) $= 3.5/4.5 = 0.78$. This is much higher, but far from good enough to immediately treat her for the suspected disease. In this case, treatment requires an operation on the appendix. This is major surgery, and although pretty safe in this day and age, it is still more risky than not operating if the patient does not have appendicitis. Most surgeons want the probability of appendicitis to be over 85% before they will operate on the patient. This is called the treatment threshold.

Therefore, even with the white-cell count this high, we have not crossed the treatment threshold of 85%. This value was adopted based upon previous studies and prevailing surgical practice when it was considered important to have a negative operative rate of 15% in order to prevent missing appendicitis and risking rupture of the appendix. Therefore, if the probability of appendicitis is greater than 0.85, the patient should be operated upon.

Let's see what will happen if we lump the test results, considering a white-blood-cell count of 9000 as the upper limit of normal. Now use likelihood ratios to calculate predictive values and apply them to a population with a prevalence of 50%. For the original study patients, LR+ $= 1.66$ and LR− $= 0.34$ (Fig. 22.11). For the patient in our example, post-test odds $= 1 × 1.66 = 1.66$ and the post-test probability $= 1.66/2.66 = 0.62$. This is slightly different from the results using the interval likelihood ratio, but is still below the treatment threshold.

Fig. 22.12 2×2 table to calculate the post-test probability of a urinary tract infection using the dipstick results on urine testing for UTI. Data from K. N. Shaw et al. J. Pediatr. 1991; 118: 733–736.

$$LR+ = (36/90)/(18/910) = 20$$

$$LR- = (54/90)/(892/910) = 0.61$$

	D+	D–	
T+	36	18	54
T–	54	892	946
	90	910	1000

For the study on the use of urine-dipstick testing for UTI which we discussed earlier in this chapter, the 2 × 2 table is shown in Fig. 22.12. In the original study, the prevalence was 0.09. Using this table allows you to visualize the number of patients in each cell, and gives an idea of the usefulness of the test.

The probability of disease if a positive test occurs is 36/54 = 0.67, and the probability of disease if the text is negative is 54/946 = 0.057. These are very similar to the values calculated using the LRs. Remember, for our population we used a prevalence of 10% (not 9%).

23

Comparing tests and using ROC curves

His work's a man's, of course, from sun to sun,
But he works when he works as hard as I do –
Though there's small profit in comparisons.
(Women and men will make them all the same.)

Robert Frost (1874–1963): A Servant to Servants

Learning objectives

In this chapter you will learn:
- the dynamic relationship between sensitivity and specificity
- how to construct and interpret an ROC curve for a diagnostic test

Analysis of diagnostic test performance using ROC curves

ROC is an acronym for Receiver Operating Characteristics. It is a concept that originated during the early days of World War 2 when radar was a newly developed technology. The radar operators had to learn to distinguish true signals (enemy planes) from noise (geese or clouds). The ROC curve let them decide which signals were which. In medicine, an ROC curve tells you which test has the best ability to differentiate healthy people from ill ones.

The ROC curve plots sensitivity against specificity. The convention has been to plot sensitivity (true positive rate) against 1− specificity (false positive rate). This ratio looks like the likelihood ratio, doesn't it? The ROC curve for a particular diagnostic test tells which cutoff point maximizes sensitivity, specificity, and both. ROC curves for two tests can also tell you which test is best.

By convention, when drawing ROC curves the x-axis is the false positive rate (1 − specificity), going from 0 to 1 (0–100%), and the y- axis is the sensitivity (true positive rate), also going from 0 to 1 (0–100%). The best cutoff point for diagnosis would be the point closest to the (0,1) point. This is the point at which there is

Table 23.1. Sensitivity and specificity for each cutoff point of WBC count in appendicitis

WBC/μL	Sensitivity (95% CI)	Specificity (95% CI)	1 – specificity (95% CI)
>4000	100 (95–100)	0 (0–3)	100 (97–100)
>7000	98 (91–100)	21 (15–29)	79 (71–85)
>9000	83 (71–92)	50 (42–59)	50 (41–58)
>11 000	76 (63–86)	74 (62–84)	26 (16–38)
>13 000	39 (27–53)	87 (73–98)	13 (2–27)
>15 000	29 (18–47)	93 (78–100)	7 (0–22)
>17 000	15 (7–27)	98 (80–100)	2 (0–20)
>19 000	6 (3–19)	100 (85–100)	0 (0–15)

Source: From S. Dueholm *et al. Dis. Colon Rectum* 1989; 32: 855–859.

perfect sensitivity and specificity. It is (by definition), the gold standard. This point has 0% false positive rate and 100% sensitivity.

Let's look at our data from studies about our girl with right-lower-quadrant pain and the possibility of appendicitis (Table 23.1) and draw the ROC curve for the results (Fig. 23.1). We calculated the sensitivity and specificity for each cutoff point as a different dichotomous value.

Comparing diagnostic tests

ROC curves can help determine which of two tests is better for a given purpose. First, examine the ROC curves for the two tests. Is one clearly better (closer to the upper left corner) than the other? For the hypothetical tests A and B depicted in Fig. 23.2 it is clear that test A outperforms test B over the entire range of lab values. This means that for any given cutoff point, the sensitivity and specificity of test A will always be better than for the corresponding point for test B.

We can compare tests even if their ROC curves overlap. This is illustrated in Fig. 23.2(b), where the curves for tests C and D overlap. We can always chose a single point cutoff for the point closest to the (0,1) point on the graph. This will always be the best single point for diagnosis.

Another approach uses the concept of area under the curve (AUC). A test whose ROC curve is the diagonal from the upper right (point 1,1) to the lower left (point 0,0) is a worthless test. At any given point, it's sensitivity and false positive rate are equal, making diagnosis using this test a coin toss for all cutoff points. The AUC for this curve is 0.5. Similarly the gold-standard test will have an AUC of one (1.0).

ROC curves that are close to the imaginary diagonal line are poor tests. We say that the AUC is only slightly greater than 0.5. Obviously, ROC curves that are under

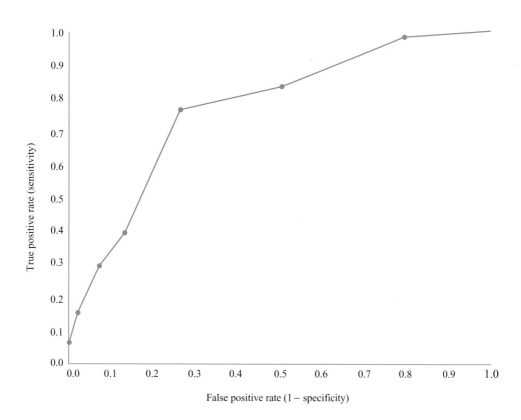

False positive rate (1 − specificity)

this line are such poor tests that they are worse than flipping a coin. We can use AUC to statistically compare the area under two ROC curves.

The AUC has an understandable meaning. It answers the two alternative-forced choice (2AFC) problem. This means that "given a normal patient chosen at random from the universe of normal patients, and an abnormal patient, again chosen at random, from the universe of abnormal patients, the AUC describes the probability that one can identify the abnormal patient using this test alone."[1]

There are several ways to measure the AUC for an ROC curve. The simplest is to count the blocks (med-student level). A minimally more complex method is to calculate the trapezoidal area (high-school-geometry level). The most complex way is to use the technique of smoothed area using maximum likelihood estimation techniques (computer-analysis level).

The probability of alcohol abuse or dependence among patients in one adolescent clinic was reported as about 0.33. A study looked at using the CAGE questionnaire as a screening tool for alcoholism among adult patients in the outpatient medical practice of a university teaching hospital. In this population, the sensitivity of an affirmative answer to one or more of the CAGE questions (Table 23.2)

Fig. 23.1 ROC curve for white blood cell count in appendicitis, based on data in Table 23.1.

[1] Michigan State University, Department of Internal Medicine. *Power Reading: Critical Appraisal of the Medical Literature.* Lansing, MI: Michigan State University, 1995.

Table 23.2. Results of CAGE questions using different cutoffs

Numbers of questions answered affirmatively	Alcoholic	Non-alcoholic	Sensitivity (TPR)	1 – specificity (FPR)
>3	56/294	56/527	0.19	0.00
>2	130/294	516/327	0.44	0.02
>1	216/294	482/527	0.73	0.09
>0	261/294	428/527	0.89	0.19

Source: Data from D. G. Buchsbaum, R. G. Buchanan, R. M. Centor, S. H. Schnoll & M. J. Lawton. Screening for alcohol abuse using CAGE scores and likelihood ratios. *Ann. Intern. Med.* 1991; 115: 774–777.

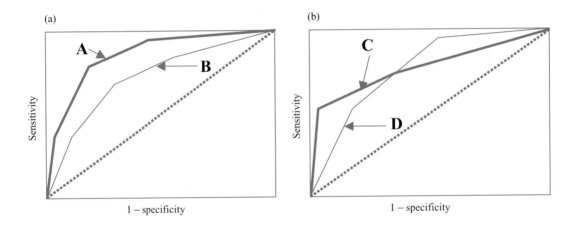

(a)   (b)

Fig. 23.2 ROC curves of four hypothetical tests A, B, C and D.

was about 0.9 and the specificity was about 0.8. Although one could consider the CAGE "positive" if a patient has one or more answers in the affirmative, in reality the CAGE is more "positive" given more affirmative answers on the four component questions (each answer can be given one point to make a score):

Have you ever felt you should **Cut down** on your drinking?

Have people **Annoyed** you by criticizing your drinking?

Have you ever felt bad or **Guilty** about your drinking?

Have you ever had a drink first thing in the morning to steady your nerves or get rid of a hangover (**Eye-opener**)?

We actually have the choice of considering the CAGE questionnaire "positive" if the patient answers all four, three or more, two or more, or one or more of the component questions in the affirmative. Moving from a more stringent to a less stringent cutoff tends to sacrifice specificity (1 – FPR) for sensitivity (TPR).

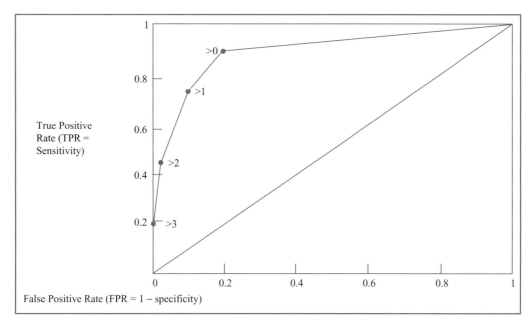

Fig. 23.3 ROC curve of CAGE
question data from
Table 23.2.

By convention, ROC curves start at the FPR = 0, TPR = 0 point. The CAGE here is always considered negative regardless of patients' answers. There are no false positives, but no alcoholics are detected. ROC curves end at the FPR = 1.0, TPR = 1.0 point. The CAGE is always considered positive regardless of patients' answers. The test has perfect sensitivity but all non-alcoholics are falsely identified as positives.

The area under this curve is 0.89 units (standard error 0.13 units); we'd expect randomly selected alcoholic patients from the sample population to have a higher CAGE score than randomly selected non-alcoholic patients about 89% of the time. Computers can be used to compare ROC curves by calculating the AUCs. Another study of the CAGE questionnaire was done by Mayfield[2] on psychiatric inpatients whereas Buchsbaum's study (Table 23.2 and Fig. 23.3) used general-medicine outpatients. The Mayfield study had an AUC of 0.9 with a standard error of 0.17. Using a statistical test, these two study results are not statistically different, validating the result.

[2] D. Mayfield, G. McLeod & P. Hall. The CAGE questionnaire: validation of a new alcoholism screening instrument. *Am. J. Psychiatry.* 1974; 131: 1121–1123.

24

Incremental gain and the threshold approach to diagnostic testing

Science is the great antidote to the poison of enthusiasm and superstition.
Adam Smith (1723–1790): The Wealth of Nations, 1776

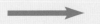

Learning objectives

In this chapter you will learn:
- how to calculate and interpret the incremental diagnostic gain for a given clinical test result
- the concept of threshold values for testing and treating
- the use of multiple tests and the effect of independent and dependent tests on predictive values
- how predictive values help make diagnostic decisions in medicine and how to use predictive values to choose the appropriate test for a given purpose
- how to apply basic test characteristics to solve a clinical diagnostic problem

Revising probabilities with sensitivity and specificity

Remember the child from Chapter 18 with a sore throat? Let's revisit our differential diagnosis list (Table 24.1). Since strep and viruses are the only strong contenders on this list, we would hope that a negative strep test would mean that the likelihood of viruses as the cause of strep throat is high enough to defer antibiotic treatment of this disease. We only need to rule out strep. Therefore, we decide to do a rapid strep test. It comes up positive. We look up the sensitivity and specificity of this test, and find that they are 0.9 and 0.9 respectively. Now the pretest probability is 0.5 (50%). We can solve this in two ways: likelihood ratios and predictive values.

Table 24.1. Pretest probability: sore throat

Streptococcal infection	50%
Viruses	75%
Mononucleosis	5%
Epiglottitis	<1%
Diphtheria	<1%
Gonorrhea	<1%

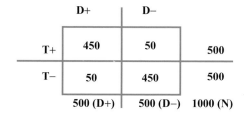

	D+	D−	
T+	TP	FP	
T−	FN	TN	
	500 (D+)	500 (D−)	1000 (N)

If: Sensitivity = 0.9
        Specificity = 0.9
Then:
TP = D+ × sens. = 500 × 0.9 = 450
TN = D− × spec. = 500 × 0.9 = 450

Fig. 24.1 Set up the 2×2 table using a population of 1000 patients and an estimated clinical prevalence of strep throat infection of 0.5. Calculate the values of TP and TN as shown.

	D+	D−	
T+	450	50	500
T−	50	450	500
	500 (D+)	500 (D−)	1000 (N)

PPV = 450/500 = 0.9

NPV = 450/500 = 0.9

FAR = 1 − PPV = 0.1

FRR = 1 − NPV = 0.1

Fig. 24.2 Write the values of TP, TN, FP and FN into the 2×2 table. Calculate PPV, NPV, FAR, and FRR as shown.

Using likelihood ratios

LR+ = sensitivity/(1 − specificity) = 0.9/0.1 = 9
LR− = (1 − sensitivity)/specificity = 0.1/0.9 = 0.11

Pretest probability of disease is 50%, so the pretest odds are 1.
Applying Bayes' theorem:
    For a positive test, post-test odds = LR+ × 1 = 9, so post-test probability = 0.9, the positive predictive value.
    For a negative test, post-test odds = LR− × 1 = 0.11, so post-test probability (FRR) = 0.1 and the negative predictive value = 0.9 (1 − 0.1).

Using predictive values

The method is shown in Figs 24.1 and 24.2. Whichever way we do the calculations, the positive predictive value is 0.9 and the negative predictive value is also 0.9.

Fig. 24.3 Results of calculating the values of the 2 × 2 table for a population of 1000 patients (N) and a clinical prevalence of strep throat infection that is low or 0.1 (100 out of 1000). Calculations for PPV and NPV are shown.

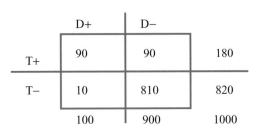

$$\text{PPV} = 90/180 = 0.5$$

$$\text{NPV} = 810/820 = 0.987$$

Therefore, with a positive test result, we would accept this diagnosis, and realize that we might have over-treated 50 out of 500 children (or 1 in 10) without strep. But the cost of that is low enough that we decide we need not worry about it. We base this on the risks of antibiotic treatment causing rare allergy to antibiotics in children with a positive test. This balances against the benefit of treatment, a one-day shorter course of symptoms and some decrease in very rare sequellae of infection (abscess and acute rheumatic fever).

Similarly, if the test had come up negative, we would throw out the likelihood of strep and accept that we might falsely reassure 10% (50 out of 500) of children with this type of sore throat. However, we have to look at the risks of not treating the patient. In this case they are small. Rheumatic fever, once a common complication of strep throat, is now extremely rare. Much less than 1% of strep infections lead to this and the rate is even lower in most populations.

Bacterial resistance from overuse of antibiotics is the only other problem left, and for now we decide that this will not deter us from prescribing antibiotics. We decide to defer a decision based on this problem to high-level government policy panels, and vow that for ourselves we will try to use antibiotics only when reasonably indicated (for a positive strep test and not for things like a common cold). We are willing to wait for a blue-ribbon panel to look at all the evidence and make a clinical guideline (algorithm or practice guideline) on when to treat and when to test for strep throat.

If the pretest probability of strep based upon signs and symptoms was much lower (say 10%), this equation will change (Fig. 24.3). We can use likelihood ratios to get the same results by starting with the pretest probability of disease, which is now 10%. The pretest odds are 0.11 and applying Bayes' theorem for a positive test results in post-test odds (= LR+ × 0.11) of 0.99. This makes the post-test probability (0.99/1.99) = 0.497. This is the positive predictive value and is pretty close to the 0.5 that was obtained using the 2 × 2 table. Similarly, for a negative test, the post-test odds (= LR− × 0.11) are 0.0121. Therefore, the post-test probability if the test is negative (equivalent to the false reassurance rate or FRR) is 0.0121 and the negative predictive value (1− FRR) is 0.988.

The PPV for a positive test is now 50%. You now decide that the benefit of antibiotics (one day less of symptoms) is not worth the excess antibiotic use (treat one without strep for every one with strep), and you will withhold treatment. In the case of a pretest probability of 10%, you can then decide not to do the test in the first place. If you practiced in a community with a high incidence of acute rheumatic fever after strep throat infections, it may still be reasonable to test since it would be worthwhile treating all the positives to prevent this more serious sequella. Over-treating one child for every one correctly treated is a small price to pay for the prevention of rheumatic fever.

Incremental gain

Incremental gain is the expected increase in diagnostic certainty of a diagnosis after the application of a diagnostic test. It is the change in the pretest estimate of a given diagnosis. Mathematically it is $PPV - P$ or positive predictive value minus pretest probability. For a negative test, it would be $(1 - P) - NPV$. For incremental gain of a negative test, begin with the prevalence of no disease $(1 - P)$ and go up to the NPV. It simply tells you how much bang (increased probability of disease) you got for your buck (using a diagnostic test). This is one measure of the usefulness of a diagnostic test. By convention we use absolute value so that all the incremental gains are positive numbers. They are all improvements on the previous level of probability.

For a given range of pretest probability, what is the diagnostic gain from doing the test? Using the example of strep throat in a child, we began with a pretest probability of 50% and after doing the test our new probability of disease was 90%. This represents an incremental gain of 40% $(90 - 50)$. For a negative test the incremental gain would also be 40% $(50 - 90)$. We can do these same calculations for a patient with a higher pretest probability of disease, but in whom we weren't certain of strep on clinical grounds. Here we would say that the pretest probability was between a coin toss (50%) and certainty (100%) so we will put it at about 75%. How would that change the incremental gain? Fig. 24.4 shows the 2×2 table and the calculations based on predictive values. Using likelihood ratios we start with the pretest probability of disease, which is now 75%. The pretest odds are 3 and the post-test odds for a positive test $(= LR+ \times 3)$ are 27. This makes the post-test probability $(27/28) = 0.964$. Similarly, for a negative test, the post-test odds $(= LR- \times 3)$ are 0.33, so the post-test probability if the test is negative (the FRR) is 0.25 and the negative predictive value $(1 - FRR)$ is 0.75.

Now the post-test probability of disease is more certain (96.4%), but if the test is negative we will be wrong more often (25%). The incremental gain is now only 21.4% for a positive test $(96.4 - 75)$ and up to 50% for a negative test $(75 - 25)$.

Fig. 24.4 Results of calculating the values of the 2×2 table for a population of 1000 patients (N) and a clinical prevalence of strep throat infection that is moderately high or 0.75 (750 out of 1000). Calculations for PPV, NPV, FAR, and FRR are shown.

	D+	D−	
T+	675	25	700
T−	75	225	300
	750	250	1000

PPV = 675/700 = 0.964

NPV = 225/300 = 0.750

FAR = 1 − PPV = 0.036

FRR = 1 − NPV = 0.250

Fig. 24.5 Results of calculating the values of the 2 × 2 table for a population of 1000 patients (N) and a clinical prevalence of strep throat infection that is very high or 0.9 (900 out of 1000). Calculations for PPV, NPV, FAR, and FRR are shown.

	D+	D−	
T+	810	10	820
T−	90	90	180
	900	100	1000

PPV = 810/820 = 0.988

NPV = 90/180 = 0.50

FAR = 1 − PPV = 0.012

FRR = 1 − NPV = 0.50

We can do the same for a pretest probability of 90% (almost certainty) (Fig. 24.5). Or, using likelihood ratios, the pretest probability of disease is now 90%, so the pretest odds are 9 and the post-test odds for a positive test (= LR + ×9) are 81. The post-test probability is therefore 0.987. For a negative test, the post-test odds (= LR− × 9) are 1, so the post-test probability (the FRR) is 0.5 and the negative predictive value (1− FRR) is 0.5.

The incremental gains are now:

Positive test: 98.8 − 90 = 8.8

Negative test: 50 − 10 = 40

Since we gain so little (8.8%), and lose a lot (40%) if the test is negative (more false negatives), we would probably choose not to do the test if we were this certain (high pretest probability based on signs and symptoms) that the child had strep throat. We can put all of these results in a table (Table 24.2) and compare results.

In general, the greatest incremental gain occurs when the pretest probability is in an intermediate range, usually between 20% and 70%. Notice also that as the pretest probability increased the number of false negatives also increased and the number of false positives decreased.

We will see this in operation when doing some problems with a screening test. At what level of clinical certainty (pretest probability) should a given test be done? This depends on the situation and the test. The use of threshold values can assist the clinician in making this judgment.

Table 24.2. Incremental gains for rapid strep throat tests

Pretest probability	Incremental gain T+	FN	Incremental gain T−	FP
10%	40 (10 to 50)	10/1000	8.8 (90 to 98.8)	90/1000
50%	40 (50 to 90)	50/1000	40 (50 to 90)	50/1000
75%	21.4 (75 to 96.4)	75/1000	50 (25 to 75)	25/1000
90%	8.8 (90 to 98.8)	90/1000	40 (10 to 50)	10/1000

Threshold values

Incremental gain tells us how much a diagnostic test increases the value of our pretest probability based upon the characteristics of the test and the prevalence of disease in the population from which the patient is drawn. This simply tells us the amount of certainty we gain by doing the test. We can decide not to do the test if the incremental gain is very small since we would feel that very little is gained clinically. The midrange of pretest probability yields the highest incremental gain.

Another way to look at the process of deciding whether to do a test is using the method of threshold values. In this process we want to find the probability of disease above which we will treat no matter what, and conversely the level below which we would never treat, and wouldn't even test. Once these have been determined, we can use our test characteristics and incremental gain to decide if it will be worthwhile to do a diagnostic test.

We can determine threshold values by calculating PPV and NPV for many different levels of pretest probability. At each step we would ask if we still wanted to treat based upon a positive result. Decision trees are also used to determine the threshold values. We will learn about decision trees in Chapter 29. An alternative method uses a simple balance sheet to approximate the threshold values. An explanation for this can be found in Appendix 6.

In practice, clinicians use their clinical judgment to determine the threshold values for each clinical situation. This is part of the "art of medicine" or that part of EBM based upon clinical experience. Clinicians ask themselves "will I gain any additional useful clinical information by doing this test?" If the answer to this question is no, they shouldn't do the test. They already know enough about the patient and would either treat or not treat regardless of the test result, since no useful additional information is gained by performing the test.

The **treatment threshold** is the value at which the clinician asks "do I know enough about the patient to begin treatment, and would treat regardless of the results of the test?" If the answer to this question is yes, the test shouldn't be done.

This occurs at high values of pretest probability. If a test is done, it ought to be one with high specificity, which can be used to rule in disease. But if you get a negative test result you must do a confirmatory test or the gold-standard test to avoid missing a person with a false-negative test.

The **testing threshold** is the value at which the clinician asks "is the likelihood of disease so low that even if I got a positive test I would still not treat the patient?" If the answer to this question is yes, the test shouldn't be done. This occurs at low values of pretest probability. If a test is done, it ought to be one with high sensitivity, which can be used to rule out disease. But, if you get a positive test result you must do a confirmatory test or the gold-standard test to avoid over-treating a person with a false-positive test.

Both of these threshold levels depend not only on the test characteristic (sensitivity and specificity) and prevalence, but also on the risks and benefits associated with treatment or non-treatment. The values of probability of disease for the treatment and testing thresholds should be established before doing the test. The clinician selects a pretest probability of disease, and determines whether performing the test will result in placing the patient above the treatment threshold or below the testing threshold. If it won't, the test is probably not worth doing.

At pretest probabilities above the treatment threshold, testing may produce an unacceptable number of false negatives in spite of a high PPV. Some patients would be denied the benefits of treatment, perhaps more than would benefit from treatment. The pretest probability of disease is so great that you should treat regardless of the results of the test. This is because you won't believe that the results of a negative test are a true negative. If you get a negative result, it is probably a false negative and could miss someone with the disease. You must be ready to do a confirmatory test here, possibly the gold standard. Similarly, you should be more willing to treat someone who does not have the disease (false positive) than to miss treating someone who is a false negative. This may not be true if treatment involves a lot of risk and suffering (e.g., an operation).

At pretest probabilities below the testing threshold, testing would lead to an unacceptable number of false positives (high FAR). Patients would be unnecessarily exposed to the side effects of further testing or treatment. The likelihood of disease in someone with a positive test is so small that you would not treat even if the test is positive, since it is too likely that a positive test will be a false positive. You must again be ready to do a confirmatory test. This approach is summarized in Fig. 24.6.

For our child with a sore throat this testing threshold is a pretest probability of strep throat below 10%. Below this level, applying the test (rapid strep antigen) and getting a positive result would still not increase the probability of disease enough to treat the patient and we are certain enough that disease is not present. Similarly, the treatment threshold is a pretest probability of strep throat above 50%. Above this level, applying the test (rapid strep antigen) and getting a negative result

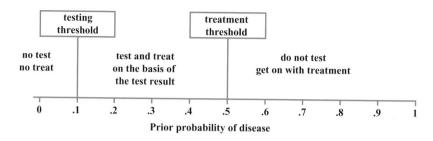

Fig. 24.6 Thresholds for strep throat example.

would still not decrease the probability of disease enough to refrain from treating the patient and we are certain enough that disease is present. Between these values of pretest probability (10–50%) do the test. Test first and treat only if the test is positive, since the post-test probability then increases above the treatment threshold.

In our example of the child with a sore throat, almost all clinicians agree that if the pretest probability is 90% (sore throat, large lymph nodes, pus on the tonsils, bright red tonsils, fever, and no signs of a cold) the child ought to be treated without doing a test. You will still incorrectly diagnose 10% of strep throats with the test. In general, as the probability of disease increases, the absolute number of missed strep throats will increase. In fact, most clinicians agree that if the post-test probability is greater than 50%, the child ought to be treated. This is the treatment threshold.

Similarly, if the probability of strep throat was 10% or less (mild sore throat, slight redness, minimal enlargement of the tonsils, no pus, minimally swollen and non-tender lymph nodes, no fever, and signs of a cold), half of all positives will be false positives. We would treat too many children. We don't gain much from a negative test, since almost all children are negative before we do the test. For a pretest probability of 10%, the PPV (as calculated before) is 50%. This is not above the treatment threshold value of 50%. The addition of the test is not going to help in differentiating the diagnosis of strep throat from that of viral pharyngitis. Therefore one should not do the test if this is the pretest probability of disease. This is the testing threshold.

If the pretest probability is between 10% and 50%, we will choose to do a test, probably the rapid strep test. This is a test that can be done quickly and will give an instant result. We choose to treat all children with a positive test. But we then have to decide what to do with a negative test. We can choose not to treat. We can also choose to do a gold-standard test on all those children with a negative test and with a moderately high pretest probability (say 50%). In this case we would do a throat-culture test. It is about five times more expensive and takes longer (two days as opposed to ten minutes) than the rapid strep test. We will save having to do the gold-standard test on half of the patients.

In the example of strep throat, the "costs" of doing the test (relatively inexpensive), of missing a case (uncommon complications), and of treatment reactions (allergies and side effects) are relatively low. Therefore the threshold for treatment would be pretty low, as will the threshold for testing.

This method is more important and becomes more complex in more serious clinical situations. Consider a patient complaining of shortness of breath. You suspect a pulmonary embolism (blood clot in the lungs). Should you order an expensive and potentially dangerous test in which dye is injected into the pulmonary arteries (pulmonary angiogram, the gold standard for this disease) in order to be certain of the diagnosis? The test itself is very uncomfortable, has some serious complications (about 10% major bleeding at the site of injection) and can cause death (less than 1% of the time).

Should you begin treatment based upon history, physical examination and an "imperfect" diagnostic test (ventilation–perfusion lung scan) that came up positive? There are problems with treatment. Treating with anticoagulants ("blood thinners") can cause excess bleeding (in an increasing number of patients as time on the drug increases) and the patient will be falsely labeled as having a serious disease (which could affect their future employability and insurability). These are difficult decisions and must be made considering all the options and the patient's values. They are the ultimate combination of science and art.

Finally, 95% confidence intervals should be calculated on all values of likelihood ratios, sensitivity, specificity and predictive values. The formulas for these are very complex. You can use an online calculator to do this. The best one is at the University of British Columbia website at www.healthcare.ubc.ca. Go to the Bayesian Calculator on the site. For very high or low values of sensitivity and specificity (FN or FP less than 5) you can use the rules for zero numerator to estimate the 95% CI. These are summarized in Chapter 13.

Multiple tests

The ideal test is capable of separating all normal people from people who have disease (definition of the "gold standard"). This test would be 100% sensitive and 100% specific with no false-positive or false-negative results. Few tests are both highly sensitive and specific, so it is common practice to use multiple tests in the diagnosis of disease. Using multiple tests to rule in or rule out disease changes the pretest probability for each new test when used in combination. This is because each test performed should raise or lower the pretest probability for the next test in the sequence. It is not possible to predict (a priori) how the use of multiple tests used in combination changes their operating characteristics.

This is because the tests may be dependent upon each other and measure the same or similar parts of the disease process. An example is using two different enzyme markers to measure heart-muscle cell damage in a heart attack. We say that tests are independent if they measure completely different things. An example

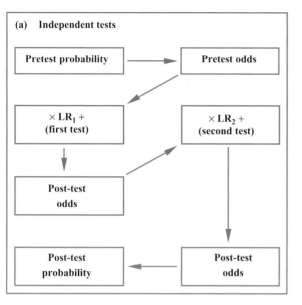

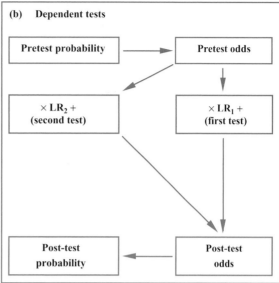

Fig. 24.7 Using multiple tests.

of this would be cardiac muscle enzymes and radionuclide scan of the heart muscle. An overview of the effects of using multiple tests is seen in Fig. 24.7.

In many diagnostic situations, multiple tests must be used to determine the final diagnosis. This is required when application of an initial test does not raise the probability of disease above the treatment threshold. If a positive result on the initial test does not increase the post-test probability of disease above the treatment threshold, a second, "confirmatory" test must be done. The expectation in this case is that a positive result on the second test will "clinch" the diagnosis (put the post-test probability above the treatment threshold).

If the second test is negative this leads to more problems. The negative result must be considered in the calculations of post-test probability. If the post-test probability after the negative second test is below the testing threshold the diagnosis is ruled out. Similarly, if the second test is positive and the post-test probability after the second test is above the treatment threshold, the diagnosis is confirmed. If the second test is negative and the resulting post-test probability is not below the testing threshold, a third test must be done. If that is positive, more testing may need to be done to resolve the discordant results on the three tests.

A complication in this process of calculation of post-test probability is that the two tests may not be independent of each other. If the tests are **independent**, they measure different things that are related to the same pathophysiological process. They both measure the same process but by different mechanisms. An example of independent tests is in the diagnosis of blood clots in the legs, deep vein thrombosis (DVT). Ultrasound testing takes a picture of the veins and blood flow through the veins using sound waves and a transducer. The serum level of d-dimer measures the presence of a byproduct of the clotting process. The two tests are complementary and independent. A positive d-dimer test is very non-specific, and a positive test does not confirm the diagnosis of DVT. A subsequent positive ultrasound virtually confirms the diagnosis. The ultrasound is not as sensitive, but is very specific. A positive test rules in the disease.

Two tests are **dependent** if they both measure the same pathophysiological process. An example would be the release of enzymes from damaged heart-muscle cells (acute myocardial infarction, AMI). The release of creatine kinase (CK) and troponin I (TropI) both occur through related pathological mechanisms. Therefore they ought to have the same characteristics (sensitivity and specificity). The two tests should give the same results when they are consecutively done on the same patient. There is a difference in the time course of release of each enzyme. Both are released early; troponin I persists for a longer time than CK. This makes the two of them useful tests when monitored over time. If a patient has an increased serum level of CK, the diagnosis of AMI is confirmed. A negative TropI may cast doubt upon the diagnosis and a positive TropI will confirm the diagnosis.

The use of multiple tests is more challenging than the use of a single test only. In general, a result that confirms the previous test result is considered confirmatory. A result that does not confirm the previous test result will most often not change the diagnosis immediately, but will only lead to questioning of the diagnosis. It then must be followed up with another test. If the pretest probability is high and the initial test is negative, or the pretest probability is low and the initial test is positive, a confirmatory test ought to be done.

If the pretest probability is high, a positive test is confirmatory (unless the specificity is very low). If the pretest probability is low, a negative test excludes disease (unless the sensitivity is very low). Obviously if the pretest probabilities are either *very high* or *very low*, the test ought not to be done and (in the case of very high pretest probability) treatment should immediately begin (without doing the test). Similarly, in the case of very low pretest probability, the test ought not to be done in the first place.

Real-life application of these principles

What happens in real life? Can these concepts be used clinically? You can do the calculations necessary to determine post-test probability. However, when you are "in the trenches," it is rarely helpful. You will most often do what you always do in a particular situation, what you have taught yourself to do through repeated similar clinical encounters. Those actions should be based on these principles of decision making. However, sometimes you will need to think about these concepts. There are some general rules that ought to be followed.

If the pretest probability of a diagnosis is high and the test result is positive there would be no question but to treat the patient. Similarly, if the pretest probability is low and the test result is negative, you would not treat the patient. However, if your disease has a high pretest probability and the test is negative, you must use a second test to confirm that the patient does not have the disease. If the second test is positive, you must do further investigation, probably the gold standard to "break the tie." Similarly, if the disease has a low pretest probability and the test is positive, you must do a second test to confirm that the patient actually has the disease. If the second test is negative, you will need to do further investigation, probably the gold-standard test.

In patients with a medium pretest probability, it may not be possible for a single test to determine the need to treat, unless that test has a very high or low likelihood ratio. In general, you can go with the result of the test if that result puts the post-test probability over the treatment threshold or under the testing threshold. The higher the LR+ of a positive test (preferably over 10 is good), the more likely it is to put the probability over the treatment threshold. The lower the LR− of a negative test (preferably under 0.1 is good) the more likely it is to put the probability under the testing threshold.

25

Sources of bias and critical appraisal of studies of diagnostic tests

It is a vice to trust all, and equally a vice to trust none.

Seneca (c.3 BC – AD 65): Letters to Lucilius

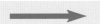

Learning objectives

In this chapter you will learn:
- the potential biases in studies of diagnostic tests
- the elements of critical appraisal of studies of diagnostic tests

Studies of diagnostic tests are unique in their design. Ideally they compare the tests in a sample of patients who have a diagnosis which we are certain is correct. The reader must be aware of potential sources of bias in evaluating these studies.

Overview of studies of diagnostic tests

In order to find bias in studies of diagnostic tests, it is necessary to know what these studies are intended to do. When evaluating studies of a diagnostic test, it is useful to use a structured approach. The first step is to formulate a four-part clinical question. In these cases, the question relates to the diagnostic test (intervention), gold standard (comparison), the patient population in whom the test would be done, and the target disorder that you are trying to diagnose.

A typical question might be framed as follows. You know that people with a blood clot in their lungs (pulmonary embolism, PE) can be diagnosed with the new-generation CT (x-ray-computed tomogram) of the chest. We want to know if this diagnostic tool is as accurate as the gold-standard pulmonary angiogram (squirting dye into the pulmonary artery and taking an x-ray) and better than the old standard test of the ventilation–perfusion (V/Q) scan of the lungs. The clinical question asks: in patients suspected of having a PE (population), does the chest

CT (intervention) diagnose definite PE (outcome as determined by angiogram) better than the V/Q scan (comparison)?

Studies of diagnostic tests should begin with a representative sample of people in whom the reasonable and average practitioner ought to be looking for the disease. This may not always be possible since studies done with different populations may result in differences in the characteristics of the test that cannot be predicted. Patient selection could limit the external validity of the test. In the ideal situation, the patients enrolled in the study are then all given the diagnostic test and the gold-standard tests without the researchers or the patient knowing the results of either test. The number of correct and incorrect diagnoses can then be computed.

As with any clinical study, there will be sources of bias in studies of diagnostic tests. Some of these are similar to biases that were presented in Chapter 8, but others are unique to studies of diagnostic tests. You ought to look for three broad categories of bias when evaluating studies of diagnostic tests. These are selection bias, observer bias, and miscellaneous biases.

Selection bias

Filter bias

Patients studied for a particular diagnostic test are selected because they possess a particular characteristic. While this should be explicit in the study methods it is often omitted. Part of the diagnostic process is selecting (or filtering out) which patients should get a particular diagnostic test done and which ones don't need it. If you as a clinician believe that a particular patient does not have the target disorder you would not order the test. Suspect this when only a portion of eligible patients are given the test. This process should be explicitly stated in any study of a diagnostic test. This way you can determine the external validity of the study. You can decide for yourself if your patient actually is similar enough to the patients in the study for you to order the test and expect results to be similar to those found in the study.

We will use our example of the study of patients with suspected PE. If only half of the eligible patients (only those strongly suspected of PE) are enrolled in the study and there is no clear-cut and reproducible way that they were selected, it is possible that an unknown filter was applied to them. Although this filter could be applied in an equitable and non-differential manner, it can still cause bias since its effect may be different in the groups of patients with and without the disease. This may make the test work better than it will in the community situation. The community doctor, not knowing what that filter was, would not know which patients to select to get the CT scan.

Spectrum and subgroup bias (case-mix bias)

A test may be more accurate when given to patients with classical forms of a disease. The test is more likely to identify patients with the disease in more severe or "well-developed" cases and less likely to accurately identify the patients who present earlier in the course of the disease or in whom the disease is occult (not obvious). This is a reflection of real-life test performance. Most diagnostic tests have very little utility in the general and asymptomatic population, while being very useful in specific clinical situations.

Some patients with leaking cerebral aneurysms present with severe headaches. If only a small leak is present, the patient is more likely to present with a severe headache and no neurological deficits. In this case, the CT scan will miss the bleed almost 50% of the time. If there is a massive bleed and the patient is unconscious or has severe neurologic deficit, the CT is positive in almost 100% of cases.

In the 1950s and 1960s, the yearly "executive physical examination" (including many laboratory, x-ray, and other tests) was very popular, especially among corporate executives. The yield of these examinations was very low. In fact the results were most often normal and, when abnormal, were usually falsely positive. We are seeing a similar phenomenon today with a proliferation of private CT scanners that are advertised as generalized screening tests for anyone who can pay for them. They are touted as being able to spot asymptomatic disease in early and curable stages with testimonials given on their usefulness. We will discuss the correct use of screening tests in Chapter 26.

Verification bias

Patients are selected to receive the gold-standard test based upon the results of the diagnostic test being evaluated. Those who have negative tests don't all have the gold standard test. This will usually make the test perform better than it would if it were done on all patients who would be considered for the test in a real clinical situation. Frequently, patients with negative tests are followed clinically for a certain period of time instead of having the gold-standard test performed on them. This may be appropriate if no patients are lost to follow-up and if the presence of disease results in some measurable change in the patient over the time of follow-up. You cannot do this with silent diseases that become apparent only many years later unless you follow all the patients for many years.

Incorporation bias

The diagnostic test being studied is used as or is part of the gold standard. One diagnostic sign of interest is a reason that patients are enrolled into the study. This means that the final diagnosis of the disease is dependent on the presence of a positive diagnostic test. Ideally the diagnostic test and the gold standard should be independent of each other. This means that there is no mechanistic relationship between them.

A classic example of this type of bias occurs in studies of acute myocardial infarction (AMI). One criterion for diagnosis of AMI is the elevation of the creatine kinase enzyme (CK) in the blood of patients with AMI. This results from muscle damage as the result of an infarction. The other criterion is characteristic changes on the electrocardiogram. Studies of the usefulness of CK as a serum marker for making the diagnosis of AMI will be flawed if it is used as part of the definition of AMI. CK will be increased in all AMI patients since it is both the diagnostic test (reference or gold-standard) and the test being investigated. This will make it look better (more accurate) in the diagnosis of AMI.

In another example, patients with suspected carpal tunnel syndrome have certain common clinical signs of carpal tunnel syndrome such as tenderness over the carpal tunnel. The presence of this sign gets them into a study looking at the validity and usefulness of common signs of carpal tunnel syndrome, which are important diagnostic criteria in patients referred for specialty care. This bias makes the sign look better than it actually is in making a positive diagnosis since patients who might not have this sign, and who probably have milder disease, were never referred to the specialist and were therefore excluded from the study.

Observer bias

Absence of a definitive test (tarnished gold standard)

This is probably the most common problem with studies of diagnostic tests. The gold standard must be reasonably defined. In most cases, no true gold standard exists, and you must make do with the best that is available.

For example, patients with abdominal trauma may undergo a CT scan of the abdomen to look for internal organ damage. If the scan is positive, they are admitted to the hospital and may be operated upon. If it is negative, they are discharged and followed for a period of time to make sure a significant injury was not missed. However, if the follow-up time is too short or incomplete, there may be some patients with significant missed injuries who are not discovered and some may be lost to follow-up. The real gold standard, operating on everyone with abdominal trauma, is ethically unacceptable.

Review bias (interpretation bias)

Interpretation of a test can be affected by the knowledge of the results of other tests or clinical information. This can be prevented if the persons interpreting the test results are blinded to the nature of the patient's other test results or clinical presentation. If this bias is present, the test will appear to work better than it otherwise would in an uncontrolled clinical situation. There are two forms of review bias.

In **test review bias**, the person interpreting the tests has prior knowledge of the patient's outcome (or gold-standard test result), and therefore may be more likely to interpret the test so that it confirms the (already known) diagnosis. For example, a radiologist reading the myocardial perfusion scan (map of blood flow through the heart) of a patient whom they know to have an AMI is more likely to read an equivocal area of the scan as showing no flow and therefore consistent with an MI. This is because he or she knows that there is a heart attack in that area (i.e., an area of heart muscle with diminished blood flow), and as a result interprets the equivocal sign as definitely showing no flow.

In **diagnostic review bias**, the person interpreting the gold-standard test knows the result of the diagnostic test. This may change the interpretation of the gold standard, and make the diagnostic test look better (since it will concur with the gold standard more often). This will not occur if the gold-standard test is completely objective (e.g., totally automated or a dichotomous result) and if the interpreter is blinded to the results of the diagnostic test. For example, a patient with a positive ultrasound of the leg veins is diagnosed with deep venous thrombosis (blood clot in veins). A radiologist reading the venogram (x-ray of the veins) is more likely to read an equivocal area as one showing blockage since he or she knows that the diagnostic test showed an area of clot.

Context bias

This is a common heuristic, or thought pattern. The person interpreting the test will base their reading of the test upon known clinical information. This can be a bias when determining raw test data or in a real-life situation. Radiologists are more likely to read pneumonia on a chest x-ray if they are told that the patient has classical findings of pneumonia (cough, fever, and localized rales over one part of the lungs, etc.) on examination. In daily clinical situations, this will make the correlation between clinical data and test results seem better than they may be in a situation in which the radiologist is given much less clinical information.

Miscellaneous sources of bias

Indeterminate and uninterpretable results

Some tests have results that are not always clearly positive or negative, but may be unclear, indeterminate, or uninterpretable. If these are classified as positive or negative, the characteristics of the test will be changed. This makes calculation and manipulation of likelihood ratios or sensitivity and specificity much more complicated since categories are no longer dichotomous, but have other possible outcomes.

For example, some patients with pulmonary emboli (blood clots in the lungs) have an indeterminate lung scan (scan showing distribution of radioactive material in the lung) when tested for this condition. This means that the results are neither positive nor negative and the clinician is unsure about how to proceed. Similarly, the CT scan for appendicitis in some patients with the condition may not show the entire appendix. This is more likely to occur if the appendix lies in a retrocecal location. In cases of patients who actually have the disease, if the result is classified as positive, the patient will be correctly classified. If however, the result is classified as negative, the patient will be incorrectly classified.

Reproducibility

The performance of a diagnostic test depends on the performance of the technician and the equipment used in performance of the test. Tests that are operator-dependent are most prone to this. They may perform very well when carried out in a research setting, but when extrapolated to the community the persons performing them may never rise to the level of expertise required, either because they don't do enough of the tests to become really proficient or because of lack of enthusiasm or interest. For example, CT scans for appendicitis are harder to read than for other GI problems. When tested in a center that was doing research on this use, they performed very well. When extrapolated to the community hospital setting, they did less well.

Post-hoc selection of test positivity criteria

This situation is often seen when a continuous variable is converted to a dichotomous one for purposes of defining the cutoff between normal and abnormal. In studying the test, it is discovered that most patients with the disease being sought have a test value above a certain threshold and most without the disease have a test value below that threshold. There is statistical significance for the difference in disease occurrence in these two groups ($P < 0.05$). That threshold is therefore selected as the cutoff point.

It is possible that the researchers looked at several cutoff points before deciding on a final one. Some of them produced differences that were not statistically significant. This is a form of data dredging and could be a Type I error. A validation study should be done to verify this result. This problem can be evaluated by using likelihood ratios and sensitivity and specificity rather than statistical significance as the defining variables in test performance.

Temporal changes

Test characteristics measured at one point in time may change as the test is techni-cally improved. The measures calculated from the studies of the newer technology will not apply to the older technology. This is especially true in radiology, where new generations of MRI machines, CT scanners, and other imaging modalities are regularly introduced. The results of a study done with the latest generation of CT scanners may not be seen if your hospital is still using the older scanners. Look for this problem in the use of newer biochemical or pathological tests, as well as in questionnaire tests.

Publication bias

Studies that are positive, that find a statistically significant difference between groups, are more likely to be published than those that find no difference. Consider the possibility that there may be several unpublished negative studies "out there" when deciding to accept the results of studies of a new test.

Words of caution: the manufacturers of a new test want many physicians to use the test as much as possible and may sponsor studies that have these biases. There is lots of money to be made in the introduction of a new test, especially if it involves a new technology. For example, an MRI (magnetic resonance imaging) machine costs several million dollars, which must be justified by the performance of lots of scans. These may not be justified based on good objective evidence. As a conscientious physician, you must decide when these expensive technologies are truly useful to your patient.

Studies sponsored by the manufacturer of the test being studied are always open to extra scrutiny. Although this does not automatically make it a bad study, the authors have a financial stake in the results of the study, and often "spin" the results in the most favorable manner. Conversely, a company producing a diagnostic test will resist publication of a negative study, and this may lead to suppression of important medical information.

The ideal study

We will use the following hypothetical example of an ideal research study of a diagnostic test. The study looked at the use of head CT in predicting the compli-cations of stroke therapy with blood thinners. Patients who are having a stroke get an immediate head CT. The scan is initially read by a community radiologist (not a neuro-radiologist, a specialist in reading head CTs) who is part of the treating group. If in that radiologist's opinion the scan shows any sign of potential bleeding into the brain, that patient is excluded from the study.

This scan is then taken to two neuro-radiologists who are experts in reading head CTs. They read the scan without knowing the nature of the patient problem or each other's reading of the scan. If they disagree with each other's reading, a third radiologist is called in as a tiebreaker. All patients who are felt to be clinically eligible for the drug are given either the drug or placebo. The rate of resolution of symptoms and the percentage of patients who make full recovery, do worse, and die are measured for each group.

The reference standard is the reading of the two blinded radiologists, or majority in the case of disagreement. This is not perfect, but mirrors the best that could be done in the community. The outcome should then be judged by a clinician (probably a neurologist in this case) who is also blinded to the results of the CT and the group to which the patient was randomized. Although not perfect, and no study is, there are adequate safeguards to ensure the validity of the results. The inclusion criteria are specified and the filter for which patients are chosen is explicit. The biggest problem with this study is that patients who are excluded by the initial reading of the CT may in fact have been eligible for the treatment. However, in a real-life situation, this is what would occur, so the results are generalizable to the setting of a community hospital.

The gold standard is clearly defined and about as good as it gets. The test (CT read by community radiologist) and gold standard (CT read by neuro-radiology specialist) are independent of each other and read in a blinded manner since the two groups of radiologists are not communicating with each other. A more perfect gold standard could be MRI (magnetic resonance imaging) of the brain. All patients would need to have both the diagnostic test and the gold-standard test. The follow-up period must be made sufficiently long. There is not a significant problem here as all patients can be observed immediately for the outcome. The outcome is being measured by a clinician who is blinded to the results of the gold-standard test and the treatment given to the patient.

How to evaluate research studies of diagnostic tests: putting it all together

As a practicing physician, you will be faced with being able to order an ever-increasing number of diagnostic tests. Many of these will have only theoretical promise and may not have been tested very thoroughly in clinical practice. You must be able to critically evaluate the studies of diagnostic tests and determine for yourself whether the test is appropriate to use in your particular clinical setting. The criteria discussed in this chapter are taken (with permission) from the series called Users' guides to the medical literature, published in *JAMA* (see Bibliography).

Are the results valid?

(1) Was there an independent, blind comparison with a reference (gold) standard of diagnosis?

Diagnostic test studies measure the degree of association between the predictor variable (test result) and the outcome (disease). The presence or absence of the outcome is determined by the result of a reference or gold-standard test. The presence of absence of disease is determined by the gold standard. The diagnostic test under study cannot be used to determine the presence or absence of the disease (incorporation bias).

The term "normal" must be sensibly defined. How this term is arrived at (Gaussian, percentile, risk factor, culturally desirable, diagnostic, or therapeutic) must be specified. If prolonged follow-up of apparently well patients is used to define the absence of disease, the period of follow-up must be reasonable so that any latent cases of the disease in question can be identified.

Both the diagnostic test being studied and the gold standard must be applied to the study and control subjects in a standard and blinded fashion. This should be done following a standardized protocol and using trained observers to improve reliability. Comparing the new test to the gold standard assesses accuracy and validity. Blinding reduces measurement bias. Ideally, the test should be automated (not operator-dependent), multiple measurements made, and at least two investigators involved. One will apply or interpret the new diagnostic test to the subjects while the second will apply the gold standard to the subjects.

(2) Was the study test described adequately?

The test results should be easily reproducible (reliability) and easy to interpret (low inter-observer variation). Enough information should be present in the Methods section to perform the diagnostic test, including any special requirements, dosages, precautions, and timing sequences. An estimated cost of performing the test should be included, including reagents, physician or technician time, specialty care, and turn-around time. Long and short-term side effects and complications associated with the test should be discussed. The test parameters may be very variable in different settings because test reliability varies. For "operator-dependent tests" the level of skill of the person performing the test should be noted.

(3) Was the diagnostic test evaluated in an appropriate spectrum of patients?

In order to reduce sampling bias, the study patients should be adequately described and representative of the population likely to receive the test. The distribution of age, sex, and spectrum of other medical disorders unrelated to the outcome of interest should be representative of the population in whom the test will ultimately be used. The spectrum of disease should be wide enough to represent all the outcomes of interest, including early disease, late disease, classical cases, and difficult-to-diagnose cases (i.e., those commonly confused with other disorders). If only very classical cases are studied, the diagnostic test may perform better than it would for less characteristic cases (spectrum bias).

Frequently research studies of diagnostic tests are done at referral centers that see many cases of severe, classical, or unmistakable disease. This may not correlate with disease seen in physicians' offices or community hospitals (referral or sampling bias). Investigators testing a new test often choose a sample of subjects that have a higher-than-average prevalence of disease. This may not represent the prevalence of disease in the population. If the study is a case–control study or retrospective study, typically 50% of the subjects will have disease and 50% will be normal.

There should be no evidence that any kind of selection filter was used to preselect some people (who are eligible for the test) to be in the diseased group as opposed to others (who should also be eligible for the test). The control patients should be similar in every way to the diseased subjects except for the presence of disease. You cannot use only young healthy volunteers for this! The similarity of study and control subjects increases the possibility that the test is measuring differences due to disease and not age, sex, general health, or other disease conditions.

(4) Was the reference standard applied regardless of the diagnostic test result?

The choice of a reference or diagnostic standard (gold standard) may be very difficult. The diagnostic standard test may be invasive, painful, costly, and possibly even dangerous to the patient, resulting in morbidity and even mortality. Obviously taking a biopsy is a very good reference standard, but it may involve major surgery for the patient. For this reason, for many diseases, prolonged follow-up of affected patients is an acceptable standard. How and for how long this follow-up is done will often determine the internal validity of the study. The study should be free of verification and other forms of review bias (test review and context).

(5) Has the utility of the test been determined?

If the test is to be used (or the investigator desires that it be used) as part of a battery or sequence of tests, the contribution of this test to the overall validity of the battery or sequence must be determined. Is the patient better off for having the test done? Is the diagnosis made earlier, the treatment made more effective, the diagnosis made more cheaply, or more safely?

What is the impact of the results?

The study results must be important. This means you must evaluate the likelihood ratios of the test. In most studies you will wind up doing this by calculation from the sensitivity and specificity. If these are reasonably good, you can go on to the next step, deciding if the results can be applied to your patients. Confidence intervals should be given.

Can the results be applied to my patients?

Consider the population tested and the patient whom you are evaluating. The answer to the question of generalizability or particularizability depends on how similar your patient is to the study population. You have to ask whether he or she would have been included in the study. Ideally we want the answer always to be yes. But sometimes there are reasons for using a particular population. For example, studies done at the Veterans Affairs Hospital System will be mostly of men. This does not automatically disqualify your female patient from having the test done for the target disorder. There ought to be a good reason to exclude the results. Perhaps there is some hormonal effect on the results of the test. However, you must use your best clinical judgment to be able to determine whether the results of the study can be used in your patient. Other factors which might affect the characteristics of the test in your patient, include age and ethnic group.

(1) Is the diagnostic test available, affordable, accurate and precise in my setting?

You must know the capabilities of your lab or diagnostic center. This is a function of the type of equipment used and the operator-dependency of the test. The estimated costs of false-positive and false-negative test results should be addressed, including the cost of repeat testing or further diagnostic procedures for false-positive results and of a missed diagnosis due to false-negative results. The cost of the test should be given, as well as the cost of following up on false-positive tests and missing some patients with false-negative tests.

(2) Can I come up with a reasonable pretest probability of disease for my patient?

This was addressed earlier, and although small deviations from the true pretest probability are not important, large variations are. You do not want to be very far off (say you estimate 10% and the true probability is 90%) or you will miss the ability to diagnose the problem. The data come from several sources. These include published studies of symptoms, your personal experience, the study itself (if the sample is reasonably representative of the population of patients from which your patient comes), and clinical judgment. If none of these gives a reasonable pretest probability, you ought to consider getting some help. A colleague (consultant) will probably help here.

(3) Will the post-test probability change my management of this patient?

This is the most important question to ask about the usefulness of a diagnostic test, and will determine whether you do the test or not. The first issue is a mathematical one. Will the resulting post-test probability move the probability across the testing or treatment threshold? If not, either do not do the test, or be prepared to do a second (or third) test to confirm.

Next, is the patient interested in having the test done and are they going to be "part of the team?" If the patient is not a willing partner in the process, you might as well not begin. You must be able to give the information to your patients in a manner they can understand and then ask them if they want to go through with the testing. They ought to know the risks of disease, and of correct and incorrect results of testing, and the ramifications of a positive and negative test. Incorporated in this is the question of ultimate utility of the test.

Finally, how will a positive or negative result help your patient reach his or her goals for treatment? If the patient has "heartburn" and you no longer suspect a cardiac problem, but suspect gastritis or peptic ulcers, will doing a test for *Helicobacter pylori* infection (as a cause of ulcers) and specific anti-microbial treatment if positive, or symptomatic treatment if negative, satisfy the patient that he does not have a gastric carcinoma? If not, then endoscopy (the gold standard) ought to be considered without stopping for the intermediate test.

Studies of diagnostic tests should determine the sensitivity and specificity of the test under varying circumstances. The prevalence of disease in the population studied may be very different from that in most clinical practices. Therefore, predictive values reported in the literature should be reserved for validation studies and studies of the use of the test under clinical conditions.

Final thoughts about diagnostic test studies

It is critical to realize that studies of diagnostic tests done in the past were often done differently than those we recommend be done now. Many of these studies looked for the correlation between a diagnostic test and the final diagnosis. For example, a study of pneumonia might look at all physical-examination findings for patients who were subjected to chest x-rays, and determine which correlated most closely with a positive chest x-ray (the gold standard).

There are two problems with these types of studies. First, the patients are selected by inclusion criteria (got a chest x-ray), which already narrows down the probability that they have the illness. Second, correlation only tells us that you are more or less likely to find a certain clinical finding with an illness. It does not tell you what the probability of the illness is after application of that finding or test. The correlation does give some useful information in that it will tell the clinician if certain diagnostic findings correlate with the presence of illness. It will not tell you how to use the clinical finding to determine the presence of disease since the patients were screened using the clinical finding and therefore it cannot become the outcome variable of the study.

26

Screening tests

Detection is, or ought to be, an exact science, and should be treated in the same cold and unemotional manner. You have attempted to tinge it with romanticism, which produces much the same effect as if you worked a love-story or an elopement into the fifth proposition of Euclid.

Sir Arthur Conan Doyle (1859–1930): The Sign of Four, 1890

Learning objectives

In this chapter you will learn:
- the attributes of a good screening test
- the effects of lead-time and length-time biases and how to recognize them in evaluating a screening test
- how to evaluate the usefulness of a screening test
- how to evaluate studies of screening tests

Introduction

Screening tests are defined as diagnostic tests that are useful in detecting disease in asymptomatic or presymptomatic persons. The goal of all screening tests is to diagnose the disease at a stage when it is more easily curable (Fig. 26.1). This is usually earlier than the symptomatic stage and is one of the reasons for doing a diagnostic test.

Screening tests must rise to a higher level of utility since the majority of people being screened derive no utility from the test. Because the vast majority of people who are screened do not have the disease, they get minimal reassurance from a negative test. A negative test is only a small benefit since their pretest probability of disease was low to start with. However, for many people, the psychological relief in a negative test (especially for something they are really scared of) is a worthwhile positive outcome.

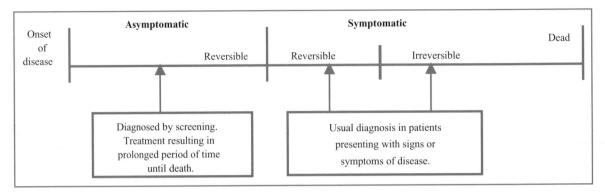

Fig. 26.1 Disease timeline and diagnosis by screening or diagnostic test. The ideal screening test.

There are three rules for diagnostic tests that must be more carefully applied to screening tests. The first rule is that there is no free lunch. As the sensitivity of a test increases to detect a greater percentage of diseased persons, the number of false positives increases and specificity falls. The second rule is that prevalence matters. As the prevalence decreases, the number of false positives increases (and relative number of true positives decreases). The final rule is that the burden of proof (regarding efficacy) depends upon the clinical context, which depends on multiple factors. If the intervention is innocuous, screening should be done more often than if the intervention is dangerous (high-risk or toxic). Similarly, if the test or treatment is very expensive, the level of proof must be greater.

During the 1950s the executive physical examination was used to screen for "all" diseases in corporate executives and other (mostly wealthy) people. It was a comprehensive set of diagnostic tests (multiple x-rays, blood tests, exercise stress tests, etc.) usually administered while the patient spent a week in the hospital. It was justified by the thought that finding disease early was good and would lead to improved length and quality of life. The more disease looked for, the more that would be found in an earlier phase, and treatment at this early stage would lead to better health outcomes. Subsequent analysis of the data from these extensive examination programs revealed no change in health outcomes as a result of these examinations. There were more people incorrectly labeled with diseases which they didn't have than diseases detected early enough to reduce mortality or morbidity. Ironically, most of the diseases that were identified in these programs could have been detected from a comprehensive history only.

Criteria for screening

There are five criteria that must be fulfilled before a test should be used as a screening test. These are listed in Table 26.1. Following these will prevent the abuses of screening tests that occurred in the 1950s and 1960s and which continue today.

Table 26.1. Criteria for a valid screening test

(1) Burden of suffering	The disease must be relatively common. The burden of suffering must be sufficiently great.
(2) Early detectability	The disease must be detectable at an early stage, preferably when totally curable.
(3) Accuracy and validity	The test must be accurate and valid: it must reliably pick up disease (few misses) and not falsely label too many healthy people.
(4) Acceptability	The test must be simple, inexpensive, not noxious, and easy to administer. It must be acceptable to the patient and to the health-care system.
(5) Improved outcome	There must be treatment available, which if given at the time that early disease is detected, will result in improved outcome (lower mortality and morbidity) among those patients being screened.

The disease must impose a significant burden of suffering on the population to be screened. This means either that the disease is common or that it results in serious disability. This disability may result in loss of productive employment, patient discomfort or dissatisfaction, as well as passing the disease on to others. It also means that it will cost someone a lot of money to care for persons with the disease. We hope to reduce this cost both in human suffering and in dollars by treating at an earlier stage of disease and preventing complications or early death. We depend on well-designed studies of harm (risk) to tell us which diseases are likely to be encountered in a significant part of the population in order to decide to screen for them.

For example, it would be unreasonable to screen the population of all 20-year-old women for breast cancer with yearly mammography. The risk of disease is so low in this population that even a tiny risk of increased cancer associated with the radiation from the examination may cause more cancers than the test would detect. Similarly screening for HIV in an extremely low-risk population would lead to incorrectly labeling many more people as being HIV-positive who were not affected (false positives). This would lead to a lot of psychological trauma and require lots of confirmatory testing in these positives, which would cost a huge amount of money to find one true case of HIV.

The screening test must be a good one. It must accurately detect disease in the population of people who are in the presymptomatic phase of disease (high sensitivity). It should also reliably exclude disease in the population without disease (high specificity). Of the two, the specificity must be extremely high so that only a few people without disease are mislabeled (high positive predictive value, PPV). A confirmatory test must be available that will more accurately discriminate between those people with a positive screening test who do and don't have the disease. This confirmatory test ought to be not only acceptable (not uncomfortable or causing serious side effects) to most people, but also reasonably priced.

A screening test will be unacceptable if it produces too many false positives since those people will be falsely labeled as having disease, a circumstance which could lead to insurance or employment discrimination or social conflicts. False labeling has a deleterious effect on most people. Several studies have found significant increases in anxiety, which interferes with life activities, in persons who were falsely labeled as having disease on a screening test. This is an especially serious issue with genetic tests in which a positive test does not mean the disease will express itself, but only that a person has the gene for the disease.

There are practical qualities of a good screening test. The cost ought to be low so it can be economically done on large populations. It should be simple to perform with good accuracy and reliability. And finally, it must be acceptable to the patient. For screening tests, most people will tolerate only a low level of discomfort either from the test procedure itself or from the paperwork involved in getting the test done. People are more willing to have a test performed to detect disease when they are symptomatic than when they are well. People would much rather have their blood pressure taken to screen for hypertension than have a colonoscopy to look for early signs of colon cancer.

The mechanics of a screening program must be well planned. We are giving a huge number of people a diagnostic test. If the test is too complex (e.g., screening colonoscopy for colon cancer) most people would not be willing to have it done. A test that is very uncomfortable (e.g., digital rectal exam for prostate or rectal cancer) may be refused by a large proportion of patients. Both examples also require more complex logistics (individual examining rooms and sedation for the colonoscopy) than a screening test such as blood pressure. Screening tests must also be well advertised so that people will know why and how to have the test done.

Pitfalls in the screening process

Simply diagnosing the disease at an earlier stage is not helpful unless the prognosis is better if treatment is begun at that earlier stage of the illness. The treatment must be acceptable and more effective before people will be willing to accept treatment at an asymptomatic stage of illness. Why should someone take a drug for hypertension when that drug can cause significant side effects and must be taken for a lifetime, if they have no signs or symptoms of the disease?

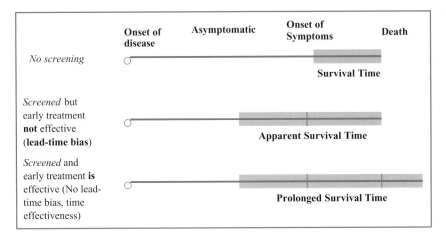

Fig. 26.2 Lead-time bias.

During the 1960s and 1970s, lung cancers were detected at an earlier stage by routine screening chest x-rays. However, immediate treatment of these cancers did not result in increased survival, and caused increased patient suffering due to serious side effects of the surgery and drugs. Therefore, even though cancers were detected at an earlier stage, mortality was the same.

You can determine the validity of a screening test from the evidence in the literature. Screening tests must balance the need to learn something about a patient (diagnostic yield) with the ability to actively and effectively intervene in the disease process at an earlier stage.

There are three significant problems of studies of screening tests. These are **lead-time, length-time**, and **compliance biases**. Lead-time bias results in over-optimistic results of the screening test in the clinical study. The patients seem to live longer but this is only because their disease is detected earlier. In this case, the total time from onset of illness to death is the same in the screened (and treated early) group and the unscreened group. The lead time is the time from diagnosis of disease by screening test to the appearance of symptoms. The time from appearance of symptoms to death is the same whether the disease was detected by the screening test or not. The total life span of the screened patient is no different than that of the unscreened patient. The time between early diagnosis with the screening test and appearance of symptoms (the lead time) will now be spent undergoing treatment (Fig. 26.2). This could be very uncomfortable (from side effects of treatment) or dangerous (if treatment can result in death) for the patient.

Length-time bias is much more likely to occur in observational studies. Patients are not randomized and the spectrum of disease may be very different in the screened group as compared to the unscreened group. A disease that is indolent and slowly progressive is more likely to be detected than one that is rapidly progressive and quickly fatal. Patients with aggressive cancers are more likely to

Fig. 26.3 Length-time bias.

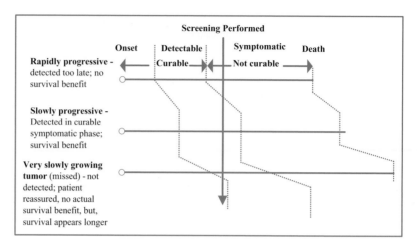

die shortly after their cancer is detected. Those with slow growing indolent tumors are more likely to be cured of their disease after screening and will live a long time until they die of other causes. There are some whose disease is too early to detect and who will be missed by screening. Without screening, his or her disease will be detected when it becomes symptomatic, which will be at a later stage. This problem can be reduced in large population studies by effective randomization that ensures a similar spectrum of disease in screened and unscreened patients. This is illustrated in Fig. 26.3.

Compliance bias occurs because patients who are compliant with therapy (in general) do better than those who are not, regardless of the therapy. Compliant patients may have other characteristics that lead to better outcomes (for example they may be more health-conscious). Studies of screening tests often compare a group of people who are in a screening program with people in the population who are not in the screening program. They are usually not randomized to be in either group. Therefore, the screened group is more likely to be composed of people who are more compliant, since they took advantage of the screening test in the first place. This will make it more likely that the screened group will do better since they are the compliant patients. This bias can be avoided if patients in these studies are randomized before being put through the screening test.

Effectiveness of screening

Another problem with screening tests revolves around their overall effectiveness. For example, consider the use of mammograms for the early detection of breast cancer in young women. Women aged 50–70 in whom the cancer is detected at an early stage do appear to have better outcomes. The use of mammography for screening younger women (age 40–50) is still controversial. In studies of this

Table 26.2. Screening 40—50-year-old women for breast cancer using mammography

	Screened	Not screened
Total population	1000	1000
Positive mammogram	300	—
Biopsies (invasive procedures)	150	—
New breast cancers	15	15
Deaths from breast cancer	5–8	7–8

Source: From: D. Eddy. *Clinical Decision Making.* Sudbury, MA: Jones & Bartlett, 1996.

group, it made very little difference in ultimate survival if the woman was screened. Early detection in this population resulted in a large number of false-positive tests requiring biopsy and unnecessary worry for the women affected. It also resulted in an increased exposure to x-rays among these women and increased the cost of health care for everyone in the society.

A convenient concept to use in the calculation of benefit is the number needed to screen (NNS). Like the number needed to treat (NNT), it is simply 1/ARR. ARR is the absolute risk reduction or the difference in percentage response between the screened and unscreened groups. The ideal number to use here is the percentage of women who die from their cancer in the screened (EER) and unscreened (CER) groups. The NNS can be used to balance the positive and negative effects of screening. For example, in the case of using mammograms to screen for breast cancer in women at age 40, we can make the spreadsheet in Table 26.2.

On the benefit side, there is the prevention of at most three deaths per 1000 women screened. This leads to a large NNS = 333. This means that 333 women must be screened to prevent one death from breast cancer.

$$CER = 8/1000 \quad EER = 5/1000 \quad ARR = (8/1000 - 5/1000) = 3/1000$$

$$NNS = 1/ARR = 1/(3/1000) = 1/0.003 = 333$$

If the tests actually result in the same number of deaths from breast cancer (8% in both groups), the NNS will be infinite and there will be no benefit of screening.

Typical acceptable NNS for currently used screening modalities are in the 100–1000 range. If the test is relatively benign or treatment is very easy and the expected outcome is very good in the screened population a much larger NNS is acceptable. More randomized clinical trials of screening tests are needed to determine acceptable levels of NNS.

The United States Public Heath Service (USPHS) has published a set of criteria for an acceptable screening test. The test must be able to detect the target condition earlier than without screening and with sufficient accuracy to avoid producing large numbers of false-positive and false-negative results (accuracy of diagnostic test). Screening for and treating persons with early disease should improve the likelihood of favorable health outcomes (e.g., reduced disease-specific mortality or morbidity) compared to treating patients when they present with signs or symptoms of the disease (effectiveness of early detection). These criteria come from the USPHS *Guide to Clinical Preventive Services*, which also contains a compendium of recommendations for the use of the most important screening tests.[1] There are also very effective evidence-based guidelines for screening put out by the Agency for Healthcare Research and Quality.[2]

Critical appraisal of studies of screening tests[3]

(1) **Are the recommendations valid?**

  (a) Is there randomized-trial evidence that earlier intervention works?

   Most screening strategies are based upon observational studies. Ideally, the intervention should be shown to be effective in a well-done RCT. The overall screening strategy should also be validated by RCT, unless the intervention is so dramatic (and most aren't) that there is no question about its efficacy. Observational studies of screening are weaker than a well-done randomized clinical trial. If there is a randomized trial of the screening modality, it should be first analyzed using the *Users' guide* for studies of therapy.

  (b) Were the data identified, selected, and combined in an unbiased fashion?

   Look for potential confounding factors when subjects are recruited or identified for inclusion in a study of screening. These may easily result in serious bias. Innate differences between the screened and not-screened groups should be aggressively sought. Frequently these differences are glossed over as being insignificant and they often are not.

(2) **What are the recommendations and will they help me in caring for my patients? What are the benefits?**

  (a) What are the benefits?

   You should be able to calculate the NNS (number needed to screen). The beneficial outcomes that the results refer to should be important for the patient. The confidence intervals should be narrow.

---

[1] US Preventive Services Task Force. *Guide to Clinical Preventive Services*. 2nd edn. Washington, DC: USPHS, 1996. Available online through the National Library of Medicine's HSTAT service at hstat.nlm.nih.gov.

[2] Agency for Healthcare Research and Quality. www.ahrq.gov.

[3] Adapted with permission from the Users' Guides to the Medical Literature, published in *JAMA* (see Bibliography).

(b) What are the harms?

There are several potential harms. Persons who are labeled with the disease and who are really disease-free will be inconvenienced and may require additional testing that is not benign, or at least have increased anxiety until the final diagnosis is made. Early treatment may result in such severe side effects that patients may not want the treatment. You should be able to calculate the NNH of these based upon the study data. This should be done with confidence intervals so you can see the precision of the results.

(c) How do these compare in different people and with different screening strategies?

All possible screening strategies should be looked at when evaluating screening. Different strategies may result in different outcomes either in final results or patient suffering, depending upon the population screened and the strategy employed.

(d) What is the impact of people's values and preferences?

There ought to be an evaluation of this as part of the study. If this is missing, you ought to be suspicious about the acceptability of the screening strategy. The study should be asking patients how they feel about screening and being falsely labeled.

(e) What is the impact of uncertainty?

A sensitivity analysis (described in Chapter 28) should accompany the analysis. There is uncertainty associated with any study result and the confidence intervals should be given.

(f) What is the cost-effectiveness?

This should be done, and should consider all the possible costs associated with the screening, including (but not limited to) setting up the program, advertising, following up positives, and excess testing and treatment of positives. A more complete guide to cost-effectiveness analysis is found in Chapter 29.

27

Practice guidelines and clinical prediction rules

Any fool can make a rule
And every fool will mind it.

Henry David Thoreau (1817–1862): Journal, 1860

Whoever controls guidelines controls medicine

D. Eddy, JAMA, 1990; 263: 877–880

Learning objectives

In this chapter you will learn:
- the reasons for and origins of practice guidelines
- the problems associated with practice guidelines and the process by which they are developed
- how to evaluate practice guidelines and how they are actually used in practice
- the process of clinical prediction rule development
- the significance of different levels of prediction rules

What are practice guidelines?

Practice guidelines have always been with us. They are present in the "diagnosis" and "treatment" sections in medical textbooks. Unfortunately, published practice guidelines are not always evidence-based. As an example, for treatment of frostbite on the fingers a surgical textbook says that operation should wait until the frostbitten part falls off, yet there are no studies backing up this claim. Treatment guidelines for glaucoma state that treatment should be initiated if the intraocular pressure is over 30 mm Hg or over a value in the middle 20 mm Hg range if the patient has two or more risk factors. It then gives a list of over 100 risk factors but gives no probability estimates of the increase in rate of glaucoma attributable to any risk factor. Clearly these are not evidence-based or particularly helpful.

Practice guidelines are simply a set of steps which when followed will result in the best outcome. In the past, they have been used for good (hand washing before vaginal delivery to prevent childbed fever, puerperal sepsis) and bad (frontal lobotomies to treat schizophrenia). In some cases they are promulgated as a result of political pressure. One recent example is breast-cancer screening with mammograms in women between 40 and 50 years old. This has been instituted in spite of lack of good evidence of improved outcomes. This particular program can cost a billion dollars a year without saving very many lives and can irrationally shape behavior for years.

A physician in 1916 said "once a Caesarian section, always a Caesarian section," meaning that if a woman required a Caesarian section for delivery, all subsequent deliveries should be by Caesarian section. As a result of this one statement, the practice became institutionalized. This particular "guideline" was based on a bad outcome in just a few patients. It may have been valuable 85 years ago, but with modern obstetrical techniques it is less useful. Many recent studies had cast doubts on the validity of this guideline, but a new study suggests that there is a slightly increased risk of rupture and poor outcome for mother and baby if this is not done. Clearly the jury is still out on this one, and it is up to the individual patient with her doctor's input to make the best decision for her and her baby.

Practice guidelines are used for a variety of purposes. Primarily they ought to be used as a template for optimal patient care. This should be the best reason for their implementation and use in clinical practice. When evidence-based practice guidelines are written, reviewed, and based upon solid high-quality evidence, they should be implemented by all physicians. A good example of an evidence-based clinical guideline in current use is weight-based dosing of heparin (an anticoagulant) for the treatment of deep venous thrombosis (DVT). When the guideline is used, there are fewer adverse effects of treatment (treatment failure or bleeding) and better outcomes (more rapid resolution of the DVT).

However, there are "darker" consequences that accompany the use of practice guidelines. They can be used as means of accreditation or certification. Currently several specialty boards use chart-review processes as part of the specialty recertification process. Managed care organizations (MCOs) can develop accreditation rules that depend on physician adherence to practice guidelines in the majority of their patients with a given problem. Performance criteria can be used as incentives in the determination of merit pay or bonuses.

In the last 30 years there has been an increase in the use of (practice) guidelines in determining the proper utilization of hospital beds. Utilization review has resulted in the reduction of hospital stays, in most cases without any increase in mortality or morbidity. The process of utilization review is strongly supported by managed-care organizations and third-party payors. The guidelines upon which these rules are based ought to be evidence-based.

Development of practice guidelines

How should practice guidelines be developed? The process of guideline development should be evidence-based. Ideally a panel of interested physicians is assembled and collects the evidence for and against the use of a particular set of diagnostic or therapeutic maneuvers. Some guidelines are simply consensus- or expert-based and the results may not be consistent with the best available evidence.

When evaluating the guideline, you ought to be able to determine the process, and there are several steps you should look at when appraising the validity of that practice guideline. First, the appropriate and important health outcomes must be specified. They should be those outcomes that will matter to patients, and all relevant outcomes should be included in the guideline. These include pain, anxiety, death, disfigurement, disability, but not chemical or surrogate markers of disease. Next, the evidence must be analyzed for validity and the effect of these interventions on the outcomes of interest. This must include explicit descriptions of the manner in which the evidence was collected, evaluated, and combined.

The magnitudes of benefits and risks should be estimated and benefits compared to harms. This must include the interests of all parties involved in providing care for the patient. These are the patient, health-care providers, third-party payors, and society at large. The preferences assigned to the outcomes should reflect those of the people (patients) who will receive those outcomes.

The costs (both economic and non-economic) should be estimated and the net health benefits compared to the costs of providing that benefit. Alternative procedures should be compared to the standard therapies in order to determine the best therapy. Finally, the analysis of the guideline must incorporate reasonable variations in care provided by reasonable clinicians. A sensitivity analysis accounting for this reasonable variation must be part of the guideline.

Once a guideline is developed, physicians who will use this guideline in practice must evaluate its use. If the guideline is not acceptable for the practitioner, it will not be used. For example, in 1992 a clinical guideline was developed for the management of children aged 3 to 36 months with fever but no source, to detect and treat occult bacteremia. This guideline was published simultaneously in the professional journals *Annals of Emergency Medicine* and *Pediatrics*. Today, this guideline is only selectively used by pediatricians, but almost universally used by emergency physicians. Why? The patients seen in pediatricians' offices are significantly different than those seen in emergency departments (ED). Sicker kids are sent to the ED by the pediatricians for further evaluation. The pediatricians are able to closely follow their febrile kids while emergency physicians are unable to do this. The emergency physicians feel better doing more testing and

Table 27.1. Desirable attributes of a clinical guideline

(1) **Accurate**	the methods used must be based on good-quality evidence
(2) **Accountable**	the readers (users) must be able to evaluate the guideline for themselves
(3) **Evaluable**	the readers must be able to evaluate the health and fiscal consequences of applying the guideline
(4) **Facilitate resolution of conflict**	the sources of disagreement should be able to be identified, addressed, and corrected
(5) **Facilitate application**	the guidelines must be able to be applied to the individual patient situation

treating of febrile children in the belief that they will prevent serious sequelae. Finally, testing is easier to do in an ED than in a pediatrician's office.

Even if a practice guideline is validated and generally accepted by most physicians, there may still be a delay in the general acceptance of this guideline. This is mostly because of inertia. Physicians' behavior has been studied and certain interventions have been found to change behavior. These include direct intervention such as reminders on a computer or ordering forms for drugs or diagnostic tests, follow-up by allied health-care personnel, and education from opinion leaders in their field. One of the most effective interventions involved using prompts on a computer when ordering tests or drugs. These resulted in improved drug-ordering practices and long-term changes in physician behavior. Less effective were audits of patient care charts and distributed educational materials. Least effective were formal continuing medical education (CME) presentations especially if they were of brief duration (less than one day). In some cases, these very short presentations actually produced negative results leading to lower-quality use of evidence in physician practices.

Practice guidelines should be developed using a preset process called the evidence- and outcomes-based approach. Separate the main steps (outcome and desirability) of the policy-making process. First estimate the outcomes (specific outcomes and probability of each) of the proposed intervention, then make judgments about the desirability of the outcomes. Explicitly estimate the effect of the intervention on all outcomes that are important to patients. To the extent necessary to tailor a policy, estimate how the outcomes vary with different patient characteristics. To the greatest extent possible, base the estimates of outcomes on the highest-quality experimental evidence available. To the extent necessary to estimate outcomes accurately, use formal methods to analyze the evidence and estimate the outcomes. To the extent necessary to understand patient preferences accurately, use actual assessments of patients' preferences to determine the desirability of the outcomes.

Critical appraisal of clinical practice guidelines[1]

(1) Are the recommendations valid?
  (a) Were all important options and outcomes considered? These must be considered from the perspective of the patient as well as the physician. All reasonable physician options should be considered including comments on those options not evidence-based but in common practice.
  (b) Was a reasonable, explicit, and sensible process used to identify, select, and combine evidence? This must be reproducible by anyone reading the paper outlining how the guideline was developed. Explicit rationale for choice of studies should be done. Evidence should be presented and graded by quality indicators.
  (c) Was a reasonable, explicit, and sensible process used to consider the relative value of different outcomes? The different outcomes should be described explicitly and the reasons why each outcome was chosen should be given. Patient values should be used where available.
  (d) Is the guideline likely to account for recent developments of importance? The bibliography should include the most recent evidence regarding the topic.
  (e) Has a peer-review and testing process been applied to the guideline? Ideally, clinicians who are expert in the area of the guideline should develop and review the guideline. It should be tested in various settings to determine if physicians are willing to use it and to ensure that it accomplishes its stated goals.
(2) What are the recommendations?
  (a) Are practical and clinically important recommendations made? The guidelines should be simple enough and make enough sense for most clinicians to use them.
  (b) How strong are the recommendations? The evidence for the guideline should be compelling with large effect sizes to back up the use of the evidence.
  (c) How much uncertainty is associated with the evidence and values used in the guideline? It should be clear from the presentation of the evidence how uncertainty in the evidence has been handled. Some sort of sensitivity

---

[1] Adapted with permission from the Users' Guides to the Medical Literature, published in *JAMA* (see Bibliography).

analysis should be included. What happens when basic assumptions are changed within the limits of the 95% CI?

(3) Will the recommendations help me in caring for my patients?

(a) Is the primary objective of the guideline important clinically? The guidelines ought to meet your needs for improving the care of the patient you are seeing. They should be consistent with your patient's health objectives.

(b) How are the recommendations applicable to your patients? The patient must meet the criteria for inclusion into the guideline. Patient preferences must be considered after a thorough discussion of all the options. You must be able to provide the needed follow-up and support for patients who require the recommended health care.

Clinical prediction rules

Physicians are constantly looking for sets of rules to assist them in the diagnostic process. Prediction rules are more specific than clinical guidelines for certain diagnoses. The definition of clinical prediction rules is that they are a decision-making tool for helping to make a diagnosis, derived from original research and incorporating three or more variables into the decision process.

The Ottawa ankle rules

The Ottawa ankle rules were first developed in the early 1990s and are now in universal use in most ED and primary-care practices. Their development is an excellent model for how prediction rules should be created. The main reason for developing this rule was to attempt to decrease the number of ankle x-rays ordered for relatively minor trauma. The rule has been successfully applied in various settings and that resulted in decreased use of ankle x-rays. This has become the prototype for the development of clinical prediction rules.

The first step in the development of these rules was to determine the underlying processes in making a particular diagnosis and initiating a particular treatment modality. In the case of the Ottawa ankle rules, this involved defining the components of the ankle examination, determining whether physicians could accurately assess them, and attempting to duplicate the results in a variety of settings. In the case of the ankle rules, it was found that only a few physical examination findings could be reliably and reproducibly assessed. Surprisingly, not all physicians reliably documented findings as apparently obvious as the presence of ecchymosis. For some of the physical-exam findings the kappa values were less than 0.6. This level was considered to be the minimum acceptable level of agreement.

The next step was to take all these physical-examination variables and apply them to a group of patients with the complaint of traumatic ankle pain. The authors determined which of these multiple variables were the most predictive of an ankle fracture. These variables were then applied to a group of patients and a statistical model was used to determine the final variables in the rule. When combined, these gave the rule the best operating characteristics. This means that when these variables are correctly applied to a patient they have the best sensitivity and specificity for diagnosing ankle fractures. In this case the rule creators decided that they wanted 100% sensitivity and were willing to sacrifice some specificity in the attempt. This is pure and simple data dredging. The results of this study were the derivation set for the prediction rule. This is defined as a Level-4 prediction rule. It is developed in a derivation set and ready for testing prospectively in the validation set.

Following this the rules were applied to another group, the validation set. The same specific rules were applied to a new population in a prospective manner. In this case the rule functioned perfectly. This raised the rule to a Level-2 rule, since it had been validated in a different study population. If the rule were only valid in a small sub-population, it would be a Level-3 rule. In this case, the rule was tried in a cross-section of the population that included men and women of all ages. There was not a large ethnic mix in the population, but this is a relatively minor point in this disease since there is no a-priori reason to think that African-Americans or other non-Caucasian ethnic groups will react differently to the examination than Caucasians.

Finally, a Level-1 rule is one that is ready for general use and has been shown to work effectively in many clinical settings. It should also show that the savings predicted from the initial study were maintained when the rule was applied in other clinical settings. This is now true of the Ottawa ankle rules.

There are some published standards for clinical prediction rules. Wasson and others developed these in 1985, and a modified version was published in *JAMA* in 2000 (Table 27.2).

Methodological standards for developing clinical decision rules

The clinical problem addressed should be a fairly commonly encountered condition. It will be very difficult if not impossible to determine the accuracy of the examination or laboratory tests for uncommon or rare illnesses. The clinical predicament should have led to variable practices by physicians in order to support the need for a clinical prediction rule. This means that physicians act in very different ways when faced with several patients who have the same set of symptoms. There should also be general agreement that the current diagnostic practice is not fully effective, and a desire on the part of many physicians for this to change.

Table 27.2. Levels of clinical decision rules

Level 1	Rule that can be used in a wide variety of settings with confidence that it can change clinician behavior and improve patient outcomes. At least one prospective validation in a different population and one impact analysis demonstrating change in clinician behavior with beneficial consequences.
Level 2	Rule that can be used in various settings with confidence in its accuracy. Demonstrated accuracy in at least one prospective study including a broad spectrum of patients and clinicians or validated in several smaller settings that differ from one another.
Level 3	Rule that clinicians may consider using with caution and only if patients in the study are similar to those in the clinician's clinical setting. Validated in only one narrow prospective sample.
Level 4	Rule that is derived but not validated or validated only in split samples, large retrospective databases, or by statistical techniques.

Source: From T. G. McGinn *et al.* Users' guides to the medical literature. XXII. How to use articles about clinical decision rules. *JAMA* 2000; 284: 79–84. Used with permission.

There must be an explicit definition of findings used to predict the outcome. Ideally the inter-observer agreement should be able to be determined. Only those with a high enough inter-observer reliability (high kappa value) should then be used as part of the final rule. There are several versions of the kappa test. For most dichotomous data the simple kappa is used. Other statistical methods are used for more complex data such as ordinal data (weighted kappa) and continuous interval data (intra-class correlation coefficient). Once tested, only those predictor variables with good agreement across various levels of physician experience should be used in the final rule.

These are also called the predictor variables. All the important predictors must be included in the derivation process. These predictors are the components of the history and physical exam that will be in the rule to be developed. If significant components are left out of the prediction rule, physicians are less likely to use the rule, as it will not have face validity for them. The predictor variables all must be present in a significant proportion of the study population or they are not likely to be useful in making the diagnosis.

Next, there should be an explicit definition of the outcomes. They must be easily understandable by all physicians and be clinically important to the patient. Finding people with a genetic defect that is not clinically important may be interesting for physicians and researchers, but may not directly benefit patients.

Therefore, most physicians will not be interested in this outcome and will not seek to accomplish it.

The outcome event should be assessed in a blinded manner to prevent bias. The persons observing the outcome should be different from those recording and assessing the predictor variables. In cases where the person assessing the predictor variable is also the one determining the outcome, observation bias can occur. This occurs when the people doing the study are aware of the assessment and the outcome and may change their definitions of the outcome or the assessment of the patient.

The subjects should be carefully selected. There should be a range of ages, ethnic groups, and genders of patients. The selection of a sample should include the process of selection, inclusion and exclusion criteria, and the clinical and demographic characteristic of the sample. Patient selection should be free of bias and there should be a wide spectrum of patient and disease characteristics. The study should determine the population of patients to which this rule will be applied. This gives the clinician the parameters for application of the rule. In the Ottawa ankle rules, there were no children (under age 18) and therefore initially the rule could not be applied to them. Subsequent studies found that the rule applied equally well in children as young as 12.

The setting should also be described. Studies that are done only in a specialized setting will result in referral bias. In these cases, the rules developed may not apply in settings where physicians are not as academic or where the patient base has a broader spectrum of the target disorder. A rule that is validated in a specialized setting must be further validated in more diverse settings. The original Ottawa ankle rule was derived and validated in both a university-teaching-hospital emergency department and a community hospital. The results were the same in both settings.

The sample size and number of outcome events should be large enough to prevent a Type II error. If there are too few outcome events, the rule will not be particularly accurate. As a rule of thumb, there should be at least 10–20 desired outcome events for each independent variable. For example, if we want to study a prediction rule for cervical spine fracture in injured patients and have five predictor variables, we should have at least 50 (and preferably 100) significant cervical spine fractures. If the rule worked perfectly, it would have a sensitivity of 100% (definition of perfect rule). However since the sample size (those 50 with cervical spine fractures) was pretty small, the confidence intervals on this would go from 94% to 100%. If the outcome is not too bad, this will be a reasonable rule. However if the outcome were possible paralysis, missing up to 6% of the patients with a potential for this outcome would be disastrous.

The mathematical model used to create the rule should be adequately described. The most common methods are recursive partitioning and classification and regression trees (CART) analysis. In each of these, the various predictor variables are modeled to see how well they can predict the ultimate outcome. In the recursive-partitioning method, the most powerful predictor variable is tested to see which of the positive patients are identified. They are then removed from the analysis and the rest are tested with the next most powerful predictor variable. This is continued until all patients with the desired outcome are identified. The CART methodology, a form of logistic regression analysis, is much more complex and beyond the scope of this text.

There must be complete follow-up of all patients (ideally 100%) enrolled in the study. If fewer patients are followed to completion of the study, the effect of loss of patients should be assessed. This can be done with a best case/worst case analysis. This will give a range of values of sensitivity and specificity within which the rule can be expected to operate.

The rule should be sensible. This means it must be clinically reasonable, easy to use, and with a clear-cut course of action if the rule is positive or negative. A nine-point checklist for determining which heart-attack patient should go to the intensive care unit and which can be admitted to a lower level of care is not likely to be useful to most clinicians. There are just too many variables for anyone to remember. One way of making it useful is to incorporate it into the order form for admitting patients to these units, or creating a clinical pathway with a written checklist that incorporates the rule.

For most physicians, rules that give probability of the outcome are less useful than those that tell the physician there are specific things that must be done when a certain outcome is achieved. However, future physicians, who will be better versed in the techniques of Bayesian medical decision making, will have an easier time using rules that give probability of disease rather than specific outcome actions. They will also be better able to explain the rationale for a particular decision to their patients. The Wells criteria for risk-stratifying patients in whom you suspect deep vein thrombosis (DVT) are an example of probabilities as the outcome of the rule.[2] The final outcome classifies patients into high, moderate, and low levels of risk for having a DVT.

The rule should be tested in a prospective manner. Ideally this should be done with a population and setting different than that used in the derivation set. This is a test for misclassification when the rule is put into effect prospectively. If the rule still functions in the same manner that it did in the derivation set, it has passed the test of applicability. This is where physician training in the use of the rule can be studied. How long does it take to learn to use the rule? If it takes too long, most physicians in community settings will be reluctant to take the time to learn it. They will feel that the rule is something that will be only marginally useful in a few instances. Physicians who have a stake in development of the rule are more

[2] P. S. Wells *et al.* Value of assessment of pretest probability of deep-vein thrombosis in clinical management. *Lancet* 1997; 350: 1795–1798.

likely to use it better and more effectively than those who are grudgingly goaded into using it by an outside agency.

It must still be tested in other sites and with other practitioners in order to determine the effect of clinical use in other sites. This testing should be done in a prospective manner. As part of this testing, the use of the rule should be able to reduce unnecessary medical care. This should result in automatic cost-effectiveness of the rule. A rule designed to reduce the number of x-rays taken of the neck, if correctly applied, will result in less x-rays ordered. There is no question that there will be an overall cost saving. Of course, if there is a complex and lengthy training process involved some of the cost savings will be transferred to the training program, making the rule less effective. Of course, if the rule doesn't work well, it may lead to malpractice suits (because of error in patient care) making it even more expensive.

Critical appraisal of prediction rules[3]

(1) Is the study valid?
   (a) Were all important predictors included in the derivation process? The model should include all those factors that physicians might take into account when making the diagnosis.
   (b) Were all important predictors present in a significant proportion of the study population? The predictor variables should be those that are common. No specific percentage is required, but clinical judgment should decide this.
   (c) Were all the outcome events and predictors clearly defined? The description of the outcomes and predictors should be easily reproducible by anyone in clinical practice.
   (d) Were those assessing the outcome event blinded to the presence of the predictors and those assessing the presence of predictors blinded to the outcome event?
   (e) Was the sample size adequate and did it include adequate outcome events? There should be at least 10–20 cases of the desired outcome, patients with a positive diagnosis, for each of the predictor variables being tested.
   (f) Does the rule make clinical sense? The rule should not fly in the face of current clinical practice otherwise it will not be used.
(2) What are the results?
   (a) How well do clinicians agree on the presence or absence of the findings incorporated into the rule? Inter- and intra-rater agreement and kappa values with confidence intervals should be given.

---

[3] Adapted with permission from the Users' Guides to the Medical Literature, published in *JAMA* (see Bibliography).

(b) What is the sensitivity and specificity of the prediction rule? The rule should lead to a high LR+ (ideally > 10) and low LR− (ideally < 0.1).

(c) How well does the rule predict the outcome? Depending on the severity of the outcome, the rule should find patients with the desired outcome almost all of the time. Is the post-test probability for the rule high in all clinical scenarios?

(3) How can I apply the results to my patients?

(a) Are the patients in the study similar enough to my patient?

(b) Can I efficiently and effectively use the rule in my patients?

28

Decision analysis and quantifying patient values

Chance favors only the prepared mind.

Louis Pasteur (1822–1895)

Learning objectives

In this chapter you will learn:
- the function of each part of a decision tree
- how to use a decision tree in conjunction with the uncertainties of a diagnostic test to assist in decision making for patients
- different ways of quantifying patient values
  - linear rating scale
  - time trade-off
  - standard gamble
- how to define and use QALYs

Introduction

How do physicians choose between various treatment options? For the individual physician treating a single patient, it is a matter of obtaining the relevant clinical information to make a diagnosis. This is followed by treatment as set down in some sort of clinical guideline or from a well-done RCT. However, these results may have a high degree of uncertainty (large 95% CI) and may not consider the patient's preferences or values. To help deal with these issues there are some statistical techniques that quantify the process.

To put the concept of risk into perspective, we must briefly go back a few hundred years. Girolamo Cardano (1545) and Blaise Pascal (1660) noted that in making a decision that involved any risk there were two elements that were completely unique and yet both were required to make the decision. These were the objective facts about the likelihood of the risk and the subjective views on the part of the risk taker about the utility of the outcomes involved in the risk (usefulness or expected value). This involved weighing the gains and losses involved in taking each of these risks. Pascal created the first recorded decision tree when deciding whether or not to believe in God.

The Port Royal text on logic (1662) noted that people who are "pathologically risk-averse" make all their choices based only upon the consequences and will refuse to make a choice if there is even the remotest possibility of an adverse consequence. They do not consider the statistical likelihood of that particular consequence in making a decision. Later, in the early eighteenth century, Daniel Bernoulli noted that those who make choices based only upon the probability of an outcome without any regard for the quality of the risk involved with that particular outcome would be considered foolhardy. Most of us are somewhere in between. This takes us to the modern era in medical decision making.

There is a systematic way in which the components of decision making can be incorporated to make a clinical decision and determine the best course of therapy. This statistical method for determining the best path to diagnosis and treatment is called expected-values decision making. Given the probability of each of the risks and benefits of treatment, which strategy will produce the greatest overall benefit for the patient? The theory of expected-values decision making is based on the assumption that there is a risk associated with every treatment option and uncertainty associated with each risk.

By using the technique of instrumental rationality the clinician can calculate the treatment strategy which will produce the most benefit for the average or typical patient. The clinician quantifies each treatment strategy by assigning a numerical value to each outcome (**utility**) and multiplying that value by the **probability** of occurrence of that outcome. The utilities and probabilities can be varied to account for variation in patient values and likelihood of outcomes.

The vocabulary of expected-values decision making: expected value = utility × probability

The probability is a number from 0 to 1 that represents the likelihood of a particular outcome of interest. You must know as much about each outcome of the various treatment options as possible. The probability of each outcome (P) comes from clinical research studies of patient populations with the same or similar characteristics as your patient or population. These can also come from systematic reviews of many clinical studies or a meta-analysis. They are usually not exact, but are only a best approximation, and ought to come with 95% confidence intervals attached.

You must then assign each outcome a value or utility (U) that tells how desirable or undesirable that outcome is. A utility of 1 is assigned to a perfect outcome, usually meaning a complete cure or perfect health. A utility of 0 is a totally un-acceptable outcome, usually reserved for death. Intermediate utility values are assigned to other outcomes. The quality of life resulting from each intermediate outcome will be less than expected with a total cure. This outcome state may be wholly or partially unbearable due to treatment side effects or adverse effects of the illness. A numerical value for utility between 1 and 0 is then assigned to this outcome. Recent studies of patient values for outcomes of cardiopulmonary resuscitation (CPR) revealed that some patients will give negative scores to out-comes they consider worse than death such as surviving in a persistent vegetative state and being maintained on a ventilator.

A decision tree illustrating treatment options can then be constructed, as seen from the following clinical example. Thrombolytic therapy (clot-dissolving med-ication called t-PA) can be used to treat acute embolic or thrombotic cerebrovas-cular accident (CVA or stroke due to a blood clot in the brain). Your patient is a 60-year-old man with sudden onset of weakness of the right arm and leg associ-ated with inability to speak. You suspect a stroke and want to try a new form of treatment to dissolve the suspected clot in the artery supplying the left parietal area of the brain. A CT scan shows no apparent bleeding in the brain. There are two options for your patient. You can give the thrombolytic therapy (t-PA) or treat using traditional methods of anticoagulation and intensive physical therapy.

First you must list the possible outcomes for each therapy. For purposes of the exercise we will simplify this process and assume that there are only two possible outcomes. Thrombolytic therapy can result in a cure (complete resolution of the symptoms) or death from intracranial hemorrhage (bleeding in the brain). Traditional medical therapy will result in some but not complete improvement in the clinical picture in all patients.

Next, find the probabilities of each of the outcomes. Outcome probabilities are obtained from studies of populations of patients with similarities for both the stroke and risk factors for bleeding. The probability of death from thrombolyic therapy is P_d, for complete cure it is P_c (which is equal to $1 - P_d$), and for partial improvement with medical therapy in this example the probability is 1.

Finally, assign a utility to each of the outcomes. The utility of cure is 1, death is 0, and the unknown, U_x, for chronic or residual disability. These values are obtained from studies of patient attitudes towards each of the outcomes in question and will be discussed in more detail later.

Mechanics of constructing a decision tree

There are three components to any decision tree. Nodes are junctures where something happens. There are three types of nodes: decision, probability (or chance), and stationary. A decision node is the point where the clinician or

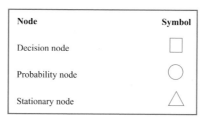

Fig. 28.1 Symbols used in a decision tree.

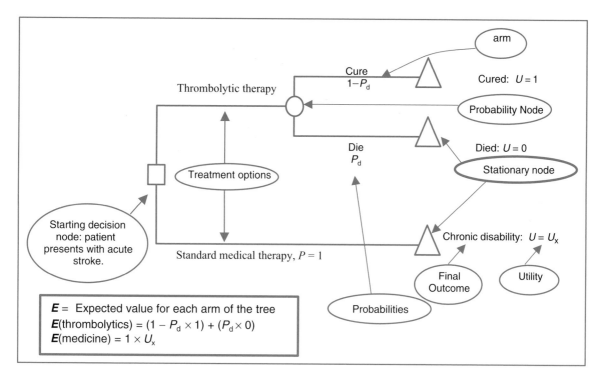

Fig. 28.2 Decision tree for thrombolytic therapy.

patient must choose between two or more possible options. A probability node is the point where one of two or more possible outcomes can occur by chance. A stationary node is the point where the patient starts (initial presentation) or finishes (ultimate outcome). The symbols for the nodes are shown in Fig. 28.1.

Arms connect the nodes. Each arm represents one treatment or management strategy. Fig. 28.2 shows a simple decision tree for our problem. In this simplified decision tree for stroke, one arm represents thrombolytic therapy and the other represents standard medical therapy.

In the simplified stroke-therapy example we can calculate the expected values in each arm by multiplying the utility and probability and summing their values around each node. Therefore, for thrombolytic therapy the expected value E will equal $1(1 - P_d) + 0(P_d)$. For standard medical therapy, since the utility of chronic residual disability is U_x and since all patients have this intermediate outcome,

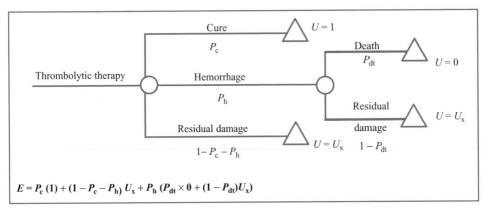

$$E = P_c \, (1) + (1 - P_c - P_h) \; U_x + P_h \, (P_{dt} \times 0 + (1 - P_{dt}) U_x)$$

Fig. 28.3 Expanded decision tree for thrombolytic therapy.

the expected value E is U_x. Since the patient should always prefer the strategy that leads to the highest expected value, here they would always choose standard treatment for stroke if the expected value for this arm is 100% (i.e., if $U = 1$) and for the thrombolytic arm it is $100\% - P_d$.

For purposes of this example, let's assume the value of a lifetime of chronic neurological disability is 0.9. This means that living with chronic neurological disability is somehow equated with living 90% of a normal life. Recalculating the expected value of each arm will determine what probability of death from thrombolytics would result in wanting to choose thrombolytics over medical therapy. We must solve the equation $1 - P_d = 0.9$. Since the value of E for the medicine arm is now 0.9, this will occur as long as $P_d < 0.10$.

Disagreeable events such as side effects may reduce the value of a given arm. For example, since the experience of getting thrombolytics may be unpleasant, we may want to introduce a utility reduction of 0.01, changing the expected value of that arm to $1 - 0.01 - P_d$. In our example, and with a U_x of 0.9, thrombolytics would still be favored as long as $P_d < 0.09$.

In reality, there are more outcomes than shown in this example. For the thrombolytic-therapy arm, the clot can be dissolved successfully, there can be residual deficit, or the patient may have an intracranial bleed resulting in death, or have partial improvement but be left with a residual deficit. The thrombolytic arm of the decision tree would then look as shown in Fig. 28.3 (where P_c is the probability of cure and P_h the probability of hemorrhage). The probability of death due to hemorrhage is P_{dt}. For residual damage we will use the same utility, U_x as in the previous example for the standard-therapy arm. Fig. 28.3 shows the thrombolytic therapy arm of our decision tree with these new constraints.

Similarly, standard medical treatment can result in spontaneous cure or death. This will result in that side of the decision tree looking like Fig. 28.4. Here P_c is the probability of complete resolution and P_{dm} the probability of death.

The reason we need this decision tree at all is because while there is an increase in complete cures with thrombolytic therapy there is also an increase in bleeding

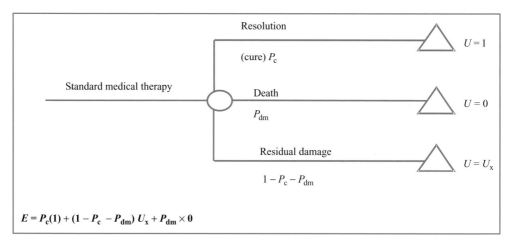

$$E = P_c(1) + (1 - P_c - P_{dm})\, U_x + P_{dm} \times 0$$

(intracranial hemorrhage) leading to residual damage or death. Simply balancing the two, using NNT for cure and NNH for death due to hemorrhage, ignores the patient's values for each of these outcomes. This is especially true when one of the alternative outcomes is a lifetime of disability.

Fig. 28.4 Expanded decision tree for standard medical therapy.

Sensitivity analysis

Sensitivity analysis is a way to deal with imprecision in the data used to create the decision tree. As you already know, this is true of almost all data obtained from the medical literature. The sensitivity analysis tests the "robustness" of the conclusions over a range of different values of probabilities for each branch of the decision tree. Sensitivity analysis asks what would happen to the expected value of thrombolytics against standard medical management if we varied the probability of any of the outcomes. The probabilities used usually come with 95% confidence intervals and these are the extreme values used in the sensitivity analysis.

If there is very little difference between the expected values of two treatments, then a slight change in the probabilities assigned to each arm could easily alter the direction of the decision. In that case, if our probabilities are off by just a little bit, the entire result will change and the patient and physician will have little useful information regarding the relative merits of the two treatments.

Sensitivity analysis determines how much variation in the final outcome will result from plausible variations in each of the input variables. One-way sensitivity analysis changes only one parameter at a time (Fig. 28.5, 28.6). Multi-way sensitivity analysis looks for the variable that causes the biggest change in overall model. Then the analysis changes all those assumptions that are "very sensitive" to see what happens to the model. Finally, a curve is drawn to show what happens to the expected values when the two most "sensitive" variables are changed (Fig. 28.7).

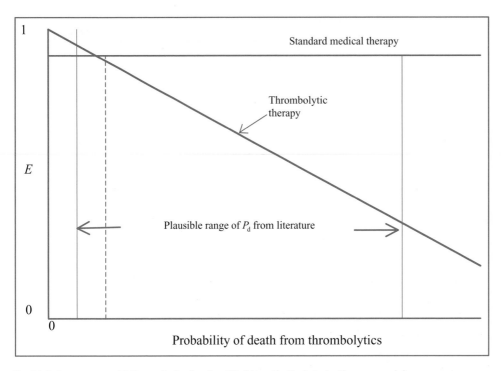

Fig. 28.5 One-way sensitivity analysis of a simplified hypothetical stroke therapy model.

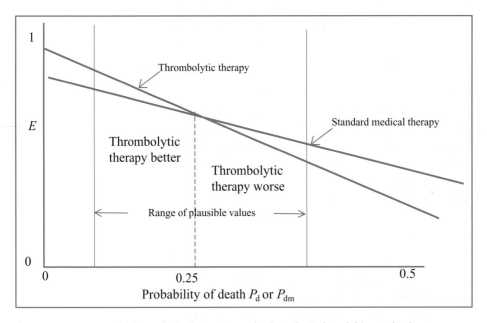

Fig. 28.6 One-way sensitivity analysis of a more complex hypothetical model for stroke therapy.

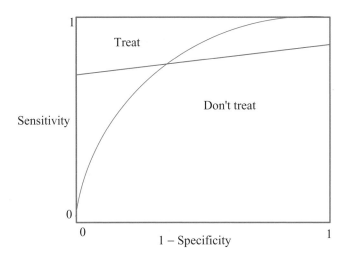

Fig. 28.7 Two-way sensitivity analysis of a complex model of treatment for stroke based on the results of the CT scan. (Yes, the graph of sensitivity vs. 1 − specificity is the ROC curve.)

The results of a sensitivity analysis can be graphed, showing the effect on the final outcomes with a change in each of these values. We usually express the expected values for each branch of the decision tree as quality-adjusted life years (QALYs). QALY equals $E \times$ life expectancy (where E is the expected value from a decision tree).

Adding the uncertainty associated with the results of a CT scan which checks for early signs of intracranial bleeding as the cause of the stroke complicates the previous example of thrombolytic therapy in stroke. This is because the presence of a small amount of bleeding is difficult to diagnose, and if thrombolytic therapy is given in the presence of a bleed (even a very small one) the likelihood of a serious and possibly fatal intracranial hemorrhagic stroke increases. Since the presence of a bleed is not always detected, the CT is not always a valid test. You must consider the possibilities of incorrect interpretations of the CT.

Using a decision tree, you can now determine the probability of giving thrombolytic therapy when there actually is a bleed (false-negative CT), and of not giving the therapy when there is truly no bleed and yet one is read on the CT scan (false-positive CT). The ultimate decision should be based on whichever strategy gives the highest final expected utility. Fig. 28.8 shows this more complex but also more realistic decision tree of thrombolytic therapy in stroke.

Reality check! (disclaimer)

This is not a model of what doctors actually do now. It is a mathematical modeling technique that can help doctors and patients find the best possible way of making decisions. In actuality, physicians have trouble applying decision analysis to individual patients even when there is a clearly superior treatment. Also, the

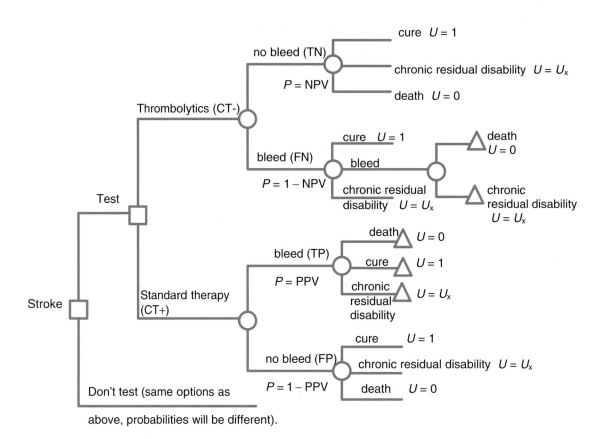

Fig. 28.8 Complex decision tree incorporating the use of CT scans in decision making for stroke. The probabilities have been omitted for clarity.

model requires you to put outcomes into a few discrete categories when in fact there are many outcomes that are not clear-cut.

Thrombolytic therapy complications can vary from serious to mild. Chronic disability can also vary from a mild to a constant disabling deficit. It can be very severe for a brief period of time and then spontaneously resolve. Standard medical treatment may actually result in more patients having only a small amount of residual deficit. On the other hand, thrombolytic treatment may result in more cases with increased residual deficit or death (both unsatisfactory outcomes). This can occur even if a "cure" is obtained in a few more patients in the thrombolytic group, making this a more realistic model of the situation.

Computers can be used to show patients how their personal values for each outcome will change the expected value of each treatment. There are some commercially available programs to assist patients in making difficult decisions about whether or not to have prostate surgery. This is clearly a direction for future research in decision-making theory. The development of user-friendly computerized interfaces will help improve the quality of our decisions. This will never make the doctor obsolete. We must continue to be able to educate our patients about the consequences of each action and describe for them the objective reality of each disease state, so that they can make appropriate decisions on the utility they want to assign to each outcome.

Threshold approach to decision making

Earlier, in Chapter 24, we talked about the treatment and testing thresholds. The threshold approach to testing and treatment can use decision trees to determine when diagnostic testing should be done. Consider the situation of a patient complaining of shortness of breath in whom you suspect a pulmonary embolism (blood clot in the lungs). Should you order a test in which dye is injected into the pulmonary arteries (pulmonary angiogram)? The test itself is very uncomfortable, causes some complications, and can cause death. There are basically three options:

(1) You can treat based on clinical examination (give the patient an anticoagulant) without doing the test
(2) You can test first and treat only if the test is positive
(3) You can neither test nor treat (if you are very sure that disease is not present)

The treatment threshold is the probability of disease above which we should initiate treatment for the disease without first doing the test for the disease. This is the level at which testing will produce an unacceptable number of false negatives and patients would then be denied the benefits of treatment. "The pretest disease likelihood is so great, I will treat regardless of the results of the test."

The testing threshold is the probability of a disease above which we should test before initiating treatment for that disease. This is the probability below which there are an unacceptable number of false positives and patients would then be exposed unnecessarily to the side effects of treatment. "The likelihood of a positive test is so small, I would not treat even if the test is positive."

If the probability of disease is higher than the treatment threshold, we should skip the test and go ahead with the treatment. If the post-test probability of disease after a positive test (positive predictive value) is still lower than the treatment threshold, we should not start treatment. If the post-test probability after a negative test (false reassurance rate) falls below the testing threshold (after doing the test), it was a worthwhile test. It took the probability of disease from a value of probability at which you would test before treating, to one at which you would neither treat nor do further tests. In essence, you have ruled out disease. Decision trees are another way for us to determine the cutoffs for testing and treating.

In order to complete the decision tree for our example of thrombolytic therapy and stroke, you need to know the posterior probability that a bleed has occurred. To find this you need to know the sensitivity and specificity of the CT scan and the prevalence of intracranial bleeding. If the post-test probability of a bleed is low, thrombolytic treatment is better as a bleed is unlikely, making standard medical therapy less beneficial. If the post-test probability of a bleed is high, standard treatment is likely to be better, since thrombolytic therapy is more likely to lead to increased bleeding rates.

These are both dependent on prevalence, or pretest probability! (Remember?) At a low pretest probability, even a positive CT ought not make a difference since there would be many false positives and you shouldn't do the test at all since you are more likely to have a false positive and unnecessarily avoid thrombolytic therapy on someone who could benefit. An example would be a person with known atrial fibrillation, not on anticoagulants, who had a sudden onset of severe left hemiparesis without a headache. Changing one fact of this pattern would change the probability of a bleed and the final decision since the consequence of giving thrombolytic therapy to someone with a bleed makes the CT worthwhile, since treating anyone with a positive scan can result in a real tragedy.

At a high pretest probability, even a negative CT should not make a difference since the clinical picture is so strong that you shouldn't do the test at all since you are more likely to have a false negative and would treat someone with a potential bleed. An example would be someone with a sudden onset of the worst headache of their life with their only deficit being slight weakness of their non-dominant hand. Here the potential of giving thrombolytic therapy to someone with a bleed is too high and the projected benefit not great enough.

Mathematical expression of threshold approach to testing

There are formulas for calculating these thresholds (don't memorize them).

Test threshold =
$$\frac{(FP\ rate)(risk\ of\ inappropriate\ Rx) + (risk\ of\ test)}{(FP\ rate)(risk\ of\ inappropriate\ Rx) + (TP\ rate)(benefit\ of\ appropriate\ Rx)}$$

Test-treatment threshold =
$$\frac{(TN\ rate)(risk\ of\ inappropriate\ Rx) - (risk\ of\ test)}{(TN\ rate)(risk\ of\ inappropriate\ Rx) + (FN\ rate)(benefit\ of\ appropriate\ Rx)}$$

Determining the risks and benefits of incorrect diagnosis will set these thresholds. A false positive resulting in unnecessary use of risky tests or treatments (e.g., cardiac catheterization or cardiac drugs) or a false negative resulting in unnecessarily withholding beneficial tests or treatments are both adverse outcomes of testing. You can substitute different values of test characteristics (different positive and negative predictive values) in a sensitivity analysis of the decision tree and determine what the effect of these changes will be on the utility of each treatment arm.

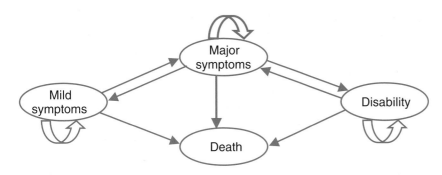

Fig. 28.9 Markov model schematic. From F. A. Sonnenberg & J. R. Beck. Markov models in medical decision making: a practical guide. *Med. Decis. Making* 1993; 13: 322–338.

Markov models

Another method of making a decision analysis is through the use of Markov models. These consider the simultaneous interaction of all possible health states. A patient can be in only one health state at a time. You must decide on the average time a given individual patient spends in each health state and then weigh this time by considering the quality of life in each state.

Ovals are states of health associated with quality measures such as death ($U = 0$), complete health or cure ($U = 1$), and other outcomes (U varies from 0 to 1). Arrows are transitions between states (or within a state) and are attached to probabilities or the likelihood of changing states or remaining in the same state. This type of model is ideal for putting into a computer to get the final expected values. A Markov model of health decision making is diagrammed in Fig. 28.9.

Ethical issues

Finally, there are significant ethical issues raised by the use of decision trees and expected-values decision making. After performing a decision tree, you must place ethical values on the decisions. Issues of morality and fairness must be considered. When there are limited resources, is it more just to spend a large amount of resources for a small gain? Do we define a small gain as one affecting only a few people or one having only a small health benefit?

The use of a decision tree in making medical decisions helps the patient, physician, and society decide which treatment modality will be most just. Look for treatments that benefit the most people or have the largest improvement in health outcome. Ethical problems arise when we must make a choice on whether to consider the best outcome from the perspective of a large population or the individual patient. If we take the perspective of the individual patient, how are we to know that the treatment will benefit that particular patient, the next patient, or the next

Table 28.1. Seigler's schema for ethical decision making in medicine

Ethical concern	Ethical principle
MEDICAL INDICATION What is the best treatment? What are the alternatives?	BENEFICENCE The duty to promote the good of the patient
PATIENT PREFERENCES What does the patient want? What outcome does the patient prefer?	AUTONOMY Respect for the patient's right to self-determination
QUALITY OF LIFE What impact will the proposed treatment or lack of it have on the patient's life?	NON-MALEFICENCE The duty not to inflict harm or injury
SOCIECONOMIC ISSUES (CONTEXTUAL FEATURES) What does the patient want within their own socioeconomic milieu? What are the needs of the patient's society?	JUSTICE The patient is given what is their "due"

Source: From A. R. Jonsen, M. Seigler & W. J. Winslade. *Clinical Ethics.* 3rd edn. New York: McGraw-Hill, 1992. pp. 1–10.

20 patients? Should we use the perspective of statistical significance ($P < 0.05$) or is it fairer to use NNT? Is the decision up to each individual or should the decision be legislated by society?

Decision trees allow the physician, society, and the patient to decide which therapy is going to be the most beneficial for the most people. Whether decision trees are a mathematical expression of utilitarianism is a hotly debated issue among bioethicists.

Siegler's schema (Table 28.1) is useful for using these models in medical and ethical decision making. The basic perspectives of medical care within the traditional patient-physician relationship include medical indications (physician-directed) and patient preferences (patient-driven), both of which are input variables in the decision tree. Current or added perspectives modify the decision. These include quality of life (considering the impact on the individual of high-technology interventions) and contextual features (cultural, societal, family, religious or spiritual, community, and economic factors). These are all part of the discussion between the doctor and the patient and form the basis of the doctor–patient relationship.

Assessing patient values

Patient values must be incorporated into medical decision making and health-care policies by physicians, government, managed care organizations, and other decision makers. The output of decision trees is variable and based on patient preferences. We can measure and quantify patient values and use them in decision trees to help patients make difficult decisions.

Using unadjusted life expectancy (e.g., life years) cannot compare various states of health in cases with the same number of years of life, and does not quantify the quality of those years. Quality-of-life scales or measures of status rated by others or by self include health status, functional status (e.g., Activities of Daily Living – ADL – or the Arthritis Activity Scale used in rheumatoid arthritis), well-being, or patient satisfaction. These are difficult to use in a quantitative manner. We will learn to use several standardized quantitative measures of patient preference that can be used to measure the relative preference that a patient has for one or another outcome.

The linear-rating-scale method utilizes a visual analog scale (VAS) (Fig. 28.10). The patient is asked "where on this scale would you rate your life if you had to live with chronic disease?" (In our example, it would be the residual stroke syndrome.) The resultant value of U is the percentage of the length of the line.

The time trade-off method asks "suppose you have 10 years left to live with chronic residual disability from the stroke. If you could trade those 10 years for x years without any residual neurological deficit, what is the smallest number of years you would trade to be deficit-free?" Since it is a direct question, there is a lot of variability attached to the answer between patients.

The standard-gamble (utility) method attempts to find out how much risk the patient is willing to take. The patient is told to consider an imaginary situation in which you will give them a potion that will instantly cure their stroke. However, there is a risk in that it occasionally causes instant but painless death. If there were 100% cure and 0% death every patient would always take the potion. On the other hand, if there were 0% cure and 100% death no one would ever take the potion (unless the patient is extremely depressed and considers their life totally worthless). Continue to change the cure-to-death ratio until the person cannot decide which course of action to take. This is the point of indifference. "At what level of certainty would you be indifferent to the outcome?" In our stroke example, the sure thing is chronic residual neurological deficit and the gamble is no deficit

Fig. 28.11 Standard gamble.

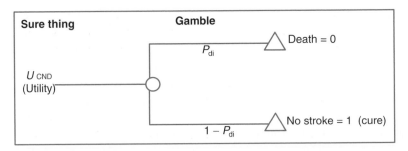

or death. Set up a "mini decision tree" and solve for the utility of living with chronic neurological deficit. This is diagrammed in Fig. 28.11, where:

P_{di} is the probability of death at the point of indifference, the information learned when using the standard gamble.

$$U_{CND} = (0 \times P_{di}) + (1 - P_{di}) \times 1 \quad \text{or}$$

$U_{CND} = 1 - P_{di}$ This is the value of living with chronic stroke syndrome that the patient assigns an outcome through a standard gamble.

QALYs are the standardized measure that combines the quality of life and life expectancy. It is the output measure that is commonly used in decision analyses. It combines total life expectancy with a quantitative measure of patient value. A decision analysis can determine how many QALYs result from each strategy. The QALY is determined by taking the normal life expectancy and multiplying it by the patient value of one year of life (utility).

Different values will be obtained from each method used to measure patient values. The linear rating scale measures the quality of functionality of life, the time trade-off introduces a choice between two certainties, and the standard gamble introduces probability and willingness to take risks into the equation.

Attitudes towards risk and framing effects

Attitudes towards risk vary with individuals and at different periods of time during their lives. Patient values can be related to special events (birth of a child, marriage, etc.), habits (smoking, drinking, etc.), or age (length of time involved in the trade-off, since a younger person may be less likely to trade off years). Also personal preferences (amount of risk a person is generally willing to take in other activities, like sky-diving, etc.) play a role in determining patient values. Since values tend to be very personal, physicians should not be the ones to assign these values. Values based on the physician's own risk-taking behavior will not accurately measure the values of the patient.

How the questions are worded or framed will influence the answer to the question. Asking what probability of death a patient is willing to accept will likely give a lower number than asking what probability of survival they are willing to accept. The framing of the questions may reflect the risk-taking attitude of the physician. A patient is more likely to prefer a treatment if told that 90% of those treated are alive five years later than if told that 10% are dead after the same time period, even though the outcome is exactly the same. The feelings aroused by the idea of death are more likely to lead to the rejection of an option framed from the perspective of death when this same option would be endorsed in the opposite framing of the choice (perspective of survival). Although apparently inconsistent and irrational, this effect is a recurrent occurrence. This irrationality is not due to lack of knowledge since physicians respond no differently than non-physician patients.

Probability means different things to different people. This is related to how individuals relate to numbers and how well people understand probabilities. In general, people (including physicians) do not understand probabilities very well. Physicians tend to give qualitative rather than quantitative expressions of risk in many different and ambiguous ways. For example, what does a "rare risk" of death mean? Does it mean 1% of the time, or one in a million? From the patient perspective, a rare event happens 100% of the time if it happens to them.

Finally, patient values change when they have the disease in question as opposed to when they do not. Patients who are having a stroke are much more willing to accept moderate disability than well persons who are asked about the abstract notion of disability if they were to get a stroke. This means that stroke patients assign a higher value to the utility (U) of residual deficit than well people asked in the abstract. Most clinical studies of these issues that are now being done have quality-of-life and patient-preference measures attached to possible outcomes. They should help clarify the effects of variations in patient values on the outcomes of decision trees.

29

Cost-effectiveness analysis

When gold argues the cause, eloquence is important.

Publilius Syrus (first century BC): Moral Sayings

 Learning objectives

In this chapter you will learn:
- the process of evaluating an article on cost-effectiveness
- the concepts of marginal cost and marginal benefit
- how to use these tools to help make medical decisions for a population
- how to calculate a simple cost-effectiveness problem and evaluate the cost-effectiveness of a specific therapy

The cost of medical care is constantly rising. The physician of the future will seek to use the most cost-efficient methods to care for her or his patients. We can use cost-effectiveness analysis to help choose between treatment options for an individual patient or for large populations. Governments and managed care organizations use cost-effectiveness techniques to justify their coverage for various health-care "products." Drug companies often produce cost-effectiveness studies to show that their more expensive drugs are actually cheaper in the long run. Physicians and insurance-plan administrators must be able to evaluate the validity of these claims.

How do we decide if a test or treatment is worth it?

If one treatment costs less and is clearly more effective than the alternative option there is no question about which treatment to use. We would treat our patient with the most effective treatment and be glad we are saving money in the process. More often than not, however, we are faced with a situation in which one therapy costs much more and is marginally more effective than a much less expensive therapy. Cost-effectiveness analysis gives us the data to answer the question "how much more will this extra effectiveness cost?"

This is a serious ethical issue for society. If one very expensive treatment is beneficial for a few people and we pay for that treatment, we will be unable to afford other equally or more effective treatments that may help more people. There is only so much money to go around and you can't spend the same dollar twice! If we fund bone marrow transplants for questionable indications, we may not be able to pay for hypertension screening leading to treatment that could prevent the need for certain other organ transplants (kidneys and hearts) in the future. A bone marrow transplant may prolong one life by six years, yet result in loss of funds for hypertension screening and treatment programs which could prevent six new deaths from uncontrolled hypertension in that same period.

Cost rationing has always been present in medicine. The wealthy can get any medical procedure done regardless of efficacy or cost while the poor must wait for available services. This is known as de-facto rationing and is manifested by long waiting times in a municipal hospital emergency department or for an appointment to get diagnostic studies. In the USA, there may be reduced availability of certain drugs to patients in some MCOs (Managed Care Organizations), on Medicaid, and certainly to uninsured working people. The State of Oregon used a type of cost-effectiveness analysis to decide what services the State Medicaid program should cover. We are constantly making value judgments over how we as a society will spend our money. These ethical issues are left to the politicians and ethicists to discuss. This chapter will give you the tools to evaluate studies of cost-effectiveness.

Cost-effectiveness studies can be very complex to evaluate. On the most basic level, they simply add up all the costs of a particular procedure, subtract from them the cost of the comparison procedure (the one in current use) and divide by the benefit, usually the number of additional QALYs obtained by using the new procedure. However, the manner in which analysis is set up will have an enormous impact on what kind of result will be obtained. It is difficult to do a good and fair cost analysis, and relatively simple to do a bad (and often biased) one. Therefore it is up to the reader to apply a few simple rules when reading a cost analysis. If these rules are followed you can be fairly sure the analysis is relatively valid.

Guidelines for assessing an economic analysis of clinical care[1]

Was a broad enough viewpoint adopted?

Is there a specified point of view (a hospital, a ministry of health or preferably society as a whole) from which the costs and effects are being viewed? The viewpoint should be given from the perspective of who is paying for the

---

[1] Adapted with permission from the Users' Guides to the Medical Literature, published in *JAMA* (see Bibliography).

treatment and who is affected by the decision outcome of what to treat and not treat. Often these studies compare usual fee for service or third-party insurance against managed-care costs. However, the comparison may simply be for the costs of the treatments only without a specific viewpoint on whom is paying for them or how much is being reimbursed.

There is a disconnect between costs and charges in health-care finances because of the large amount of uncompensated care that is delivered. This must be considered in any economic analysis. Costs are the amount of money that is required to initiate and run a particular intervention. Charges are the amount of money that is going to be requested from the payors. It is disingenuous to use charges since they always overestimate the costs. However, when using simple costs only, the cost of treating non-insured patients must be factored into the accounting.

The different programs must be adequately described. From reading the article's methods, you should be able to set up the same program. This requires a full description of the process of setting up the program, the costs and effects of the program, and how these were measured.

Were all the relevant clinical strategies compared?

Is the analysis comparing well-defined alternative courses of action? The comparison between treatment options must be specified. Typically two treatment options or treatment as opposed to non-treatment are considered in a cost-effectiveness analysis. The treatment options ought to be those that are in common use. Using treatments that are no longer in common use will give a biased result to the analysis.

Was clinical effectiveness established?

The program's effectiveness should have been validated. There should be hard evidence from well-done randomized clinical trials to show that the intervention is effective, and this should be explicitly stated. Where not previously done, a systematic review or meta-analysis should be performed as part of the analysis. A cost-effectiveness analysis should not be done based on the assumption that because we can do something it is good. If no RCT is available that looks at the relevant clinical question, observational studies can be used, but with the caveat that they are more prone to bias.

Were the costs measured accurately?

Does the analysis identify all the important and relevant costs and effects that you think it should? Did it select credible measures for these costs and effects? On the cost side this includes the actual costs of organization (setting up a program) and continuing operations, additional costs to patient and family, costs outside the health-care system (time lost from work, decreased productivity, etc.), and intangible costs (loss of pleasure, loss of companionship, etc.). These costs must be compared for both doing the intervention program and not doing the program but doing the alternatives.

On the effect side, the analysis should include "hard" clinical outcomes: mortality, morbidity, residual functional ability, quality of life/utility, and effect on future resources. These include the availability of services and future costs of health care and other services incurred by extending life. For example, it may be fiscally better to allow people to continue to smoke since this will reduce their life span and save money on end-of-life care for those people who die prematurely. This doesn't mean we should encourage smoking.

The error made most often in performing cost-effectiveness analyses is the omission of consideration of opportunity costs. At the start of this chapter I referred to the fact that you cannot spend the same dollar twice. If you pay for one therapeutic intervention you may not be able to pay for some other one. Cost-effectiveness analyses must include an analysis of these opportunity costs so that the reader can see what equivalent types of programs might need to be cut from the health-care budget in order to finance the new (and presumably better) one. Analyses that do not consider this issue are giving a biased view of the usefulness of the new program and keeping it out of the context of the greater society.

What is the resulting cost or cost per unit health gained and is this gain impressive?

The marginal (incremental) gain for both the costs and effects (health-care gains) should be calculated. First, the degree of risk reduction is determined. A very simple way to do a quick cost-effectiveness analysis is with the number needed to treat (NNT). This is the number of patients you must treat in order to achieve the desired effect in one additional patient. It is the inverse of the attributable risk reduction (ARR) between the two therapies.

For example, in the GUSTO trial of thrombolytic therapy for myocardial infarction, a difference in outcomes was found when t-PA was used instead of streptokinase: t-PA at $2000/dose resulted in 6.5% mortality while streptokinase at $200/dose resulted in 7.5% mortality. The ARR is the difference between the two, or 1%. The NNT for t-PA is 100 (1/ARR) and this is how many patients must be treated with t-PA instead of streptokinase to prevent one additional death. The marginal or incremental cost per life saved is then $180 000 [($2000 − $200) × 100 lives].

The prices used to calculate costs should be appropriate to the time and place. The use of US dollars in studies on Canadian health-care resources will not

Table 29.1. Comparing inpatient vein stripping (IP Stripping) to outpatient injection (OP Injections) of varicose veins

Treatment	Outcomes			
	Cost to hospital per patient (indexed)	No further treatement needed	Support stockings needed	Further treatment needed
OP injections	9.77	78%	9%	13%
IP stripping	44.22	86%	11%	3%

Table 29.2. Comparing doxycycline to azithromycin for *Chlamydia* infections

Treatment	Outcomes			
	Cost to hospital per patient	No further treatement needed	Adverse effects	Compliance rate
Doxycycline	3	77%	29%	70%
Azithromycin	30	81%	23%	100%

Source: Data extracted from A. C. Haddix *et al.* The cost effectiveness of azithromycin for *Chlamydia trachomatis* infections in women. *Sex. Transm. Dis.* 1995; 22: 274–280.

translate into a credible cost analysis. Also, the effects measured should include lives or years of life saved, improvement in level of function, or utility.

There are several different ways to analyze costs and effects. In a cost-minimization analysis only costs are compared. This works if the effects of the two interventions are equal or minimally different. For example, when comparing inpatient vein stripping to outpatient injection of varicose veins, the results in Table 29.1 were obtained. Here the cost is so different that even if 13% of outpatients require additional hospitalization (and therefore we must pay for both procedures) you will still save money by performing outpatient injections.

Another analysis compared doxycycline (100 mg twice a day for seven days) to azithromycin (1 g given as a one-time dose) for the treatment of *Chlamydia* infections in women. It found that some patients do not complete the full seven-day course for doxycycline and then need to be retreated, and can infect other people (Table 29.2). The cost of azithromycin that would make the use of this drug cost-effective for all patients can then be calculated. In this case, the drug company making azithromycin actually lowered their cost for this product based on the analysis to a level that would make azithromycin more cost-effective.

Table 29.3. Cost-effectiveness of strategy A vs. strategy B

	Outcome	Cost
Strategy A	15 QALY	$10 000
Strategy B	20 QALY	$110 000

In a cost-effectiveness analysis the researcher seeks to determine how much more has to be paid in order to achieve a benefit of preventing death or disability days. Here, the effects are unequal and all outcomes must be compared. These include costs, well years, total years, and utility or benefits. The outcome is expressed as incremental or marginal cost over benefit. Commonly used units are additional dollars per QALY or life saved.

The first step in a cost-effectiveness analysis is to determine the difference in the benefits or effects of the two treatment strategies or policies being compared. This gives the incremental or marginal gain expressed in QALYs or other units of utility. It is possible that one of the tested strategies may do very little and yet be overall more cost-effective than others, which can be more effective but are very much more expensive.

Next the difference in cost of the two treatment strategies or policies must be determined, to get the incremental or marginal cost. The cost-effectiveness is the ratio of the incremental cost to the incremental gain. Consider the example of two strategies, A and B. In the first (A), the quality-adjusted life expectancy is 15 QALYs and the cost per case is $10 000. In the second (B), the life expectancy is 20 QALYs, a definite improvement, but at a cost of $110 000 per case. The results can be summarized as shown in Table 29.3.

The cost-effectiveness of B as compared to A is the difference in cost divided by the difference in effects. This is $(110\,000 - 10\,000)/(20 - 15) = \$20\,000/\text{QALY}$ gained. Note that if the more effective treatment also costs less, you should obviously do it unless it has serious drawbacks. Calculate this only when the more effective treatment strategy or policy is also more costly.

Are the conclusions unlikely to change with sensible changes in costs and outcomes?

Since most research on a given therapy is done at different times, changes over time must be accounted for. This process is called discounting and considers inflation and depreciation. It takes into account that inflation occurs and that instead of paying for a program now, you can invest the money now and pay for solving the problem later. For example, you can pay $200 a year for 10 years or $2000 in 10 years. The future costs are usually expressed in current dollars since

$200 in the future is equivalent to less than $200 today. Actuarial and accounting methods used should be specified in the methods section of the analysis.

Setting up a program is usually a greater cost than running it as initial costs are usually amortized over several decades. Discounting the value side of the equation considers that the value of a year of life saved now may be greater than a year saved later. Adding a year of life to someone at age 40 may mean more to them than adding a year of life to a 40-year-old but only when they reach age 60. This was considered in the discussion on patient preferences and values (Chapter 28).

As with any other clinical research study, the numbers used to perform the analysis are only approximations and have 95% confidence levels attached. Therefore, a sensitivity analysis should always be done to check on the assumptions made in the analysis. This is a process by which the results of the analysis are changed based on reasonable changes in costs or effects that are statistically expected based upon the 95% CI values.

Are the estimates of the costs and outcomes appropriately related to the baseline risk in the population?

There may be various levels of risk within the population. What is cost-effective in one subgroup may not be in another. The study should attempt to identify such subgroups and assign individual cost-effectiveness analyses to each of them. For example, if we look at the cost-effectiveness of positive isotropic agents in the treatment of heart failure, it may be that for severe heart failure their use is cost-effective, while for less severe cases it is not. The use of beta-blocker drugs in heart failure has been studied and the cost-effectiveness is much greater when the drug is used in high-risk patients than in low-risk patients. However, it is above the threshold for saving a life in both circumstances.

Final comments: ethical issues

How much are we willing to spend to save a life? What is an acceptable cost per QALY gained? A commonly accepted figure in the decision-analysis literature is $40 000 to $50 000 per QALY, approximately the cost to maintain a person on dialysis for one year. There are multiple ethical issues involved in the use of cost-effectiveness analyses. The physician is being asked to take sides with the option that will cost the least, or at least be the most cost-effective. This may not be the best option for each patient. Cost-effectiveness analyses are really more useful as political tools than for daily use in bedside clinical decision making.

There are some cases when cost-effectiveness is the best thing to do for the individual patient. Universally these situations occur when the best practice is the cheapest. One example is the use of antibiotics for treating urethral *Chlamydia* infections that was mentioned earlier. More importantly, you must be able to understand the issues involved in cost-effectiveness analyses when these come up in health policy areas. Pharmaceutical and medical instrument and device manufacturers and some specialty physicians are constantly trying to assert that their service, product, or procedure is the best and most cost-effective because, although it is more expensive now, it will lead to savings later. This can occur because of the "spin" that is put on their cost-effectiveness analysis. To be able to pick up the inconsistencies and omissions from a cost-effectiveness analysis is very difficult. However, you ought to be able at least to understand the analysis and subsequent comments made by people who are more highly trained in evaluating this type of study.

One current debate is over the use of chest pain evaluation units (CPEU) in emergency departments (ED) of acute care hospitals. These are for patients who are at low risk of having a myocardial infarction and for whom a stay of 48 hours in an intensive care unit is probably unnecessary. In this discussion, it is assumed that discharge home from the ED is not safe as up to 4% of acute MIs are missed by emergency physicians. Proponents of these CPEUs point out that a lot of money will be saved if these low-risk patients are put into the CPEU rather than the acute-care hospital bed. They have done cost-effectiveness analyses that show only a slight overall increase in costs. However, if all the very low-risk patients, even those who have almost no risk, are admitted to the CPEU, the overall admission rate may actually increase, resulting in markedly increased costs. Clearly there must be a search for some other method of dealing with these patients, which will be cost-effective and result in decreased hospital-bed utilization. The methods of cost-effectiveness analysis must look at all eventualities.

30

Outcome analysis

He ended; and thus Adam last replied:
How soon hath thy prediction, seer blest,
Measured this transient world, the race of time,
Till time stand fixed! Beyond is all abyss,
Eternity, whose end no eye can reach.

John Milton (1608–1674): Paradise Lost

Learning objectives

In this chapter you will learn:
- how to describe various outcome measures
- the ways outcomes may be compared
- the steps in reviewing an article which measures outcomes

One of the most important pieces of information that patients want is to know what is going to happen to them during their illness. The clinician must be able to provide information about prognosis to the patient in all medical encounters. You need to tell patients the details of the outcomes they can expect from their disease and treatment. Evaluation of the clinical research literature on prognosis is a required skill for the physician of the future. Outcome analysis looks at the interplay of three factors: the patient, the intervention, and the outcome. We want to know how long a patient with the given illness will survive if given one of two possible treatments. These treatments can be two active therapies or therapy and placebo. Studies of outcomes (or prognosis) should clearly define these three elements.

The patient: the inception cohort

To start an outcome study, an appropriate inception cohort must be assembled. The disease must be identified at a uniform point in the course of the disease (inception). This can be at the appearance of the first unambiguous sign or symptom of a disease or at the first application of testing or therapy. Ideally this should be as early in the disease as possible. However, it should be at a stage where most reasonably prudent physicians can make the diagnosis, not sooner. Collection of the cohort after the occurrence of the outcome event and looking backwards will distort the results either in a positive or negative way if some patients with the disease die before diagnosis or commonly have spontaneous remissions soon after diagnosis. A study of survival of patients with acute myocardial infarction who are studied from the time they arrive in the coronary care unit will miss those who die either suddenly before seeking care or in the emergency department.

Incidence/prevalence bias can be a fatal flaw in the study if the inception cohort is assembled at different stages of illness. This confuses new from ongoing cases of the illness. There may be very different prognoses for patients at these stages of illness. Lead-time and length-time bias occurring as the result of screening programs should be avoided by proper randomization. These were discussed in detail in Chapter 26 on screening tests.

Diagnostic criteria, disease severity, referral pattern, comorbidity, and demographic details for inclusion must be specified. Patients referred from a primary-care center may be different than those referred from a tertiary-care center. Termed referral filter bias, this is due to an over-representation of patients with later stages of disease or more complex illness. They are more likely to have poor results. Centripetal bias is another name for cases referred to tertiary-care centers because of the need for special expertise. Popularity bias occurs when more challenging and interesting cases only are referred to the experts in the tertiary care center. The results of these biases limit external validity in other settings where most patients will present with earlier or milder disease.

All members of the inception cohort should be accounted for at the end of the study and their outcomes known. There are non-trivial reasons why patients drop out of a study. These include recovery, death, refusal of therapy due to the disease, side effects of therapy, loss of interest, or moving away. One study showed that patients in a study who were harder to track had a higher mortality rate.

There are several rules of thumb to use in determining the effect of incomplete follow up. First, identify the outcome of most interest to you and determine the fraction of patients who had this outcome. Then add the patients "lost to follow-up" to both the numerator and the denominator, which gives the result if all patients lost had the outcome of interest. Now add the patients lost to follow-up to only the denominator, giving the lowest result if no patient lost had the outcome of interest. Compare these two results. If they are very close to each other, the result is useful. If not the result of the study may be useless. In the example in Table 30.1, the difference in relapse rates is minor while the difference in mortality is quite large. As a general rule, the lower the rate of an outcome, the more likely it is to be affected by patients lost to follow-up.

Table 30.1. A study of 71 patients 6 of whom were lost to follow-up

	Original study	"Highest" case	"Lowest" case
Relapse rate	$39/65 = 60\%$	$45/71 = 63\%$	$39/71 = 55\%$
Mortality rate	$1/65 = 1.5\%$	$7/71 = 10\%$	$1/71 = 1.4\%$

The intervention

There should be a clear and easily reproducible description of the intervention being tested. All details of a therapeutic program should be given. A reader should be able to duplicate the results at another institution. All the interventions tested or compared should be those that make a difference. Testing a drug against placebo may not be as important or useful as testing it against the favorite currently used drug. Most of these issues have been discussed in the chapter on randomized clinical trials in Chapter 15.

The outcome

The outcome criteria should be objective, reproducible, and accurate. The outcome assessment should be done in a blinded manner to avoid diagnostic suspicion and expectation bias in the assessment of patient outcomes.

There can be significant bias introduced into the study if the outcomes are not measured in a consistent manner. Ideally, the outcome measures should be ones that are unmistakably objective. Death or life are clear and easily measured outcome variables and admission to the hospital is clear and objective. However, outcomes such as "full recovery at home" or "feeling better" have a degree of subjectivity associated with them. Even cause of death as measured on a death certificate is not always a reliable outcome measure of the actual cause of death.

There should be adjustment for extraneous prognostic factors. The researcher should determine whether the prognostic factor is merely a marker or actually part of the causation. This determines whether or not there are alternative explanations for the outcomes. Although you can count on the article being reviewed by a statistician who can determine that the authors used the correct statistical analysis, your job is to decide whether the correct adjustment for extraneous factors was done at all. If the authors suggest that a group of signs, symptoms, or diagnostic tests accurately predict an outcome, look for a validation sample in a second study which attempts to verify that indeed these results occurred because of a causal relationship and not just by chance. Look for at least 10 and preferably 20 patients with the outcome of interest for each prognostic factor that is evaluated to give clinically and statistically significant results. Chapter 14 has a discussion of multivariate analysis.

Most often outcomes are expressed as a dichotomous nominal variable (e.g., dead or alive, disease or no disease, a patent or occluded bypass, improved or worse, it works or it doesn't, etc.). We are interested in the association of an independent variable (e.g., drug use, therapy, risk factor, diagnostic test result, tumor stage, age of patient, blood pressure, etc.) with the dependent or outcome variable.

Diagnostic-suspicion bias occurs when the physician caring for the patient knows the outcomes being measured and changes the care or observation of the patient. Expectation bias occurs when the person measuring the outcome knows the clinical features of the case or the results of a diagnostic test and alters their interpretation of the outcome event. This is less likely when the intervention and outcome measures are clearly objective. Ideally blind diagnosis, treatment, and assessment of all the patients going through the study will prevent these biases.

Another problem in the outcomes selected occurs when multiple outcomes are lumped together. Many more studies of therapy are comparing two groups for several outcomes at once. These are also called composite outcomes. Commonly used measures of heart therapies might include death (important outcome), non-fatal myocardial infarction, and need for revascularization procedure (maybe less important). The use of these measures can lead to over-optimistic conclusions regarding the therapy being tested. If each outcome were measured alone, none would have statistical significance (possible Type II error). When combined, multiple or composite outcomes may then show statistical significance.

One example is the recent CAPRIE trial of clopidogrel (a new antiplatelet agent) against aspirin. The primary outcome measures were overall number of deaths, and of deaths due to stroke, myocardial infarction, or vascular causes. The definition of vascular causes was not made clear. The end result was that there were no decreases in death from stroke or myocardial infarction, but a 20% reduction in deaths in the patients with peripheral arterial disease. The absolute reduction was 1.09% (from 4.80% to 3.71%, giving an NNT of 91). If these patient outcomes were considered as separate groups, the differences would not have been statistically significant. Another danger is that some patients may be counted several times because they have several of the outcomes. Finally, the clinical significance of the combined outcomes is unknown.

There are basically three types of data that are used to indicate risk of an outcome. Interval data is usually considered to be normally distributed and measured on a continuous scale (e.g., blood pressure). Nominal data is categorical (e.g., tumor type or treatment options) and often dichotomous like alive and dead or positive and negative test results. Ordinal data is also categorical but with some relation between the categories (e.g., tumor stage). There are three types of analyses applied to this type of problem: frequency tables, logistic analysis, and survival analysis. Decision theory uses probability distributions to estimate the probability of an outcome. A loss function measures the relative benefit or utility of that outcome.

Frequency tables

Frequency tables use a chi-square analysis to compare the association of the outcome with risk factors that are nominal or ordinal. For the chi-square analysis, data are usually presented in a table where columns are outcomes, rows are risk factors and the frequencies appear as table entries. The observed data are compared with the data that would be expected if there were no association. The analysis results in a P value which indicates the probability that the observed outcome could have been obtained by chance when it was really no different from the expected value (Type I error). Fisher's exact test is used when the observed value of any cell is less than 5.

Logistic analysis

This is a more general approach to measuring outcomes than using frequency tables. Logistic regression estimates the probability of an outcome based on one or more risk factors. The risk factors may be interval, ordinal, or nominal variables. Results of logistic regression analysis are often reported as the odds ratio or relative risk. For one independent variable (interval-type data and relative risk) this method tells us how much of an increase in the risk of the outcome occurs for each incremental increase in the exposure to the risk factor. An example of this would answer the question "how much additional risk of stroke will occur for each increase of 10 mm Hg in systolic blood pressure?" For ordinal data the analysis calculates the probability of an outcome based on the stage of disease (i.e., recurrence of a stage 4 compared to a stage 2 tumor).

For multiple variables, we want to know if there is some combination of risk factors that will better predict an outcome than one risk factor alone. We also want to know which risk factors best predict that outcome. The identification of significant risk factors can be done using multiple regressions or stepwise regression analyses as we discussed in Chapter 27 on clinical prediction rules.

Survival analysis

In the real world the ultimate outcome is often not known (e.g., dead vs. so far, so good). It would be difficult to justify waiting until all patients in a study die so that survival in two treatment or risk groups can be compared. Another common problem with comparing survival occurs in trying to determine what to do with patients who are doing fine but die of an incident unrelated to their medical problem (e.g., a bypass graft is patent for 15 years and the patient then dies in

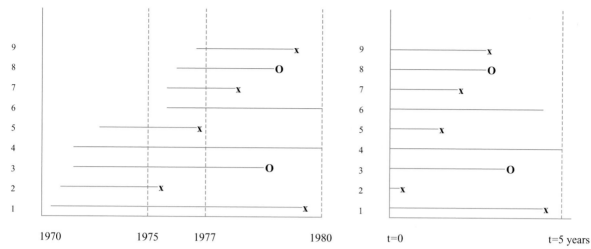

Fig. 30.1 Censoring. Patients are enrolled in a study over a two-year period (1975–1977). All are followed until 1980 and patients who die are marked with an x. Some patients (2 and 5) are enrolled at a late stage of their disease. Their inclusion will bias the cohort towards poorer survival. Two patients (4 and 6) are still alive at the end of the observation period. Patient 1 lived longer than everyone except patient 4, although it appears that patient 1 didn t live so long, since their previous survival (pre-1975) does not count in the analysis. We don't know how long patient 4 will live since he or she is still alive at the end of the observation period and their data is censored at t = 5 years. Two other patients (3 and 8) are lost to follow-up and their data is censored early (o).

a motor-vehicle accident). This will alter the information used in the analysis of time to occlusion with two different types of bypasses. Finally, how should we handle the patient who simply moves away and is lost to follow-up?

The situations described above are examples of **censored** data. The data consist of a time interval and a dichotomous variable indicating status, either failure (dead, graft occluded, etc.) or censored (i.e. success so far). In the latter case, the patient may still be alive, have died but not from the disease of interest, or been alive when last seen but could not be located again.

A potential problem in these analyses is the definition of the start time. Early diagnosis may automatically confer longer survival if the time of diagnosis is the start time. This is also called lead-time bias, as discussed in Chapter 26. Censoring bias occurs when one of the treatment groups is more likely to be censored. If certain patients are lost as a result of treatment (e.g., harmful side effects) their chances of being censored are not independent of their survival times. A survival analysis initially assumes that any patient censoring is independent of the outcome. Fig. 30.1 shows an example of the effects of censoring on a hypothetical study.

Survival curves

The distribution of survival times is most often displayed as a survivor function (also called a survival curve). This is a plot of the proportion of subjects surviving versus time. It is important to note that "surviving" may indicate things other than actual survival (i.e., life vs. death), such as success of therapy (i.e., patent vs. non-patent coronary bypass grafts). These curves can be deceptive since the number of individuals represented by the curve decreases as time increases. It is key that a statistical analysis is applied at several times to the results of the

Fig. 30.2 Kaplan—Meier survival curve.

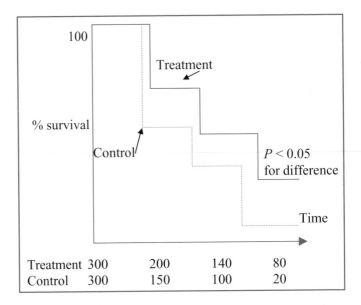

curves. The number of patients at each stage of the curve should also be given. The Kaplan-Meier curve is the one most commonly used.

There are two methods for plotting and analyzing survival curves. In the actuarial-life-table method, the length of time from the moment the patient is entered into the study until failure occurred is plotted. In the product-limit (also known as Kaplan–Meier) method, the analysis looks at the period of time (month, year, etc.) in which the failure occurred. A typical Kaplan–Meier curve is shown in Fig. 30.2.

There are several tests of equality of these survivor functions (curves) that are commonly performed. One of the most popular is the Mantel–Cox (also known as log-rank) test. The Cox proportional-hazard model uses interval data as the independent variable determining how much the odds of survival are altered by each unit of change in the independent variable (e.g., how much is the risk of stroke increased with each increase of 10 mm Hg in mean arterial blood pressure?). Further discussion of survival curves and outcome analysis is beyond the scope of this book. Two of the Users' Guides articles provide more detail.[1,2]

[1] A. Laupacis, G. Wells, W. S. Richardson & P. Tugwell. Users' guides to the medical literature. V. How to use an article about prognosis. *JAMA* 1994; 272: 234–237.
[2] C. D. Naylor & G. H. Guyatt. Users' guides to the medical literature. X. How to use an article reporting variations in the outcomes of health services. *JAMA* 1996; 275: 554–558.

31

Meta-analysis and systematic reviews

Common sense is the collection of prejudices acquired by age eighteen.

Albert Einstein (1879–1955)

Learning objectives

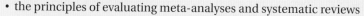

In this chapter you will learn:

- the principles of evaluating meta-analyses and systematic reviews
- the concepts of heterogeneity and homogeneity
- the use of L'Abbé and funnel plots
- measures commonly used in systematic reviews: odds ratios and effect size
- how to review a published meta-analysis and use the results to solve a clinical problem

Background and rationale for performing meta-analysis

Over the past 50 years there has been an explosion of research in the medical literature. In the worldwide English-language medical literature alone, there were 1300 biomedical journals in 1940, while in 2000 there were over 14 000. It has become almost impossible for the individual practitioner to keep up with the literature. This is more frustrating when contradictory studies are published about a given topic. Meta-analyses and systematic reviews are relatively new techniques used to synthesize and summarize the results of multiple research studies on the same topic.

A primary analysis refers to the original analysis of research data as presented in an observational study or randomized clinical trial (RCT). Secondary analysis is a re-analysis of the original data either using another statistical technique or answering new questions with previously obtained data.

The traditional review article is a qualitative review. It is a summary of all primary research on a given topic, and it may provide good background information that is more up to date than a textbook. But review articles have the disadvantage of being somewhat subjective and reflecting the biases of the author. One must be knowledgeable of the literature being reviewed in order to evaluate this type of article critically.

Meta-analysis is more comprehensive or "transcends" traditional analysis of data. Typically, a meta-analysis looks at data from multiple studies of the same clinical question and uses a variety of statistical techniques to integrate their findings. It may be called a quantitative systematic review and represents the rigorous application of research techniques and statistical analysis to present an overview of a given topic.

A meta-analysis is usually done to reconcile studies with different results. It can look at multiple negative studies to uncover Type II errors or at clinical problems where there are some negative and some positive studies to uncover Type I or Type II errors. It can help uncover a single study which has totally different results because of systematic error or bias in the research process. Large confidence intervals in some studies may be narrowed by combining them. For example, multiple small trials done before 1971 showed both positive and negative effects of light therapy (phototherapy) on hyperbilirubinemia in newborns. A meta-analysis in 1985 showed an overall positive effect.

Occasionally a large trial shows an opposite effect from that found in multiple small trials. This is often due to procedural or methodologic study design difference in the trials. However, as a general rule, correctly done large cooperative trials are more reliable than meta-analysis of many smaller trials. For example a meta-analysis of multiple small trials of magnesium in acute myocardial infarction (AMI) showed a positive effect on decreasing mortality. The ISIS-4 trial, a large multicenter study where magnesium was given (although later in the course of the AMI), showed no benefit. The disparity of study methodologies in this case required a new multicenter study (called MAGIC and now in progress) to be done. The use of meta-analysis does not reduce the need for large well-done studies of primary clinical modalities.

Guidelines for evaluation of systematic reviews[1]

Were the question and methods clearly stated, and were the search methods used to locate relevant studies comprehensive?

In meta-analysis, the process of article selection and analysis should proceed by a preset protocol. By not changing the process in mid analysis the author's bias and retrospective bias are minimized. This means that the definitions of outcome and predictor (or therapy) variables of the analysis are not changed in mid-stream.

---

[1] Adapted with permission from the Users' Guides to the Medical Literature, published in *JAMA* (see Bibliography).

The research question must be clearly defined, including a defined patient population and clear and consistent definitions of the disease, interventions, and outcomes.

A carefully defined search strategy must be used to detect and prevent publication bias. This bias occurs because trials with positive results and those with large sample sizes are more likely to be published. Sources should include conference proceedings, Dissertation Abstracts and other databases, as well as the usual search of MEDLINE. A manual search of relevant journals may uncover some additional studies. The bibliographies of all relevant articles found should be checked to find any misclassified articles that were missed in the original search.

The authors must cite where they looked and should be exhaustive in looking for unpublished studies. Not using foreign studies may introduce bias since some foreign studies are published in English-language journals while others may be missed. The authors should also contact the authors of all the studies found and ask them about other researchers working in the area who may have unpublished studies available. The Cochrane Collaboration maintains a register of controlled trials called CENTRAL, which attempts to document all current trials regardless of result.

Were explicit methods used to determine which articles to include in the review, and were the selection and assessment of the methodologic quality of the primary studies reproducible and free from bias?

Objective selection of articles for the meta-analysis should be clearly laid out and include inclusion and exclusion criteria. The objectives and procedures must be defined ahead of time. This includes a clearly defined research and abstraction method and a scoring system for assessing the quality of the included studies. For each study several factors ought to be assessed. The publication status may suggest stronger studies in that those that were never published or only published in abstract form may be significantly deficient in methodological areas.

The strength of the study design will determine the ability to prove causation. RCTs are the strongest study design. A well-designed observational study with appropriate safeguards to prevent or minimize bias will also give very strong results. The methods of meta-analysis include ranking or grading the quality of the evidence. Appendix 1 gives the criteria for grading various levels of evidence.

The study sites and patient populations of the individual studies may limit generalizability of the meta-analysis. The interventions or exposures should be similar between studies. Finally, the studies should be measuring the same or very similar outcomes. We will discuss issues of how to judge homogeneity and combine heterogeneous studies.

Independent review of the methods section looks at inclusion and exclusion criteria, coding, and replication issues. There must be accurate and objective abstraction of the data, ideally done by blinded abstracters. Two abstracters should gather the data independently and the author should check for inter-rater agreement. The methods and results sections should be disguised to prevent reviewers from discovering the source of the research. Inter-rater reliability of coders should be maximized with a minimal level of 0.9 on the kappa statistic. Once this has been established, a single coder can code all the remaining study results.

Were the differences in individual study results adequately explained and were the results of the primary studies combined appropriately?

Studies may be homogeneous or heterogeneous. There are both qualitative and quantitative measures of homogeneity. Testing for homogeneity of the studies is done to determine if the studies are qualitatively similar enough to combine. The tests for homogeneity include the Mantel–Haentszel chi-squared test, the Breslow–Day test, and the Q statistic by the DerSimonian and Laird method. They all suffer from low power (Type II error). If the test statistic is statistically significant ($P < 0.05$), the studies are likely to be heterogeneous. However, the absence of statistical significance does not mean homogeneity.

The presence of heterogeneity among the studies analyzed will result in erroneous interpretation of the statistical results. If the studies are very heterogeneous, one strategy for analyzing them is to remove the study with most extreme (outlier) results and recalculate the statistic. If the statistic is no longer statistically significant, you may assume that the outlier was responsible for all or most of the heterogeneity. That study should then be examined more closely to determine what about the study design might have caused the observed extreme result. This could be due to differences in the population studied or systematic bias in the conduct of the study.

Analysis and aggregation of the data can be done in several ways, but should consider sample sizes and magnitude of effects. A simple vote count in which the number of studies with positive results is directly compared with the number of studies with negative results is not an acceptable method since neither effect size nor sample size are considered. Pooled analysis or lumped data add numerators and denominators to produce a new result. This is better than a vote count, but still not acceptable. That process ignores the confidence intervals for each study and allows errors to multiply in the process. Simple combination of P values is not acceptable because this does not consider the direction of the effect or magnitude of the effect size.

Weighted outcomes compare small and large studies, analyze them as equals, and then weight the results by size of sample. This involves adjusting each outcome by a value that accounts for the sample size and variation. Confidence intervals should be applied to the mean results of each study evaluated. Aggregate study and control-group means and confidence intervals can then be calculated. Subgroups should be analyzed where appropriate. There are two standard measures for doing this: the odds ratio and the effect size.

The odds ratio (OR) is the most common way of combining results in meta-analysis. The odds ratio can be calculated for each study showing whether the intervention increases or decreases the odds of a favorable outcome. These can then be combined statistically and the 95% confidence intervals calculated for all the odds ratios. If we are looking at a positive outcome (e.g., % alive) an OR > 1 favors the experimental treatment. If looking at a negative outcome (e.g., mortality rates) an OR < 1 favors the experimental treatment.

The effect size (= d or δ), a standard metric compared across studies, is a relative and not an absolute value. The equation for effect size is $d = (m_1 - m_2)/SD$, where m_1 and m_2 are the means of the two groups being studied and SD is the standard deviation of either sample population. A difference (δ) in SD units of 0.2 SD is a small effect, 0.5 a moderate effect, and >0.8, a large effect. If the data are skewed, it is better to use median rather than mean of the data to calculate the effect size, but this requires the use of other statistical methods to accomplish the analysis.

The statistical analytic procedures usually employed in systematic reviews are far too complex to discuss here. However, there are important distinctions, which the reader should be aware of, between the methods used in the presence and in the absence of heterogeneity of the results of the studies. If the data are relatively homogeneous, a fixed-effects model can be used. This assumes that all the studies can be (statistically) analyzed as equals. However, if the data are very heterogeneous, a random-effects model should be used. This is more complex and takes into account that the various studies are part of a population of studies of the events. The result is the presence of wider confidence intervals. Unfortunately, the methods used for the random-effects model give more weight to the smaller studies. Frequently, a single meta-analysis will use both methods to determine statistical significance. If the two methods give the same result, the statistical significance is more "powerful" than if one method finds statistical significance and the other does not.

There are two graphic techniques that can be used to look at the overall data. Both of these can demonstrate the effect of the problem of publication bias. Large studies or those showing positive effects are more likely to be published. It is very likely that if one small study showed a positive effect it would be published. Conversely if a small study showed a negative effect (no difference between the groups) it is less likely to be published. It is important to be able to estimate the effect of this phenomenon on the results of the meta analysis.

Graphic displays are a powerful tool to show the difference in study results. The most common way of graphing meta-analysis results is to show the results

Fig. 31.1 Hypothetical meta-analysis. Initial studies (except one) lacked power to find a difference. A difference was found when all studies were combined.

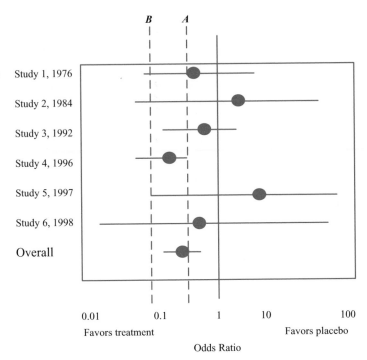

of each study as a point estimate for the rate, risk difference, or ratio (odds ratio, relative risk, or effect size) and a line for the 95% confidence intervals on this point estimate. A log scale is commonly used so that the reciprocal values are an equal distance from 1 (Fig. 31.1). Always be careful to check the scales. It is easy to see if the confidence interval crosses the point of no significance, 0 (for differences) or 1 (for ratios).

There is a visual guide that can suggest heterogeneity in this type of a plot. Simply draw a perpendicular from the higher end of the 95% CI for the study with the lowest point value. In Fig. 31.1 this is line A drawn through the higher end of the 95% CI of study 4. Draw a similar line through the lower end of the 95% CI of the study with the highest point value. Here it is line B, through the lower point of study 5. If the confidence intervals of all of the studies appear in the space between these two lines, the studies are probably not heterogeneous. Any study outside this area may be the cause of significant heterogeneity in the aggregate of the studies.

The L'Abbé plot (Fig. 31.2) is used to show how much each individual study contributes to the outcome. The two possible outcome rates (control and intervention) are plotted on the x- and y-axis respectively. A circle, the diameter of which is proportional to the sample size, represents each study. A key to the sample size is given with the plot.

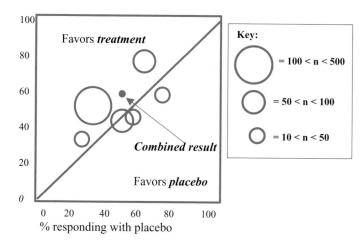

Fig. 31.2 L'Abbé plot of a hypothetical meta-analysis. The largest studies showed the most effect of the treatment, suggesting that the smaller studies lacked power.

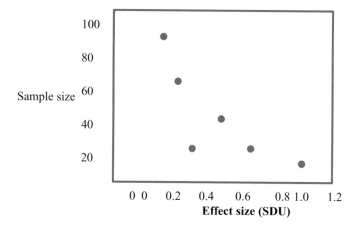

Fig. 31.3 Funnel plot of six studies. Notice that the largest effect sizes were found in the smallest studies. A plot with this configuration suggests publication bias.

A funnel plot (Fig. 31.3) is another way to show the effect of sample size on the effect size. This is a plot of effect size (δ) on the x-axis and sample size on the y-axis. If there are many small studies with large effect sizes, the resulting plot will look like an asymmetric triangle or half of an upside-down funnel. This suggests that the overall result of the meta-analysis is being unduly influenced by these many, very positive, small studies. This could be due to publication bias or they may have similar and perhaps fatal flaws in their execution.

Were the reviewers' conclusions supported by the data cited?

A sensitivity analysis should be done to address the possibility of publication bias (also called the file-drawer effect). Negative and unpublished studies are frequently small and usually won't be able to drastically change the results of the meta-analysis. Using the funnel or the L'Abbé plots and other methods will help alert the reader to the potential presence of publication bias.

There is a way of calculating the potential effect of publication bias. Fail-safe N is an estimate of the number of negative studies you would need in order to eliminate the difference you have found. This can mean to reverse the δ value or increase the overall probability of finding a difference when one doesn't exist to a value higher than the δ level (i.e., $P > 0.05$). If a large part of the effect found is due to a few small and very positive studies, it is possible that there are also a few small and clearly negative studies that because of publication bias have never been published. If the fail-safe N is small only a few studies would be needed to reverse the finding, and this is a plausible occurrence. But if fail-safe N is big, it is unlikely that there are that many negative studies "out there" that have never been published and you would accept the results.

Some common problems with meta-analyses are that they may be comparing diverse studies with different designs or over different time periods. There may be excessive inter-observer variability in deciding on which trials to evaluate, and how much weight to give each trial. These issues ought to be addressed by the authors and difference in the results explained. In many cases, the methodologies will contribute biases that can be uncovered in the meta-analysis process.

Cumulative meta-analysis is meta-analytic approach that doesn't look at each study individually, but looks at them cumulatively. There are two ways of doing this. In one, the studies are looked at chronologically. Each study's results are combined with the ones done before to give a new estimate of the effect size. You can look and see where in the progression of these studies the results became statistically significant.

Another way of doing this is by beginning with the study with smallest sample size and then successively adding larger ones. This is a good way to uncover Type II errors. You can see where in the progression of studies the results become statistically significant. If they only become statistically significant after the vast majority of the studies had been done, the results are not as strong as if they had become statistically significant after only a few studies. The chronological cumulative meta-analysis by Lau and colleagues of therapeutic trials of streptokinase in myocardial infarction shows statistical significance after the sixth trial (of a total of 33 studies) was done (Fig 31.4).

A recent addition to the quantitative (systematic) review literature comes from the Cochrane Collaboration. Begun in the United Kingdom in 1992 and named after Archie Cochrane, this is a worldwide network of interested clinicians, epidemiologists, and scientists who perform systematic reviews and meta-analyses of clinical questions. Their reviews are standardized, of the highest quality, and updated regularly as more information becomes available. These systematic reviews are available online in the Cochrane Library (see Chapter 5).

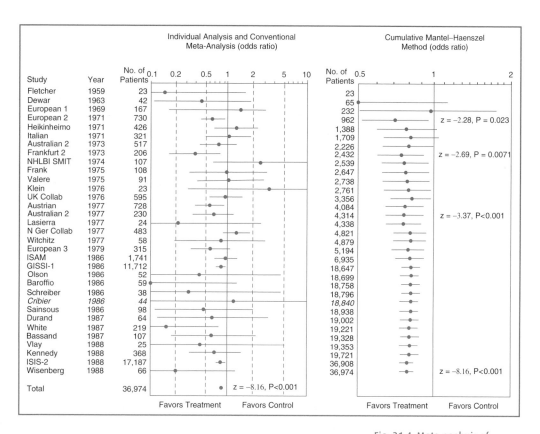

Fig. 31.4 Meta-analysis of therapeutic trials for myocardial infarction. From J. Lau *et al.* Cumulative meta-analysis of therapeutic trials for myocardial infarction. *N. Engl. J. Med.* 1992; 327: 248–254. Used with permission.

Additional guidelines for meta-analysis

There are some additional guidelines for creating and reviewing meta-analyses that were published in 1985 by Green and Hall and are still very useful to follow.[1]

The inclusion and exclusion criteria for the relevant studies should be defined and reported. This may lead to substantive and conceptual issues such as how to handle a study with missing or incomplete data. The coding categories should be developed in a manner that will accommodate the largest proportion of the identified literature. Over-coding of characteristics of studies is better than under-coding. The following characteristics should be coded: type and length of the intervention, sample characteristics, research design characteristics and quality, source of study (e.g., published, dissertation, internal report, and the like), date of study, and so on. The reliability of the coders should be checked with the kappa statistic.

Multiple independent and dependent variables should be separately evaluated using a sensitivity analysis. Interactions between variables outside the principal

[1] B. Green & J. Hall. Quantitative methods for literature review. *Annu. Rev. Psychol.* 1984; 35: 37–53.

relationship being reviewed should be looked for. The distribution of results should be examined and graphed. Look at outliers more closely. Perform statistical tests for the heterogeneity of results. If the studies are found to be heterogeneous, a sensitivity analysis should be performed to identify the outlier study. The effect size should be specified and level of significance or confidence intervals given. Effect sizes should be recalculated to give both unadjusted and adjusted results. Where necessary, nonparametric and parametric effect size estimates should be calculated.

In the conclusions, the authors should examine other approaches to the same problem. Qualitative evaluation of all studies should be combined with quantitative reviews of the topic. This should look at the comparability of treatment and control groups from study to study. They should also look at other potentially interesting and worthwhile studies that are not part of the quantitative review. Finally, the limitations of the review and ideas for future research should be discussed. For the reader, it is well to remember that "data analysis is an aid to thought, not a substitute."[2]

The same is true of evidence-based medicine in general. It should be an aid to thought, and an encouragement to integrate the science of medical research into clinical practice, but it is not a substitute for critical thinking and the art of medicine. There is a great tendency to accept meta-analyses as the ultimate word in evidence. The results of such an analysis are only as good as the evidence upon which it is based. Then again, this statement can apply to all evidence in medicine. We will always be faced with making difficult decisions in the face of uncertainty. In that setting, it takes our clinical experience, intuition, common sense, and good communications with our patients to decide upon the best way to use the best evidence.

[2] B. Green & J. Hall. *Ibid.*

Appendix 1 Levels of evidence and grades of recommendations

Adapted and used with permission from the Oxford Centre for Evidence-Based Medicine *Levels of Evidence* (May 2001), available at www.cebm.net/levels_of_evidence.asp.

Levels of evidence

Level	Therapy/Prevention, Etiology/Harm	Prognosis	Diagnosis	Differential diagnosis/Symptom prevalence study	Economic and decision analyses
1a	SR (with homogeneity) of RCTs[a]	SR (with homogeneity) of inception cohort studies; CDR validated in different populations[d]	SR (with homogeneity) of Level 1 diagnostic studies; CDR with 1b studies from different clinical centres	SR (with homogeneity) of prospective cohort studies	SR (with homogeneity) of Level 1 economic studies
1b	Individual RCT (with narrow confidence interval)	Individual inception cohort study with ≥80% follow-up; CDR validated in a single population	Validating cohort study with good reference standards; or CDR tested within one clinical centre[g][h]	Prospective cohort study with good follow-up[j]	Analysis based on clinically sensible costs or alternatives; systematic review(s) of the evidence; and including multi-way sensitivity analyses
1c	All or none[b]	All-or-none case series	Absolute SpPins and SnNouts[i]	All-or-none case series	Absolute better-value or worse-value analyses[k]
2a	SR (with homogeneity) of cohort studies	SR (with homogeneity) of either retrospective cohort studies or untreated control groups in RCTs	SR (with homogeneity) of Level >2 diagnostic studies	SR (with homogeneity) of 2b and better studies	SR (with homogeneity) of Level >2 economic studies
2b	Individual cohort study (including low-quality RCT; e.g., <80% follow-up)	Retrospective cohort study or follow-up of untreated control patients in an RCT; Derivation of CDR or validated on split-sample only[e]	Exploratory cohort study with good reference standards; CDR after derivation, or validated only on split-sample or databases	Retrospective cohort study, or poor follow-up	Analysis based on clinically sensible costs or alternatives; limited review(s) of the evidence, or single studies; and including multi-way sensitivity analyses

Level					
2c	"Outcomes" research; ecological studies	"Outcomes" research		Ecological studies	Audit or outcomes research
3a	SR (with homogeneity) of case–control studies		SR (with homogeneity) of 3b and better studies	SR (with homogeneity) of 3b and better studies	SR (with homogeneity) of 3b and better studies
3b	Individual case–control study		Non-consecutive study; or without consistently applied reference standards	Non-consecutive cohort study, or very limited population	Analysis based on limited alternatives or costs, poor quality estimates of data, but including sensitivity analyses incorporating clinically sensible variations.
4	Case series (and poor-quality cohort and case–control studies)^c	Case series (and poor-quality prognostic cohort studies)^f	Case–control study, poor or non-independent reference standard	Case series or superseded reference standards	Analysis with no sensitivity analysis
5	Expert opinion without explicit critical appraisal, or based on physiology, bench research or "first principles"	Expert opinion without explicit critical appraisal, or based on physiology, bench research or "first principles"	Expert opinion without explicit critical appraisal, or based on physiology, bench research or "first principles"	Expert opinion without explicit critical appraisal, or based on physiology, bench research or "first principles"	Expert opinion without explicit critical appraisal, or based on economic theory or "first principles"

Users can add a minus sign to denote the level of that fails to provide a conclusive answer because of:

• EITHER a single result with a wide confidence interval (such that, for example, an ARR in an RCT is not statistically significant but whose confidence intervals fail to exclude clinically important benefit or harm)

• OR a systematic review with troublesome (and statistically significant) heterogeneity.

Such evidence is inconclusive, and therefore can only generate Grade D recommendations.

^{a} By homogeneity we mean a systematic review that is free of worrisome variations (heterogeneity) in the directions and degrees of results between individual studies. Not all systematic reviews with statistically significant heterogeneity need be worrisome, and not all worrisome heterogeneity need be statistically significant. As noted above, studies displaying worrisome heterogeneity should be tagged with a "−" (minus sign) at the end of their designated level.

(Continued)

Levels of evidence (*continued*)

[b] All or none: met when *all* patients died before the therapy became available, but some now survive on it; or when some patients died before the therapy became available, but *none* now die on it.

[c] By poor-quality *cohort* study we mean one that failed to clearly define comparison groups and/or failed to measure exposures and outcomes in the same (preferably blinded) objective way in both exposed and non-exposed individuals and/or failed to identify or appropriately control known confounders and/or failed to carry out a sufficiently long and complete follow-up of patients. By poor-quality *case–control* study we mean one that failed to clearly define comparison groups and/or failed to measure exposures and outcomes in the same (preferably blinded) objective way in both cases and controls and/or failed to identify or appropriately control known confounders.

[d] CDR: Clinical Decision Rule. These are algorithms or scoring systems which lead to a prognostic estimation or a diagnostic category.

[e] Split-sample validation is achieved by collecting all the information in a single group, then artificially dividing this into "derivation" and "validation" samples.

[f] By poor-quality prognostic cohort study we mean one in which sampling was biased in favour of patients who already had the target outcome, or the measurement of outcomes was accomplished in <80% of study patients, or outcomes were determined in an unblinded, non-objective way, or there was no correction for confounding factors.

[g] Validating studies test the quality of a specific diagnostic test, based on prior evidence. An exploratory study collects information and trawls the data (e.g., using a regression analysis) to find which factors are "significant."

[h] *Good* reference standards are independent of the test, and applied blindly or objectively to all patients. *Poor* reference standards are haphazardly applied, but still independent of the test. Use of a non-independent reference standard (where the "test" is included in the "reference", or where the "testing" affects the "reference") implies a level 4 study.

[i] An "Absolute SpPin" is a diagnostic finding whose Specificity is so high that a Positive result rules-in the diagnosis. An "Absolute SnNout" is a diagnostic finding whose Sensitivity is so high that a Negative result rules-out the diagnosis.

[j] Good follow-up in a differential diagnosis study is >80%, with adequate time for alternative diagnoses to emerge (e.g., 1–6 months acute, 1–5 years chronic).

[k] Better-value treatments are clearly as good but cheaper, or better at the same or reduced cost. Worse-value treatments are as good and more expensive, or worse and equally or more expensive.

Grades of recommendation

A consistent level 1 studies

B consistent level 2 or 3 studies *or* extrapolations from level 1 studies

C level 4 studies *or* extrapolations from level 2 or 3 studies

D level 5 evidence *or* troublingly inconsistent or inconclusive studies of any level

"Extrapolations" are where data is used in a situation which has potentially clinically important differences than the original study situation.

Appendix 2   Overview of critical appraisal

Adapted from G. Guyatt & D. Rennie (eds.) *Users' Guides to the Medical Literature: a Manual for Evidence-Based Clinical Practice*. Chicago: AMA, 2002. Used with permission.

(1) Randomized clinical trials (commonly studies of therapy or prevention)
- (a) Are the results valid?
    - (i) Were the patients randomly assigned to treatment and was allocation effectively concealed?
    - (ii) Were the baseline characteristics of all groups similar at the start of the study?
    - (iii) Were the patients who entered the study fully accounted for at its conclusion?
    - (iv) Were participating patients, family members, treating clinicians, and other people (observers or managers) involved in the study "blind" to the treatment received?
    - (v) Were all measurements made in an objective and reproducible manner?
    - (vi) With the exception of the experimental intervention, were all patients treated equally?
    - (vii) Were the patients analyzed in the groups to which they were randomized?
    - (viii) Was follow-up complete?
- (b) What are the results?
    - (i) What is the treatment effect? (Absolute Rate Reduction, Relative Rate Reduction, Number Needed to Treat)
    - (ii) What is the variability of this effect? (Confidence Intervals)
- (c) Will the results help me in my patient care?
    - (i) Were all clinically important outcomes considered in the study?
    - (ii) Will the benefits of the experimental treatment counterbalance any harms and additional costs?
    - (iii) Can the results of this study be applied to most of my patients with this or similar problems?

(2) Cohort studies (commonly studies of risk or harm or etiology)
- (a) Are the results valid?
    - (i) With the exception of the risk factor under study, were all groups similar to each other at the start of the study?
    - (ii) Were all measurements (outcome and exposure) made in an objective and reproducible manner and carried out in the same ways in all groups?
    - (iii) Were all patients that were entered into the study accounted for at the end of the study and was the follow-up for a sufficiently long time?

(b) What are the results?

    (i) Is the temporal relationship between the cause and effect correct?

    (ii) Is there a dose–response gradient between the cause and effect?

    (iii) How strong is the association between cause and effect? (Relative Risk Reduction, Relative Risk, Absolute Risk Reduction, Number Needed to Harm)

    (iv) What is the variability of this effect? (Confidence Intervals)

(c) Will the results help me in my patient care?

    (i) What is the relative magnitude of the risk in my patient population?

    (ii) Can the results of this study be applied to most of my patients with this or similar problems?

    (iii) Should I encourage the patient to stop the exposure? If yes, how soon?

(3) Case–control studies (commonly studies of etiology or risk or harm)

(a) Are the results valid?

    (i) With the exception of the presence of the disease under study, were all groups similar to each other at the start of the study?

    (ii) Were all measurements (disease and exposure) made in an objective and reproducible manner and carried out in the same ways in all groups? Was an explicit chart review method used for all patients?

    (iii) Was the risk factor information obtained for all patients who were entered into the study?

(b) What are the results?

    (i) Is there a dose–response gradient between the cause and effect?

    (ii) How strong is the association between cause and effect? (Odds Ratio)

    (iii) What is the variability of this effect? (Confidence Intervals)

(c) Will the results help me in my patient care?

    (i) What is the relative magnitude of the risk in my patient population?

    (ii) Can the results of this study be applied to most of my patients with this or similar problems?

    (iii) Should I encourage the patient to stop the exposure? If yes, how soon?

    Hierarchy of relative study strength

    RCT > Cohort > Case–control > Case series

(4) Studies of diagnosis (commonly cohort or case–control studies)

(a) Are the results valid?

    (i) Were all the patients in the study similar to those patients for whom the test would be used in general medical practice?

    (ii) Was there a reasonable spectrum of disease in the patients in the study?

    (iii) Were the details of the diagnostic test described adequately?

    (iv) Were all diagnostic and outcome measurements made in an objective and reproducible manner and carried out in the same ways in all patients?

    (v) Was both the test under study and a reasonable reference standard used to test all patients?

    (vi) Was the comparison of the test under study to the reference standard done in a blinded manner?

    (vii) Did the results of the test being studied influence the decision to perform the reference standard test?

(b) What are the results?
  (i) How strong is the diagnostic test? (Likelihood Ratios, Sensitivity and Specificity)
  (ii) What is the variability of this result? (Confidence Intervals)
(c) Will the results help me in my patient care?
  (i) Can the test be used in my patient population when considering factors of availability, performance, and cost?
  (ii) Can I determine a reasonable pretest probability of disease in my patients?
  (iii) Will the performance of the test result in significant change in management for my patients?
  (iv) Will my patient be better off as a result of having obtained the test?

Appendix 3   Formulas

Descriptive statistics

Mean: $\mu = (\Sigma x_i)/n$
> where x_i-the numerical value of the i th data point, and n-the total number of data points.

Variance (s^2 or σ^2): $s^2 = (\Sigma(x_i - \mu)^2)/(n-1)$.

Standard deviation (SD, s, or σ): $s = \sqrt{s^2}$

Confidence intervals using the standard error of the mean

95% CI $= \mu \pm Z_{95\%}(\sigma/\sqrt{n})$

$Z_{95\%} = 1.96$(number of standard deviations defining 95% of the data)

SEM $= \sigma/\sqrt{n}$

95% CI $= \mu \pm 1.96$(SEM)

Basic probability

Probability that event a *or* event b will occur: $P(\text{a or b}) = P(\text{a}) + P(\text{b})$

Probability that event a *and* event b will occur: $P(\text{a and b}) = P(\text{a}) \times P(\text{b})$

Probability that *at least one* of several mutually exclusive events will occur $= 1 - P$ (none of the events will occur)
> where P(none of the events will occur) $= P(\text{not a}) \times P(\text{not b}) \times P(\text{not c}) \times \ldots$

Event rates

Control event rate $=$ CER $=$ control patients with outcome/all control patients $=$ A/CE

Experimental event rate $=$ EER $=$ experimental patients with outcome/all experimental patients $=$ C/EE

Relative rate reduction $=$ RRR $=$ (CER $-$ EER)/CER

Absolute rate reduction $=$ ARR $=$ | EER $-$ CER |

Number needed to treat $=$ NNT $=$ 1/ARR

Fig. A.3.1 Event-rate calculations: 2 × 2 table.

	Events of interest	Other events		
Control or placebo group	A	B	CE	Control group events
Experimental group	C	D	EE	Experimental group events

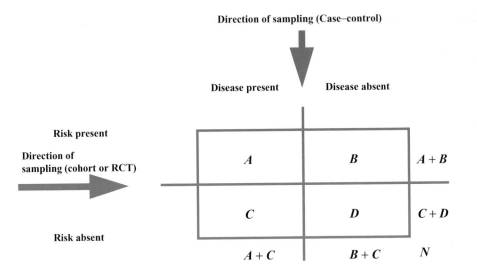

Fig. A.3.2 Relative-risk and odds-ratio calculations: 2 × 2 table.

Relative risk and odds ratio

Absolute risk of disease in risk group $= a/(a+b)$
Absolute risk of disease in no risk group $= c/(c+d)$
Relative risk of disease $=$ RR $= [a/(a+b)]/[c/(c+d)]$
Absolute attributable risk $=$ AAR $= [a/(a+b)] - [c/(c+d)]$
Attributable risk percent $= [a/(a+b) - c/(c+d)]/[a/(a+b)]$
Also called relative attributable risk
Number needed to harm $=$ NNH $= 1/\text{AAR}$
Odds of risk factor if diseased $= a/c$
Odds of risk factor if not diseased $= b/d$
Odds ratio $=$ OR $= [a/c]/[b/d] = ac/bd$

Confidence intervals

For odds ratio: Confidence Interval $=$ CI $= \exp\ln(\text{OR}) \pm 1.96\sqrt{}(1/a + 1/b + 1/c + 1/d)$
For relative risk: Confidence Interval $=$ CI $= \exp\ln(\text{RR}) \pm 1.96\sqrt{}([(1 - (a/(a+b)))/a])$
$+ [(1 - (c/(c+d))/d])$
Let the computer do the calculations!

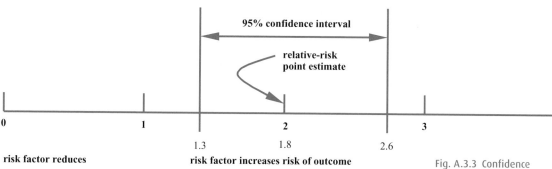

Fig. A.3.3 Confidence interval for relative risk.

		Disease: Present	Disease: Absent	
Test	Positive	TP	FP	T+
Test	Negative	FN	TN	T−
		D+	D−	

Fig. A.3.4 Diagnostic tests: 2 × 2 table.

Diagnostic tests

True positive rate = TPR = TP/D+ = sensitivity
False positive rate = FPR = FP/D− = 1 − specificity
False negative rate = FNR = FN/D+ = 1 − sensitivity
True negative rate = TNR = TN/D− = specificity

Likelihood ratio of a positive test = LR+ = sensitivity/(1 − specificity)
Likelihood ratio of a negative test = LR− = (1 − sensitivity)/specificity

Positive predictive value = PPV = TP/T+
Negative predictive value = NPV = TN/T−
False alarm rate = FAR = 1 − PPV
False reassurance rate = FRR = 1 − NPV

Bayes' theorem

Odds = probability/(1 − probability)
Probability = odds/(1 + odds)
Post-test odds = pretest odds × likelihood ratio (this is PPV if LR+ is used and FRR if LR− is used)

Appendix 4 Commonly used statistical tests

The following is a very simplistic summary of the usual tests used in statistical inference.

Descriptive statistics			
Type of variable	What is being described	Statistic	Graph
Single variable			
Ratio or interval	Central tendency	Mean	Histogram Stem–leaf plot Frequency polygon Box plot
	Dispersion	Standard deviation	
	Deviation from normality	Skew or Kurtosis	
Ranks	Central tendency	Median	Box plot (ordinal) Bar chart
	Dispersion	Range	Interquartile range
Named	Central tendency	Mode	Bar chart (nominal) Dot plot
	Dispersion	Number of categories	
Two variables			
Ratio or interval	Association	Pearson's r	Scatter plot
Nominal or ordinal	Comparison	Kappa, phi, rho Weighted kappa	Paired bar chart Scatter plot

Inferential statistics

Type of dependent variables	Number and type of independent variables	Test
Ratio or interval data		
One or two means	None	t-test or z-test ($n > 100$)
	Continuous	F-test or t-test
	Nominal	t-test
(Multiple regression)	Multiple continuous	F-test
(ANOVA)	Multiple nominal	F-test or Student Newman–Keuls test
(ANCOVA)	Multiple continuous and nominal	F-test
	Association	Pearson's r
	Predicting variable values	Regression
Ordinal data	None	Wilcoxon signed rank test
	Ordinal	Spearman's test
	Nominal	Mann–Whitney test
	Multiple ordinal	χ^2-test
	Multiple nominal	Kruskal–Wallis test
	Association	Spearman's ρ
Nominal data	None (affected by time)	Normal approximation to Poisson
	Nominal (paired)	McNemar's test
	Nominal (unpaired)	χ^2-test, normal approximation, or Mantel–Haenszel test
	Continuous	χ^2-test for trend
	Multiple continuous or nominal	χ^2-test
	Multiple nominal	Mantel–Haenszel test

Multivariate analysis

Multiple linear regression is used when the outcome variable is continuous

Multiple logistic regression is used when the outcome variable is binary event (e.g., alive or dead, disease-free or recurrent disease, etc.)

Discriminate function analysis is used when the outcome variable is categorical (better, worse, or about the same)

Proportional hazards regression (Cox regression) is used when the outcome variable is the time to the occurrence of a binary event (e.g., time to death or tumor recurrence)

Appendix 5　Proof of Bayes' theorem

For a given test with the following parameters:

Sensitivity $=$ N　Specificity $=$ S　Pretest probability (prevalence of disease) $=$ P
the 2×2 table will be as shown in Fig. A.5.1.
Using the sensitivity and specificity:

$$PPV = \frac{NP}{T+} = \frac{NP}{NP + ((1-S)(1-P))}$$

Using Bayes' theorem:

$O(\text{pre}) = P/(1-P)$ and
$O(\text{post}) = O(\text{pre}) \times LR+$
$LR+ = N/(1-S)$
$O(\text{post}) = [P/(1-P)] \times [(N)/(1-S)] = NP/((1-S)(1-P))$

$$P(\text{post}) = O/(1+O) = \frac{NP/((1-S)(1-P))}{1 + (NP/((1-S)(1-P)))}$$

Now multiply top and bottom by $(1-S)(1-P)$:

$$= \frac{NP}{((1-S)(1-P)) + NP} \quad \text{or} \quad \frac{NP}{NP + ((1-S)(1-P))}$$

The same as the PPV.

Similarly:

$$FRR = 1 - NPV = \frac{(1-N)P}{T-} = \frac{P(1-N)}{S(1-P) + P(1-N)}$$

$LR- = (1-N)/S$
$O(\text{post}) = (P/(1-P)) \times ((1-N)/S) = P(1-N)/S(1-P)$

$$P(\text{post}) = \frac{P(1-N)/S(1-P)}{1 + (P(1-N)/S(1-P))}$$

Now multiply top and bottom by $S(1-P)$:

$$P(\text{post}) = \frac{P(1-N)}{S(1-P) + P(1-N)}$$

The same as the FRR.

Fig. A.5.1 Bayes' theorem: 2×2 table.

	D+	D−	
T+	NP	$(1-S)(1-P)$	$NP + (1-S)(1-P)$
T−	$(1-N)P$	$S(1-P)$	$(1-N)P + S(1-P)$
	P	$1-P$	

Appendix 6   Using balance sheets to calculate thresholds

Strep throat

Suppose you are examining a 36-year-old white male with a sore throat and want to know whether treatment for strep throat is a good idea. Exam is equivocal with large tonsils with exudate, but no cervical nodes or scarlatiniform rash, and only slight coryza.[1]

Disease   Strep throat

Prevalence in the literature   About 20% for large tonsils with exudate. If no exudate this drops to about 10%, and if also tender cervical nodes it increases to 40%.

Estimate the treatment threshold.

Potential harm from antibiotic treatment   4–5% of patients will get a rash or diarrhea, both of which are uncomfortable but not life-threatening. Anaphylaxis (life-threatening allergy) is very rare ($< 1 : 200\,000$) and will not be counted in the analysis. Harm $= 0.05$.

Impact of this harm   Discomfort for about 2–3 days, gets about 0.1 on a 0–1 scale. It could be greater if the patient modeled swimwear and a rash would put him or her out of work for those days. Impact $= 0.1$.

Impact of improvement   Since treatment results in relief of symptoms about one day sooner, this should be similar to the harm impact, 0.1 on the 0–1 scale. Impact $= 0.1$. Improvement $= 1$ (100% get better by this 1 day).

Action or treatment threshold   (Harm $\times$ harm impact) / (improvement $\times$ improvement impact) $= (0.1 \times 0.05)/(0.1 \times 1) = 0.05$.

This is the threshold for treatment without testing.

Will a test change your mind if the pretest probability is 20%?

The sensitivity and specificity of throat culture is 0.9 and 0.85 respectively. If you apply these to a pretest probability of 20%, a negative test will result in NPV $= 0.03$ (3%). This is below the action (treatment) threshold (5%) and so treatment would not be initiated if the test were negative. Therefore it pays to do the test.

Tuberculosis

Now let's consider a different problem in an Asian man with lung lesions, fever, and cough, and let's use a slightly different methodology. The differential is between tuberculosis (highly

---

[1] From R. Gross. *Making Medical Decisions*. Philadelphia, PA: American College of Physicians, 1999.

contagious and treated with antibiotics) and sarcoidosis (not contagious and treated with steroids). The initial testing is negative for both. How should the patient be treated while waiting for the results of the culture for TB (gold standard)? Clinical probability of TB estimated at 70% before initial testing, 40% after initial testing (normal angiotensin-converting-enzyme level, negative TB skin test, noncaseating granulomas on biopsy).

> Normal angiotensin-converting-enzyme level: against sarcoidosis but poor sensitivity
> Negative TB skin test: against TB, but can be present in overwhelming TB infection (poor sensitivity)
> Noncaseating granulomas on biopsy: against TB and for sarcoidosis
> Benefit (B) = untreated TB mortality − treated TB mortality = 50% − 20% = 30%
> Risk (R) = death from hepatitis due to treatment = prevalence of hepatitis in Asian men treated with TB medications (2%) × risk for death from hepatitis (7.6%) = 0.15%

Treatment threshold = $1/(B : R + 1)$

$B : R = 30 : 0.15 = 200$

Treatment threshold = $1/201 = 0.005$

> Therefore treat with TB medications since the estimated probability of disease in this patient is 40%, greater than the treatment threshold. If B is very high and R is very low, you will almost always treat regardless of the test result. If the converse (R high and B low) you will be much less likely to treat without fairly high degree of evidence of the target disorder.

Acute myocardial infarction

In this case, you must consider how sure you are of the diagnosis to use the more expensive thrombolytic therapy (t-PA) rather than the cheaper streptokinase (SK).

> $B = 0.01 − 1\%$ (difference between the mortality of AMI with t-PA compared to SK)

> $R = 0.008 − 0.8\%$ (difference between the occurrence of acute cerebral bleed from t-PA over SK)

> Therefore $B : R = 1.2$
> B:R+1 = 2.2 and T = 1/2.2 = 0.45 and you would not initiate thrombolytic therapy unless the probability of thrombotic MI was greater than 45%.

Glossary

2AFC (two-alternative-forced-choice) problem   The probability that one can identify an abnormal patient from a normal patient using this test alone.

Absolute risk   The percentage of subjects in a group that experiences a discrete outcome.

Absolute risk (rate) reduction (ARR)   The difference in rates of outcomes between the control group and the experimental or exposed group. An efficacious therapy serves to reduce that risk. For example, if 15% of the placebo group died and 10% of the treatment group died, ARR or the absolute reduction in the risk of death is 5%.

Accuracy   Closeness of a given observation to the true value of that state.

Adjustment   Changing the probability of disease as a result of performing a diagnostic maneuver (additional history, physical exam, or diagnostic test of some kind).

Algorithm   A preset path which takes the clinician from the patient's presenting complaints to a final management decision through a series of predetermined branching decision points.

All-or-none case series   In previous studies all the patients who were not given the intervention died and now some survive, or many of the patients previously died and now none die.

Alternative hypothesis   There is a difference between groups or an association between predictor and outcome variables. Example: the patients being treated with a newer antihypertensive drug will have a lower blood pressure than those treated with the older drug.

Anchoring   The initial assignment of pretest probability of disease based upon elements of the history and physical.

Applicability   The degree to which the results of a study are likely to hold true in your practice setting. Also called **external validity, generalizability, particularizability, relevance**.

Arm (of decision tree)   A particular diagnostic modality, risk factor, or treatment method.

Assessment   Clinician's inferences on the nature of the patient's problem. Synonymous with differential diagnosis or hypotheses of cause of the underlying problems.

AUC (area under the ROC curve)   Probability that one can identify a diseased patient from a healthy one using this test alone.

Availability heuristic   The ability to think of something depends upon how recently you studied that fact.

Bayes' theorem   What we know after doing a test equals what we knew before doing the test times a modifier (based on the test results). Post-test odds = pretest odds × likelihood ratio.

Bias   Any factor other than the experimental therapy that could change the study results in a non-random way. The direction of bias offset may be unpredictable. The validity of a study is integrally related to the degree to which the results could have been affected by biased factors.

Blinding   Masking or concealment from study subjects, caregivers, observers, or others involved in the study of some or all details of the study. Process by which neither the subject nor the research team members who have contact with the subject know to which treatment condition the subject is assigned. Single-blind means that one person (patient or physician) does not know what is going on. Double-blind means that at least two people (usually patient and treating physician) don't know what's going on. Triple-blind means that patient, treating physician, and person measuring outcome don't know to which group patient is assigned. It can also mean that the paper is written before the results are tabulated. The whole point of blinding is to prevent bias.

Case–control study   Subjects are grouped by outcome, cases (having the disease or outcome of interest) and controls. The presence of the risk factor of interest is then compared in the two groups. These studies are usually retrospective.

Case report or case series   One or a group of cases of a particular disease or outcome of interest with no control group.

Clinical guideline   An algorithm used in making clinical decisions. Also called a *Practice guideline*.

Clinical significance   Results that make enough difference to you and your patient to justify changing your way of doing things. For example, a drug which is found in a megatrial of 50 000 adults with acute asthma to increase FEV1 by only 0.5% ($P < 0.0001$)

would fail this test of significance. The findings must have practical importance as well as statistical importance.

Cochrane collaboration An internationally organized effort to catalog and systematically evaluate all existing clinical studies into systematic reviews easily accessible to practicing clinicians so as to facilitate the process of using the best clinical evidence in patient care.

Cohort study Subjects are grouped by the risk factor, and those with and without the risk factor are followed to see who develops the disease and who doesn't. The occurrence of the outcome of interest is compared in the two groups. These studies can be prospective or retrospective (non-concurrent).

Cointervention A treatment that is not under investigation given to a study patient. Can be a source of bias in the study.

Competing-hypotheses heuristic A way of thinking in which all possible hypotheses are evaluated for their likelihood and final decision is based on the most likely hypothesis modified by secondary evaluations.

Confidence intervals An interval around an observed parameter guaranteed to include the true value to some level of confidence (usually 95%). The true value can be expected to be within that interval with 95% confidence.

Continuous test results A test resulting in an infinite number of possible outcome values.

Control group The subjects in an experiment who do not receive the treatment procedure being studied. They may get nothing, a placebo, or a standard or previously validated therapy.

Controlled clinical trial Any study that compares two groups for exposure to different therapies or risk factors.

Cost-effectiveness Marginal cost divided by marginal benefit. (Cost of treatment A − cost of treatment B)/(benefit of treatment A − benefit of treatment B).

Cost-effectiveness (or cost–benefit) analysis Research study which determines how much more has to be paid in order to achieve a given benefit of preventing death, disability days, or another outcome.

Cost-minimization analysis Analysis in which only costs are compared.

Criterion-based validity How well a measurement agrees with other approaches for measuring the same characteristic.

Critical appraisal The process of assessing and interpreting evidence systematically, considering its validity, results, and relevance.

Critical value   Value of a test statistic to which the observed value is compared to determine statistical significance. The observed test statistic indicates significant differences or associations exist if its value is greater than the critical value.

Critically appraised topic (CAT)   A summary of a search and critical appraisal of the literature related to a focused clinical question. Catalogue of these kept in an easily accessible place (e.g., online) can be used to help make real-time clinical decisions.

Decision analysis   Systematic way in which the components of decision making can be incorporated to make the best possible clinical decision using a mathematical model. Also known as *Expected values decision making.*

Decision node   A point on a branching decision tree at which the clinician must make a decision to either perform a clinical maneuver (diagnosis or management) or not.

Degrees of freedom (df)   A number used to select the appropriate critical value of a statistic from a table of critical values.

Dependent variable   The outcome variable that is influenced by changes in the independent variable of a study.

Descriptive research   Study which summarizes, tabulates, or organizes a set of measures (i.e., answers the questions who, what, when, where, and how).

Descriptive statistics   The branch of statistics that summarizes, tabulates, and organizes data for the purpose of describing observations or measurements.

Diagnostic test characteristics   Those qualities of a diagnostic test that are important to understand how valuable it would be in a clinical setting. These include sensitivity, specificity, accuracy, precision, and reliability.

Diagnostic tests   Modalities which can be used to increase the accuracy of a clinical assessment by helping to narrow the list of possible diseases that a patient can have.

Dichotomous outcome   Any outcome measure for which there are only two possibilities, like dead/alive, admitted/discharged, graduated/sent to glue factory. Beware of potentially fake dichotomous outcome reports such as "improved/not improved", particularly when derived from continuous outcome measures. For example, if I define a 10-point or greater increase in a continuous variable as "improved", I may show what looks like a tremendous benefit when that result is clinically insignificant. This is lesson 2a in "How to lie with statistics."

Dichotomous test results   Only two possible outcome values, yes or no, positive or negative, alive or dead, etc.

Differential diagnosis   A list of possible diseases that your patient can have in descending order of clinical probability.

Effect size The amount of change measured in a given variable as a result of the experiment. In meta-analyses when different studies have measured somewhat different things, a statistically derived generic size of the combined result.

Effectiveness How well the proposed intervention works in a clinical trial to produce a desired and measurable effect in a well-done clinical trial. These results may not be duplicated in "real life."

Efficacy How well the proposed intervention actually works in practice to produce a desired outcome in other more generalized clinical situations. This is usually the desired outcome for the patient and society.

Event rate The percentage of events of interest in one or the other of the groups in an experiment. These rates are compared to calculate number needed to treat. This is also a term for absolute risk.

Expected values (E) Probability $\times$ Utility ($P \times U$). The value of each arm of the decision tree or the entire decision tree (sum of $P \times U$).

Expected-values decision making See *Decision analysis*.

Experimental group(s) The subjects in an experiment who receive the treatment procedure or manipulation that is being proposed to improve health or treat illness.

Explanatory research – experimental Study in which the independent variable (usually a treatment) is changed by the researcher who then observes the effect of this change on the dependent variable (usually an outcome). The key here is the willful manipulation of the two variables.

Explanatory research – observational Study looking for possible causes of disease (dependent variable) based upon exposure to one or more risk factors (independent variable) in the population.

Exposure Any type of contact with a substance that causes an outcome. A drug, a surgical procedure, risk factor, even a diagnostic test can be an exposure. In therapy, prognosis, or harm studies the "exposure" is the intervention being studied.

External validity See *Applicability*.

False negative (FN) Patients with disease who have a normal or negative test.

False positive (FP) Patients without disease who have an abnormal or positive test.

FAR (false alarm rate) Percentage of patients with a positive test who don't have disease and will be unnecessarily tested or treated based on the incorrect results of a test.

Filter   A process by which patients are entered into or excluded from a study. Inclusion and exclusion criteria when stated explicitly.

FNR (false negative rate)   One minus the sensitivity (1 − sens). Percentage of diseased patients with a negative or normal test.

FPR (false positive rate)   One minus the specificity (1 − spec). Percentage of non-diseased patients with a positive or abnormal test.

Framing effect   How a question is worded (or framed) will influence the answer to the question.

FRR (False reassurance rate)   Percentage of patients with a negative or normal test result who actually have disease and will lose benefits of treatment for the disease.

Functional status   An outcome which describes the ability of a person to interact in society and carry on with their daily living activities (e.g., Activities of Daily Living (ADL) or the Arthritis Activity Scale used in Rheumatoid Arthritis).

Gaussian   Typical bell-shaped frequency curve in which normal test values are 95% (± 2SD of all tests done) of all possible values.

Generalizability   See *Applicability*.

Gold standard   The reference standard for evaluation of a measurement or diagnostic test. The "gold-standard" test is assumed to correctly identify the presence or absence of disease 100% of the time.

Harm vs. benefit   An accounting of the positive and negative aspects of an exposure (positive or negative) on the outcomes of a study.

Heuristics   Models for the way people think.

Homogeneity   Whether the results from a set of independently performed studies on a particular question are similar enough to make statistical pooling valid.

Hypothesis   An educated guess on the nature of the patient's illness, usually obtained by selecting those diseases having the same history or physical examination characteristics as the patient.

Hypothetico-deductive strategy   A diagnosis is made by advancing a hypothesis and then deducing the correctness or incorrectness of that hypothesis through the use of statistical methods, specifically the characteristics of diagnostic tests.

Incidence   The rate at which an event occurs in a defined population over time. The number of new cases (or other events of interest) divided by the total population at risk.

Incorporation bias   The test being measured is part of the gold standard or inclusion criteria for entry into a study.

Incremental gain   Amount of increase in diagnostic certainty. The change in the pretest probability of a diagnosis as a result of performing a diagnostic test.

Independent variable(s)   The treatment or exposure variable that is presumed to cause some effect on the outcome or dependent variable.

Inferential statistics   Drawing conclusions about a population based on findings from a sample.

Instrumental rationality   Calculation of a treatment strategy which will produce the greatest benefit for the patient.

Instrumentation   The process of selecting or developing measuring devices.

Instruments (measuring devices)   Something that makes a measurement, e.g., thermometer, sphygmomanometer (blood pressure cuff and manometer), questionnaire, etc.

Intention-to-treat   Patients assigned to a particular treatment group by the study protocol are retained in that group for the purpose of analysis of the study results no matter what happens.

Internal validity   See *Validity*.

Inter-observer reliability   Consistency between two different observers' measurements.

Interval likelihood ratios (iLR)   Probability of a test result in the interval among diseased subjects, divided by the probability of a test result within the interval among non-diseased subjects.

Intra-observer reliability   Ability of the same observer to reproduce a measure.

Intrinsic characteristics of a diagnostic test   See *Diagnostic test characteristics*.

Justice   Equal access to medical care for all patients who require it based only upon the severity of their disease.

Kappa statistic   A measure of inter- or intra-observer reliability.

Level of significance (confidence level)   Describes the probability of incorrectly rejecting the null hypothesis and concluding that there is a difference when in fact none exists (i.e., probability of Type I error). Many times this probability is 0.01, 0.05, or 0.10. For medical studies it is most commonly set at 0.05.

Likelihood ratio of a negative test (LR−)　The false negative rate divided by the true negative rate. The amount by which the pretest probability of disease is reduced in patients with a negative test.

Likelihood ratio of a positive test (LR+)　The true positive rate divided by the false positive rate. The amount by which the pretest probability is increased in patients with a positive test.

Likelihood ratio　A single number which summarizes test sensitivity and specificity and modifies the pretest probability of disease to give a post-test probability.

Linear rating scale　A scale from zero to one on which patients can place a mark to determine their value for a particular outcome.

Markov models　A method of decision analysis that considers all possible health states and their interactions at the same time.

Matching　An attempt in an experiment to create equivalence between the control and treatment groups. Control subjects are matched with experimental subjects based upon one or more variables.

Mean　A measure of central tendency; the arithmetic average.

Measurement　The application of an instrument or method to collect data systematically. What the use of the instrument tells us, e.g., temperature, blood pressure, results of dietary survey, etc.

Meta-analysis　A systematic review of a focused clinical question following rigorous methodological criteria and employing statistical techniques to combine data from multiple independently performed studies on that question.

Multiple-branching strategy　An algorithmic method used for making diagnoses.

N or *n*　Number of subjects in the sample or the number of observations made in a study.

Negative predictive value (NPV)　Probability of no disease after a negative test result.

Nodes　Junctures where something happens. The common ones are decision and probability nodes.

Normal　(1) A normal distribution or Gaussian distribution of variables, the bell-shaped curve. (2) A value of a diagnostic test which defines patients who are not diseased.

Null hypothesis　The assumption that there is no difference between groups or no association between predictor and outcome variables.

Number needed to follow (NNF) Number of patients who must be followed before one additional bad outcome is noted. The lower this number, the worse the risk factor.

Number needed to harm (NNH) Number of patients who must be treated or exposed to a risk factor to have one additional bad outcome. The lower this number the worse the exposure.

Number needed to treat (NNT) Number of patients who must be treated to have one additional successful outcome. The lower that number, the better the therapy.

Objective Information observed by the physician from the patient examination and diagnostic tests.

Observational study Any study of therapy, prevention, or harm in which the exposure is not assigned to the individual subject by the investigator(s). A synonym is "non-experimental" and examples are case–control and cohort studies.

Odds The number of times an event occurred divided by the number of times it didn't.

Odds ratio The ratio of the odds of an event in one group divided by the odds in another group.

One-tailed statistical test Used when the alternative hypothesis is directional (i.e., specifies a particular direction of the difference between the groups.)

Operator-dependent The results of a test are dependent on the skill of the person performing the test.

Outcome Disease or final state of patient (e.g., alive or dead).

Outcomes study The outcome of an intervention, exposure, or diagnosis measured over a period of time.

***P* value** The probability that the difference(s) observed between two or more groups in a study occurred by chance if there really was no difference between the groups.

Pathognomonic The presence of signs or symptoms of disease which can lead to only one diagnosis (i.e. they are only characteristic of that one disease).

Patient satisfaction A rating scale which measures the degree to which patients are happy with the care they received or feel that the care was appropriate.

Patient values A number, generally from 0 (usually death) to 1 (usually complete recovery), which denotes the degree to which a patient is desirous of a particular outcome.

Pattern recognition Recognizing a disease diagnosis based on a pattern of signs and symptoms.

Percentiles Cutoffs between positive and negative past result chosen within preset percentiles of the patients tested.

Placebo An inert substance given to a study subject who has been assigned to the control group to make them think they are getting the treatment under study.

Plan What treatment or further diagnostic testing is required.

Point On a decision tree, the outcome of possible decisions made by the patient and clinician.

Point estimate The exact result that has been observed in a study. The confidence interval tells you the range within which the true value of the result is likely to lie with 95% confidence.

Point of indifference The probability of an outcome of certain death at which a patient no longer can decide between that outcome and an uncertain outcome of partial disability.

Population The group of people who meet the criteria for entry into a study (whether they actually participated in the study or not). The group of people to whom the study results can be generalized.

Positive predictive value Probability of disease after the occurrence of a positive test result.

Post-test odds The odds of disease after a test has been done. Post-test odds = pretest odds × likelihood ratio.

Post-test probability The probability of disease after a test has been performed. This is calculated from post-test odds converted to probability. Also called *posterior* or *a-posteriori probability.*

Power The probability that an experimental study will correctly observe a statistically significant difference between the study groups when that difference actually exists.

Precision The measurement is nearly the same value each time it is measured. Measure of random variation or error, or a small standard deviation of the measurement across multiple measurements.

Predictive values The probability that a patient with a particular outcome on a diagnostic test (positive or negative) has or does not have the disease.

Predictor variable The variable that is going to predict the presence or absence of disease, or results of a test.

Pretest odds   The odds of disease before a test is run.

Pretest probability   The probability of disease before a test is run. This is converted to odds for use with Bayes' theorem. Also called *prior* or *a-priori probability*.

Prevalence   The proportion of people in a defined group who have a disease, condition, or injury. The numbers affected by a condition divided by the population at risk. In the context of diagnosis, this is also called "pretest probability."

Probability node   A point in the decision tree at which two or more events occur by chance.

Problem-oriented medical record (POMR)   A format of keeping medical records by which one keeps track of and updates a patient's problems regularly.

Prognosis   The possible outcomes for a given disease and the length of time to those outcomes.

Prospective study   Any study done forwards in time. Important in studies on therapy, prognosis, or harm, where retrospective studies make hidden biases more likely.

Publication bias   The possibility that studies with conflicting results (most often negative studies) are less likely to be published.

Quality of life   A composite measure of the satisfaction of a patient with their life and their ability to function appropriately.

Quality-adjusted life years (QALYs)   Standardized measure of quality and life expectancy commonly used in decision analyses. Life expectancy times expected value or utility.

Random selection or assignment   Selection process of a sample of the population such that every subject in the population has an equal chance of being selected for each arm of the study.

Randomization   A technique that gives every patient an equal chance of winding up in any particular arm of a controlled clinical trial.

Randomized clinical trial or Randomized controlled trial (RCT)   An interventional study in which the patients are randomly selected or assigned either to a group which gets the intervention or to a control group.

Receiver operating characteristic (ROC) curve   A plot of sensitivity versus one minus specificity (true-positive rate versus false-positive rate) can give the quality of a diagnostic test and determine which is the best cutoff point.

Referral bias   Patients entered into a study because they have been referred for a particular test or to a specialty provider.

Relative risk   The probability of outcome in the group with exposure divided by the probability of outcome in the group without the opposite exposure.

Reliability   Loose synonym of precision, or the extent to which repeated measurements of the same phenomenon are consistent, reproducible, and dependable.

Representativeness heuristic   The ease with which a diagnosis is recalled depends on how closely the patient presentation fits the classical presentation of the disease.

Research question (hypothesis)   A question stating a general prediction of results which the researcher attempts to answer by conducting a study.

Retrospective study   Any study in which the outcomes have already occurred before the study and collection of data has begun.

Risk   Probability of an adverse event divided by all of the times one is exposed to that event.

Risk factor   Any aspect of an individual's life, behavior, or inheritance that could affect (increase or decrease) the likelihood of an outcome (disease, condition, or injury.)

Rule in   To effectively determine that a particular diagnosis is correct by either excluding all other diagnoses or making the probability of that diagnosis so high that other diagnoses are effectively excluded.

Rule out   To effectively exclude a diagnosis by making the probability of that disease so low that it effectively is so unlikely to occur or would be considered non-existent.

Sample   That part of the population selected to be studied. The group specifically included in the actual study.

Sampling bias   To select patients for study based on some criteria that could relate to the outcome.

Screening   Looking for disease among asymptomatic patients.

Sensitivity   The ability of a test to identify patients who have disease. True-positive rate.

Sensitivity analysis   An analytical procedure to determine how the results of a study would change if the input variables are changed.

Setting   The place in which the testing for a disease occurs, usually referring to level of care.

SOAP notes Subjective, objective, assessment, and plan. The typical format for problem-oriented medical record notes.

Specificity The ability of a test to identify patients without the disease when it is negative. True-negative rate.

Spectrum In a diagnostic study, the range of clinical presentations and relevant disease advancement exhibited by the subjects included in the study.

Spectrum bias The sensitivity of a test is higher in more severe or "well-developed" cases of a disease, and lower when patients present earlier in the course of disease, or when the disease is occult.

Standard gamble A technique to determine patient values by which patients are given a choice between a known outcome and a hypothetical-probabilistic outcome.

Statistic A number that describes some characteristic of a set of data.

Statistical power See *Power*.

Statistical significance A measure of how confidently an observed difference between two or more groups can be attributed to the study interventions rather than chance alone.

Stratified randomization A way of ensuring that the different groups in an experimental trial are balanced with respect to some important factors that could affect the outcome.

Strategy of exhaustion Listing all possible diseases which a patient could have and running every diagnostic test available and necessary to exclude all diseases on that list until only one is left.

Subjective Information from the patient, the history which the patient gives you and which they are experiencing.

Surrogate marker An outcome variable that is associated with the outcome of interest, but changes in this marker are not necessarily a direct measure of changes in the clinical outcome of interest.

Survival analysis A mathematical analysis of outcome after some kind of therapy in which patients are followed for given a period of time to determine what percentage are still alive or disease-free after that time.

Systematic review A formal review of a focused clinical question based on a comprehensive search strategy and structured critical appraisal of all relevant studies.

Testing threshold Probability of disease above which we should test before initiating treatment for that disease, and below which we should neither treat nor test.

Threshold approach to decision making   Determining values of pretest probability below which neither testing nor treatment should be done and above which treatment should be begun without further testing.

Time trade-off   A method of determining patient utility using a simple question of how much time in perfect health a patient would trade for a given amount of time in imperfect health.

Treatment threshold   Probability of disease above which we should initiate treatment without first doing the test for the disease.

Triggering   A thought process which is initiated by recognition of a set of signs and symptoms leading the clinician to think of a particular disease.

Two-tailed statistical test   Used when alternative hypothesis is non-directional and there is no specification of the direction of differences between the groups.

Type I error   Error made by rejecting the null hypothesis when it is true and accepting the alternative hypothesis when it isn't true.

Type II error   Error made by not rejecting the null hypothesis when it is false and the alternative hypothesis is true.

Unadjusted life expectancy (life years)   The number of years a person is expected to live based solely on their age at the time. Adjusting would consider lifestyle factors such as smoking, risk-taking, cholesterol, weight, etc.

Uncertainty   The inability to determine precisely what an outcome would be for a disease or diagnostic test.

Utility   The measure of value of an outcome. Also whether a patient is truly better off as a result of a diagnostic test.

Validity   (1) The degree to which the results of a study are likely to be true, believable and free of bias. (2) The degree to which a measurement represents the phenomenon of interest.

Variable   Something that can take on different values such as a diagnostic test, risk factor, treatment, outcome, or characteristic of a group.

Variance   A measure of the spread of values around the mean.

Bibliography

Common medical journals

The following are the major peer-reviewed medical journals grouped by specialty. This is only a partial list. Many other peer-reviewed journals exist in all specialties.

General
New England Journal of Medicine
JAMA (Journal of the American Medical Association)
BMJ (British Medical Journal)
Lancet
Postgraduate Medicine

Emergency Medicine
Annals of Emergency Medicine
American Journal of Emergency Medicine
Journal of Emergency Medicine
Academic Emergency Medicine

Family Practice
Family Physician
Journal of Family Practice
Journal of the American Board of Family Practice
Archives of Family Practice

Internal Medicine
Annals of Internal Medicine
Journal of General Internal Medicine
Archives of Internal Medicine
American Journal of Medicine

Internal Medicine Specialties
American Journal of Cardiology
Circulation
Thorax
Annual Review of Respiratory Diseases
Gut
Gastroenterology
Nephron
Blood

Medical Education
Academic Medicine
Medical Teacher

Neurology and Neurosurgery
Annals of Neurology
Neurology
Stroke
Journal of Neurosurgery
Neurosurgery

Obstetrics and Gynecology
Obstetrics and Gynecology
American Journal of Obstetrics and Gynecology

Pediatrics
Pediatrics
Journal of Pediatrics
American Journal of Diseases of Children

Psychiatry
American Journal of Psychiatry
Journal of Clinical Psychiatry

Radiology
AJR (American Journal of Roentgenology)

Surgery
Annals of Surgery
American Journal of Surgery
Archives of Surgery
American Surgeon
Journal of the American College of Surgeons

Common non-peer-reviewed journals (also known as "throw-aways")
Hospital Physician
Resident and Physician

Books

American National Standards Institute. *American National Standard for the Preparation of Scientific Papers for Written or Oral Presentation.* ANSI Z39.16. Washington, DC: American National Standards Institute, 1972.

Bernstein, P. L. *Against the Gods: the Remarkable Story of Risk.* New York, NY: Wiley, 1998.

Bradford Hill, A. *A Short Textbook of Medical Statistics.* Oxford: Oxford University Press, 1977.

Cochrane, A. L. *Effectiveness & Efficiency: Random Reflections on Health Services.* London: Royal Society of Medicine, 1971.

Cohen, J. *Statistical Power Analysis for the Behavioral Sciences.* 2nd edn. Orlando, FL: Academic Press, 1988.

Dawes, M., Davies, P., Gray, A., Mant, J., Seers, K. & Snowball, R. *Evidence-Based Practice: a Primer for Health Care Professionals.* Edinburgh: Churchill Livingstone, 1999.

Dixon, R. A., Munro, J. F. & Silcocks, P. B. *The Evidence Based Medicine Workbook: Critical Appraisal for Clinical Problem Solving.* Oxford: Oxford University Press, 1997.

Ebell, M. R. *Evidence-Based Diagnosis: a Handbook of Clinical Prediction Rules.* Berlin: Springer, 2001.

Eddy, D. *Clinical Decision Making.* Sudbury, MA: Jones & Bartlett, 1996.

Fletcher, R. H., Fletcher, S. W. & Wagner, E. H. *Clinical Epidemiology: the Essentials.* Baltimore, MD: Williams & Wilkins, 1995.

Friedland, D. J., Go, A. S., Davoren, J. B., Shlipak, M. G., Bent, S. W., Subak, L. L. & Mendelson, T. *Evidence-Based Medicine: A Framework for Clinical Practice.* Stamford, CT: Appleton & Lange, 1998.

Gelbach, S. H. *Interpreting the Medical Literature.* New York, NY: McGraw-Hill, 1993.

Geyman, J. P., Deyo, R. A. & Ramsey, S. D. *Evidence-Based Clinical Practice: Concepts and Approaches.* Boston, MA: Butterworth Heinemann, 1999.

Glasziou, P., Irwig L., Bain, C. & Colditz, G. *Systematic Reviews in Health Care: a Practical Guide.* Cambridge: Cambridge University Press 2001.

Gray, J. A. M. *Evidence-Based Healthcare: How to Make Health Policy and Management Decisions.* Philadelphia, PA: Saunders, 2001.

Gross, R. *Making Medical Decisions: an Approach to Clinical Decision Making for Practicing Physicians.* Philadelphia, PA: American College of Physicians, 1999.

Decisions and Evidence in Medical Practice: Applying Evidence-Based Medicine to Clinical Decision Making. St Louis, MO: Mosby, 2001.

Guyatt, G. & Rennie, D. (eds.). *Users' Guides to the Medical Literature: a Manual for Evidence-Based Clinical Practice.* Chicago: AMA, 2002.

Hulley, S. B. & Cummings, S. R. *Designing Clinical Research.* Baltimore, MD: Williams & Wilkins, 1988.

Matthews, J. R. *Quantification and the Quest for Medical Certainty.* Princeton, NJ: Princeton University Press, 1995.

McDowell, J. E. & Newell, C. *Measuring Health: a Guide to Rating Scales and Questionnaires.* New York, NY: Oxford University Press, 1987.

McGee, S. R. *Evidence-Based Physical Diagnosis.* Philadelphia, PA: Saunders, 2001.

Norman, G. & Streiner, D. *Biostatistics: the Bare Essentials.* St Louis, MO: Mosby, 1994.

Riegelman, R. K., Hirsch, D. S. *Studying a Study and Testing a Test. How to Read the Medical Literature.* 4th edn. Boston, MA: Little Brown, 2000.

Sackett, D. L., Haynes, R. B., Guyatt, G. H. & Tugwell, P. *Clinical Epidemiology: a Basic Science for Clinical Medicine.* 2nd edn. Boston, MA: Little Brown, 1991.

Sackett, D. L., Straus, S. E., Richardson, W. S., Rosenberg, W. & Haynes, R. B. *Evidence Based Medicine: How to Practice and Teach EBM.* 2nd edn. London: Churchill Livingstone, 2000.

Sox, H. C., Blatt, M. A., Higgins, M. C. & Marton, K. I. *Medical Decision Making.* Boston, MA: Butterworth Heinemann, 1988.

Spencer, J. W. & Jacobs, J. *Complementary and Alternative Medicine: an Evidence-Based Approach.* St Louis, MO: Mosby, 2003.

Straus, S. E. I-Hong Hsu, S., Ball, C. M. & Phillips, R. S. *Evidence-Based Acute Medicine.* Edinburgh: Churchill Livingstone, 2001.

Tufte, E. R. *The Visual Display of Quantitative Data.* Cheshire, CT: Graphics Press, 1983.

Velleman, P. *ActivStats.* Reading, MA: Addison-Wesley, 1999.

Wulff, H. R. & Gotzsche, P. C. *Rational Diagnosis and Treatment: Evidence-Based Clinical Decision-Making.* 3rd edn. London: Blackwell, 2000.

Journal articles

General

Ad Hoc Working Group for Critical Appraisal of the Medical Literature. A proposal for more informative abstracts of clinical articles. *Ann. Intern. Med.* 1987; 106: 598–604.

Bradford Hill, A. Statistics in the medical curriculum? *Br. Med. J.* 1947; ii: 366.

Cuddy, P. G., Elenbaas, R. M. & Elenbaas, J. K. Evaluating the medical literature. Part I: abstract, introduction, methods. *Ann. Emerg. Med.* 1983; 12: 549–555.

Day, R. A. The origins of the scientific paper: the IMRAD format. *AMWA J.* 1989; 4: 16–18.

Department of Clinical Epidemiology and Biostatistics, McMaster University Health Sciences Centre. How to read clinical journals. I: why read them and how to start reading them critically. *Can. Med. Assoc. J.* 1981; 124: 555–558.

How to read clinical journals. V: to distinguish useful from useless or even harmful therapy. *Can. Med. Assoc. J.* 1981; 124: 1156–1162.

Diamond, G. A. & Forrester, J. S. Clinical trials and statistical verdicts: probable grounds for appeal. *Ann. Intern. Med.* 1983; 98: 385–394.

Elenbaas, J. K., Cuddy, P. G. & Elenbaas, R. M. Evaluating the medical literature. Part II: statistical analysis. *Ann. Emerg. Med.* 1983; 12: 610–620.

Elenbaas, R. M., Cuddy, P. G., & Elenbaas, J. K. Evaluating the Medical Literature. Part III: results and discussion. *Ann. Emerg. Med.* 1983; 12: 679–686.

Ernst, E. Evidence based complementary medicine: a contradiction in terms? *Ann. Rheum. Dis.* 1999; 58: 69–70.

Greenhalgh, T. How to read a paper: the Medline database. *BMJ* 1997; 315: 180–183.

Haynes, B., Glasziou, P. & Straus, S. Advances in evidence-based information resources for clinical practice. *ACP J. Club* 2000; 132: A11–A14.

Haynes, R. B., Mulrow, C. D., Huth, E. J., Altman, D. G. & Gardner, M. J. More informative abstracts revisited. *Ann. Intern. Med.* 1990; 113: 69–76.

Haynes, R. B., Wilczynski, N., McKibbon, K. A., Walker, C. J. & Sinclair, J. C. Developing optimal search strategies for detecting clinically sound studies in MEDLINE. *J. Am. Med. Inform. Assoc.* 1994; 1: 447–458.

Isaacs, D. & Fitzgerald, D. Seven alternatives to evidence based medicine. *BMJ* 1999; 319: 1618.

Mulrow, C. D., Thacker S. B. & Pugh J. A. A proposal for more informative abstracts of review articles. *Ann. Intern. Med.* 1987; 108: 613–615.

Rennie, D. & Glass, R. M. Structuring abstracts to make them more informative. *JAMA* 1991; 266: 116–117.

Sackett, D. L. & Straus, S. E. Finding and applying evidence during clinical rounds: the "evidence cart". *JAMA* 1998; 280: 1336–1338.

Taddio, A., Pain, T., Fassos, F. F., Boon, H., Ilersich, A. L. & Einarson, T. R. Quality of non-structured and structured abstracts of original research articles in the British Medical Journal, the Canadian Medical Association Journal, and the Journal of the American Medical Association. *Can. Med. Assoc. J.* 1994; 150: 1611–1615.

Taplin, S., Galvin, M.S., Payne, T., Coole, D. & Wagner, E. Putting population based care into practice: real option or rhetoric? *J. Am. Board Fam. Pract.* 1998; 11: 116–126.

Woolf, S. H. The need for perspective in evidence based medicine. *JAMA* 1999; 282: 2358–2365.

Cause and effect

Department of Clinical Epidemiology and Biostatistics, McMaster University Health Sciences Centre. How to read clinical journals. IV: to determine etiology or causation. *Can. Med. Assoc. J.* 1981; 124: 985–990.

Evans, A. S. Causation and disease: a chronological journey. *Am. J. Epidemiol.* 1978; 108: 249–258.

Weiss, N. S. Inferring causal relationships: elaboration of the criterion of "dose–response." *Am. J. Epidemiol.* 1981; 113: 487–490.

Study design

Bogardus, S. T., Concato, J. & Feinstein, A. R. Clinical epidemiological quality in molecular genetic research: the need for methodological standards. *JAMA* 1999; 281: 1919.

Burkett, G. Classifying basic research designs. *Fam. Med.* 1990; 22: 143–148.

Gilbert, E. H., Lowenstein, S. R., Koziol-McLain, J., Barta, D. C. & Steiner, J. Chart reviews in emergency medicine research: where are the methods? *Ann. Emerg. Med.* 1996; 27: 305–308.

Hayden, G. F., Kramer, M. S., & Horwitz, R. I. The case-controlled study: a practical review for the clinician. *JAMA* 1982; 247: 326–329.

Lavori, P. W., Louis, T. A., Bailar, J. C. & Polansky, M. Designs for experiments: parallel comparisons of treatment. *N. Engl. J. Med.* 1983; 309: 1291–1298.

Mantel, N., & Haenszel, W. Statistical aspects of the analysis of data from retrospective studies of disease. *J. Natl. Cancer Inst.* 1959; 22: 719–748.

Measurement

Department of Clinical Epidemiology and Biostatistics, McMaster University Health Sciences Centre. Clinical disagreement. I: how often it occurs and why. *Can. Med. Assoc. J.* 1980; 123: 499–504.

Clinical disagreement. II: how to avoid it and how to learn from one's mistakes. *Can. Med. Assoc. J.* 1980; 123: 613–617.

Bias

Crosskerry, P. Achieving quality in clinical decision making: cognitive strategies and the detection of bias. *Acad. Emerg. Med.* 2002; 9: 1184.

Feinstein, A. R., Sosin, D. M. & Wells, C. K. The Will Roger phenomenon: stage migration and new diagnostic techniques as a source of misleading statistics for survival in cancer. *N. Engl. J. Med.* 1985; 312: 1604–1608.

Sackett, D. L. Bias in analytic research. *J. Chronic Dis.* 1979; 32: 51–63.

Sackett, D. L. & Gent, M. Controversy in counting and attributing events in clinical trials. *N. Engl. J. Med.* 1979; 301: 1410–1412.

Schulz, K. F., Chalmers, I., Hayes, R. J. & Altman, D. G. Empirical evidence of bias: dimensions of methodological quality associated with estimates of treatments effects in controlled trials. *JAMA* 1995; 273: 408–412.

General biostatistics

Berwick, D. M. Experimental power: the other side of the coin. *Pediatrics* 1980; 65: 1043–1045.

Moses, L. Statistical concepts fundamental to investigations. *N. Engl. J. Med.* 1985; 312: 890–897.

Streiner, D. L. Maintaining standards: differences between the standard deviation and standard error, and when to use each. *Can. J. Psychiatry* 1996; 41: 498–502.

Type I and II errors

Cook, R. J. & Sackett, D. L. The number needed to treat: a clinically useful measure of treatment effect. *BMJ* 1995; 310: 452–454.

Cordell, W. H. Number needed to treat (NNT). *Acad. Emerg. Med.* 1999; 33: 433–436.

Freiman, J. A., Chalmers, T. C., Smith, H. Jr. & Kuebler, R. R. The importance of beta, the Type II error and sample size in the design and interpretation of the randomized clinical trial: survey of 71 "negative" trials. *N. Engl. J. Med.* 1978; 299: 690–694.

Todd, K. H. & Funk, J. P. The minimum clinically important difference in physician-assigned visual analog pain scores. *Acad. Emerg. Med.* 1996; 3: 142–146.

Todd, K. H., Funk, K. G., Funk, J. P. & Bonacci, R. Clinical significance of reported changes in pain severity. *Ann. Emerg. Med.* 1996; 27: 485–489.

Young, M., Bresnitz, E. A. & Strom, B. L. Sample size nomograms for interpreting negative clinical studies. *Ann. Intern. Med.* 1983; 99: 248–251.

Risk

Concato, J., Freinstein, A. R. & Halford, T. S. The risk of determining risk with multivariate analysis. *Ann. Intern. Med.* 1993; 118: 200–210.

Hanley, J. A. & Lippman-Hand, A. If nothing goes wrong, is everything all right? *JAMA* 1983; 249: 1743–1745.

Schulman, K. A., Berlin, J. A., Harless, W., Kerner, J. F., Sistrunk, S., Gersh, B. J., Dube, R., Taleghani, C. K., Burke, J. E., Williams, S., Eisenberg, J. M. & Escarce, J. J. The effect of race and sex on physicians' recommendations for cardiac catheterization. *N. Engl. J. Med.* 1999; 340: 618–626.

Schwartz, L. M., Woloshin, S. & Welch, H. G. Misunderstandings about the effects of race and sex on physicians' referrals for cardiac catheterization. (Sounding Board.) *N. Engl. J. Med.* 1999; 341: 279–283.

Clinical trials

Bailar, J. C., Louis, T. A., Lavori, P. W. & Polansky, M. Studies without internal controls. *N. Engl. J. Med.* 1984; 311: 156–162.

Elwood, J. M. Interpreting clinical trial results: seven steps to understanding. *Can. Med. Assoc. J.* 1980; 123: 343–345.

Ernst, E. & Resch, K. L. Concept of true and perceived placebo effects. *BMJ* 1995; 311: 551–553.

Ernst, E. & White A. R. Acupuncture for back pain. A meta-analysis of randomized controlled trials. *Arch. Intern. Med.* 1998; 158: 2235–2241.

Hrobjartsson, A. & Gotzsche, P. C. Is the placebo powerless? An analysis of clinical trials comparing placebo with no treatment. *N. Engl. J. Med.* 2001; 344: 1594–1602.

Louis, T. A., Lavori, P. W., Bailar, J. C. & Polancky, M. Crossover and self-controlled designs in clinical research. *N. Engl. J. Med.* 1984; 310: 24–31.

Standards of Reporting Trials Group. A proposal for structured reporting of randomized controlled trials. *JAMA* 272 (1994):1926–1931. Correction: *JAMA* 273 (1995):776.

Working Group on Recommendations for Reporting Clinical Trials in the Biomedical Literature. Call for comments on a proposal to improve reporting of clinical trials in the biomedical literature: position paper. *Ann. Intern. Med.* 1994; 121: 894–895.

Diagnostic tests

Mower WR. Evaluating bias and variability in diagnostic test reports. *Ann. Emerg. Med.* 1999; 33: 85–91.

Patterson, R. A. & Horowitz, S. F. Importance of epidemiology and biostatistics in deciding clinical strategies for using diagnostic tests: a simplified approach using examples from coronary artery disease. *J. Am. Coll. Cardiol.* 1989; 13: 1653.

Miscellaneous

Department of Clinical Epidemiology and Biostatistics, McMaster University Health Sciences Centre. How to read clinical journals. III: to learn clinical course and prognosis of disease. *Can. Med. Assoc. J.* 1981; 124: 869–872.

L'Abbé, K. A., Detsky, A. S. & O'Rourke, K. Meta analysis in clinical research. *Ann. Intern. Med.* 1987; 107: 224–233.

Olson, C. M. Consensus statements: applying structure. *JAMA* 1995; 273: 72–73.

Sonnenberg, F. A. & Beck, J. R. Markov models in medical decision making: a practical guide. *Med. Decis. Making* 1993; 13: 322.

Wasson, J. H., Sox, H., Neff, R. & Goldman, L. Clinical prediction rules: application and methodological rules. *N. Engl. J. Med.* 1985; 313: 793–799.

Users' guides to the medical literature

Barratt, A., Irwig, L., Glasziou, P., Cumming, R. G., Raffle, A., Hicks, N., Gray, J. A. & Guyatt, G. H. Users' guides to the medical literature. XVII. How to use guidelines and recommendations about screening. *JAMA* 1999; 281: 2029–2034.

Bucher, H. C., Guyatt, G. H., Cook, D. J., Holbrook, A. & McAlister, F. A. Users' guides to the medical literature. XIX. Applying clinical trial results. A. How to use an article measuring the effect of an intervention on surrogate end points. *JAMA* 1999; 282: 771–778.

Dans, A. L., Dans, L. F., Guyatt, G. H. & Richardson, S. Users' guides to the medical literature. XIV. How to decide on the applicability of clinical trial results to your patient. *JAMA* 1998; 279: 545–549.

Drummond, M. F., Richardson, W. S., O'Brien, B. J., Levine, M. & Heyland, D. Users' guides to the medical literature. XIII. How to use an article on economic analysis of clinical practice. A. Are the results of the study valid? *JAMA* 1997; 277: 1552–1557.

Giacomini, M. K. & Cook, D. J. Users' guides to the medical literature. XXIII. Qualitative research in health care. A. Are the results of the study valid? *JAMA* 2000; 284: 357–362.

Users' guides to the medical literature. XXIII. Qualitative research in health care. B. What are the results and how do they help me care for my patients? *JAMA* 2000; 284: 478–482.

Guyatt, G. & Rennie, D. (eds.). *Users' Guides to the Medical Literature: a Manual for Evidence-Based Clinical Practice.* Chicago: AMA, 2002.

Guyatt, G. H., Sackett, D. L. & Cook, D. J. Users' guides to the medical literature. II. How to use an article about therapy or prevention. A. Are the results of the study valid? *JAMA* 1993; 270: 2598–2601.

Users' guides to the medical literature. II. How to use an article about therapy or prevention. B. What were the results and will they help me in caring for my patients? *JAMA* 1994; 271: 59–63.

Guyatt, G. H., Sackett, D. L., Sinclair, J. C., Hayward, R., Cook, D. J. & Cook, R. J. Users' guides to the medical literature. IX. A method for grading health care recommendations. *JAMA* 1995; 274: 1800–1804.

Guyatt, G. H., Naylor, C. D., Juniper, E., Heyland, D. K., Jaeschke, R. & Cook, D. J. Users' guides to the medical literature. XII. How to use articles about health-related quality of life. *JAMA* 1997; 277: 1232–1237.

Guyatt, G. H., Sinclair, J., Cook, D. J. & Glasziou, P. Users' guides to the medical literature. XVI. How to use a treatment recommendation. *JAMA* 1999; 281: 1836–1843.

Guyatt, G. H., Haynes, R. B., Jaeschke, R. Z., Cook, D. J., Green, L., Naylor, C. D., Wilson, M. C. & Richardson, W. S. Users' guides to the medical literature. XXV. Evidence-based medicine: principles for applying the Users' Guides to patient care. JAMA 2000; 284: 1290–1296.

Hayward, R. S., Wilson, M. C., Tunis, S. R., Bass, E. B. & Guyatt, G. Users' guides to the medical literature. VIII. How to use clinical practice guidelines. A. Are the recommendations valid? *JAMA* 1995; 274: 570–574.

Hunt, D. L., Jaeschke, R. & McKibbon, K. A. Users' guides to the medical literature. XXI. Using electronic health information resources in evidence-based practice. *JAMA* 2000; 283: 1875–1879.

Jaeschke, R., Guyatt, G. & Sackett, D. L. Users' guides to the medical literature. III. How to use an article about a diagnostic test. A. Are the results of the study valid? *JAMA* 1994; 271: 389–391.

Users' guides to the medical literature. III. How to use an article about a diagnostic test. B. What are the results and will they help me in caring for my patients? *JAMA* 1994; 271: 703–707.

Laupacis, A., Wells, G., Richardson, W. S. & Tugwell, P. Users' guides to the medical literature. V. How to use an article about prognosis. *JAMA* 1994; 272: 234–237.

Levine, M., Walter, S., Lee, H., Haines, T., Holbrook, A. & Moyer, V. Users' guides to the medical literature. IV. How to use an article about harm. *JAMA* 1994; 271: 1615–1619.

McAlister, F. A., Laupacis, A., Wells, G. A. & Sackett, D. L. Users' guides to the medical literature. XIX. Applying clinical trial results. B. Guidelines for determining whether a drug is exerting (more than) a class effect. *JAMA* 1999; 282: 1371–1377.

McAlister, F. A., Straus, S. E., Guyatt, G. H. & Haynes, R. B. Users' guides to the medical literature. XX. Integrating research evidence with the care of the individual patient. *JAMA* 2000; 283: 2829–2836.

McGinn, T. G., Guyatt, G. H., Wyer, P. C., Naylor, C. D., Stiell, I. G. & Richardson, W. S. Users' guides to the medical literature. XXII. How to use articles about clinical decision rules. *JAMA* 2000; 284: 79–84.

Naylor, C. D. & Guyatt, G. H. Users' guides to the medical literature. X. How to use an article reporting variations in the outcomes of health services. *JAMA* 1996; 275: 554–558.

Users' guides to the medical literature. XI. How to use an article about a clinical utilization review. *JAMA* 1996; 275: 1435–1439.

O'Brien, B. J., Heyland, D., Richardson, W. S., Levine, M. & Drummond, M. F. Users' guides to the medical literature. XIII. How to use an article on economic analysis of clinical practice. B. What are the results and will they help me in caring for my patients? *JAMA* 1997; 277: 1802–1806.

Oxman, A. D., Sackett, D. L. & Guyatt, G. H. Users' guides to the medical literature. I. How to get started. *JAMA* 1993; 270: 2093–2095.

Oxman, A. D., Cook, D. J., Guyatt, G. H. Users' guides to the medical literature. VI. How to use an overview. *JAMA* 1994; 272: 1367–1371.

Randolph, A. G., Haynes, R. B., Wyatt, J. C., Cook, D. J. & Guyatt, G. H. Users' guides to the medical literature. XVIII. How to use an article evaluating the clinical impact of a computer-based clinical decision support system. *JAMA* 1999; 282: 67–74.

Richardson, W. S. & Detsky, A. S. Users' guides to the medical literature. VII. How to use a clinical decision analysis. A. Are the results of the study valid? *JAMA* 1995; 273: 1292–1295.

Users' guides to the medical literature. VII. How to use a clinical decision analysis. B. What are the results and will they help me in caring for my patients? *JAMA* 1995; 273: 1610–1613.

Richardson, W. S., Wilson, M. C., Guyatt, G. H., Cook, D. J. & Nishikawa, J. Users' guides to the medical literature. XV. How to use an article about disease probability for differential diagnosis. *JAMA* 1999; 281: 1214–1219.

Richardson, W. S., Wilson, M. C., Williams, J.W. Jr, Moyer, V. A. & Naylor, C. D. Users' guides to the medical literature. XXIV. How to use an article on the clinical manifestations of disease. *JAMA* 2000; 284: 869–875.

Wilson, M. C., Hayward, R. S., Tunis, S. R., Bass, E. B. & Guyatt, G. Users' guides to the medical literature. VIII. How to use clinical practice guidelines. B. What are the recommendations and will they help you in caring for your patients? *JAMA* 1995; 274: 1630–1632.

Websites

Free sites

Centre for Evidence-Based Medicine, Oxford University   This is the one of the oldest and best EBM sites, with many features including a toolbox, Critically Appraised Topics (CAT) maker, a glossary, and links to other sites. There is also a CAT-bank of previously prepared critical analyses. The toolbox has an all-purpose four-fold calculator, which requires Macromedia Shockwave Player.

www.cebm.net

Bandolier   This is an excellent site for getting quick information about a given topic. They do very brief summary reviews of the current literature. Sponsored by the Centre for Evidence-Based Medicine.

www.jr2.ox.ac.uk/bandolier

Evidence Based Emergency Medicine at the New York Academy of Medicine   This is an excellent site with many features including a Journal Club Bank, CAT-maker, glossary, the Users' Guides to the Medical Literature, and links to other sites.

www.ebem.org

University of British Columbia   Written by Martin Schechter, this is an excellent site for online calculations of NNT, likelihood ratios, and confidence intervals. Select Course Material Downloads, then go to the Bayesian and clinical significance calculators. Must have data in dichotomous form.

www.healthcare.ubc.ca

Evidence Based Medicine Tool Kit, University of Alberta   An excellent site to do the Users' Guides to the Medical Literature. This site has worksheets for all the guides and links to text versions of the original articles, made available by the Canadian Centres for Health Evidence.

www.med.ualberta.ca/ebm

The following websites contain excellent links and other resources for learning and practicing EBM

HealthWeb   Evidence Based Health Care.

www.healthweb.org

Evidence-Based Health Informatics   Health Information Research Unit, McMaster University.

hiru.mcmaster.ca

Health Care Information Resources   Health Sciences Library, McMaster University.

hsl.mcmaster.ca/tomflem/top.html

For the Evidence Based Health Care Practitioners links, go to hsl.mcmaster.ca/tomflem/all.html

Expert Searches as Clinical Filters.

www.urmc.rochester.edu/miner/links/ebmlinks.html

Netting the Evidence.

www.shef.ac.uk/~scharr/ir/netting

New York Academy of Medicine EBM Resource Center.

www.ebmny.org

Mount Sinai School of Medicine.

www.mssm.edu/medicine/general-medicine/ebm

StatSoft Electronic Statistics Textbook.

www.statsoftinc.com/textbook/stathome.html

Evidence-Based On-Call   contains CATs related to acute-care topics. They are excellent, but there are only about 40 of them.

www.eboncall.co.uk

TRIP Database   contains a free set of critically appraised topics and evidence-based references.

www.tripdatabase.com

BestBETs   is a free site that contains CATs, many of which are related to acute-care topics. There are also unfinished CATS and topics needing CATS, and the site developers hope that others will input their information into the site.

www.bestbets.org

Cochrane Collaboration abstracts   The abstracts of the Cochrane reviews can all be accessed here and no subscription is required to view the abstracts. The full Cochrane Library is free in many countries, but not in the USA. Many libraries have subscriptions. The abstracts are good if you want only the bottom line, but you won't get any of the details and be able to decide for yourself if the review is valid or potentially biased.

www.update-software.com/cochrane/abstract.htm

Golden Hour   is an Israeli site with many features, including links and evidence-based medical information.

www.goldenhour.co.il

NHS Centre for Reviews and Dissemination at the University of York is the sponsoring site for the Database of Abstracts of Reviews of Effects (DARE)

www.york.ac.uk/inst/crd

AHRQ (Agency for Healthcare Research and Quality) of the Department of Health and Human Services has many services relevant to EBM, including an excellent set of clinical guidelines.
www.ahrq.gov/clinic

Sites requiring subscription

InfoPOEMs is the website for family-practice-related CATs (called POEMs, or Patient-Oriented Evidence that Matters). The site has a free trial period, but requires subscription after that.
www.infopoems.com

Cochrane Collaboration main site. It contains a collection of the best and most uniformly performed systematic reviews.
www.update-software.com/cochrane

Clinical Evidence from the *British Medical Journal* (*BMJ*). This is mainly geared to internal medicine and has an accompanying book and CD-ROM.
www.clinicalevidence.com

Index